Relentless

One Woman's Story of Betrayal by the Medical System

By Stephanie Greco Larson

For those struggling to find humane treatment for an inhumane disease.

Table of Contents

Preface

"Help hurts," a poignant phrase from early in Stephanie Larson's memoir *Relentless*, evokes the pain and directness of her story. Neither a complaint (though she often referred to herself in a teasing way as "whining") nor a comforting story to tell children ("This will hurt, but it will make you much better), Stephanie's memoir reveals how the medical system failed her.

An accomplished scholar, Stephanie was a political scientist who specialized in elections and the media, though she also had forayed into critical analyses of soap operas, one of her not-so-hidden pleasures. The author of two major books, *Creating Consent of the Governed: A Member of Congress and the Local Media* and *Media and Minorities: The Politics of Race in News and Entertainment*, as well as many scholarly articles, Stephanie had an astute critical mind. She was as capable of handling quantitative data analysis with ease (another of her books was actually a workbook teaching college students to evaluate public opinion data) as she was researching representations of race and gender in everything from presidential elections to her favorite television shows.

The diagnosis of incurable cancer in 2006—when she was only 46—changed the direction of her work dramatically. She had just finished *Media and Minorities*. She and her new life partner David Srokose—who she regularly described as the "love of my life"—were on a wonderful adventure, directing Dickinson's program at the University of East Anglia in England. An emergency visit to the hospital with abdominal pain revealed that she had cancer that had metastasized. Thus began years of treatments, both in England and in the United States, with many pronouncements that she didn't have long to live. With characteristic bite, one of the titles that she considered for this memoir was *Still Dying*.

Eligible for a sabbatical research leave in 2009, Stephanie submitted her proposal to her department and the Dean of the College. For the first time in her life, Stephanie wrote that she was planning to abandon the style of political scientists, with their carefully calibrated studies and painstaking research protocols. "I had always planned to try my hand at more creative writing during retirement," she noted, continuing "Since it is clear that I will not have a retirement, I feel it's imperative to try this now." Her memoir would describe her personal medical traumas in order to "call out" the medical profession, the media, and the public for the narrow ways we understand and talk about illness and death, and for the "additional burden" these ways of thinking place on those who are seriously ill. The chair of her department, Neil Diamant, wrote that Stephanie's plan "to write a first-hand account of her interactions with the American medical system" was "unconventional [. . .] given her own positivist approach to political issues." But then he noted how very important this new work was: "Stephanie's proposal really goes to the heart of what many of us try to write about: power, vulnerabilities of sorts, institutions, bureaucracy and access to scarce resources."

Stephanie's experiences with the medical system—from her childhood in the 1960s until her death in 2011—coincided with one of the most significant social and political movements of human history: the feminist movement. She had always told me that it wasn't until she was in graduate school, and started reading more theoretical works, that she even considered herself a feminist. Ironically, however, the fact that Stephanie started challenging the authority of her doctors in the 1970s positions her as one of the early practitioners of the women's health movement, even if she didn't know it at the time. Indeed, just around the time that Stephanie was dealing with all the trauma caused from her botched appendix surgery, the Boston Women's Health Book Collective (BWHBC) was publishing its first *Our Bodies, Ourselves*. Just as the women of the BWHBC trusted the truth of their own experiences and perceptions, and believed they had the right to challenge seemingly omnipotent doctors, so did Stephanie.

Unlike the women of the BWHBC, who were young adults when they began their work, Stephanie was for the most part on her own as a young adolescent when she began her adversarial relationship with the medical profession. As she grew older, however, she did not necessarily join in with any particular political group or consumer advocacy organization, but she did "befriend" a wide range of scholars whose work—on ideology, power, and gender dynamics—fueled her critique of the objectifying gaze of science and the medical system that was continually, in Stephanie's words, "handling my conditions while ignoring me." In her memoir, she challenges the way the medical system reduced her to a set of symptoms and tests, and the way that doctors, nurses, and sometimes even other patients reacted angrily when she complained about her mistreatment or questioned the validity of the pharmaceutical or surgical companies' promises. She describes the media's collusion in the objectification of cancer sufferers, particularly the media's implication that all cancer survivors share the same qualities: positive thinking and a fighting spirit. Doesn't such a characterization of cancer survivors suggest that those who die from cancer were in some way personally inadequate? Doesn't it also vilify death? Early on in her final illness—indeed early on in her life—Stephanie came to terms with the fact of human mortality. For Stephanie, the cultural insistence on ignoring our fragility, on always being positive in the face of debilitating illness, was dangerous; it disguised both significant pain and oppressive practices. Stephanie's memoir asks us to imagine a more honest and humane medical system, one that is predicated on care—not cure at any cost.

For those who knew Stephanie well—as a good friend, a keen scholar, and a quirky, humorous, energetic and vivacious person, this memoir came as a bit of a surprise. It doesn't evoke the very full life that we knew. Stephanie found this confusing herself; as she wrote, "My medical experiences are only part of my life story. They have been the saddest parts—some of them longer than others. The rest of my life has been pretty wonderful [. . . .] Now that I have terminal cancer, the foreground of my life story seems to have become the background. It feels disorienting."

Remembering the person I had met over twenty years ago, I understood Stephanie's disorientation.

I was a first-year faculty member at Dickinson, and, as the coordinator of the women's studies program, I had been asked to meet with this woman from George Washington University who was interviewing for a position in the political science department. Stephanie came striding into my tiny office in the basement of Denny Hall—wearing a blue silk dress that was rather low cut (and this was the early 90s, pre-full cleavage days) and sat down in the chair facing my desk. We talked about her work for a while, her interest in female political candidates and representations of women on soap operas, and what classes she might cross list with women's studies. Then, she leaned over my metal desk and said, "But this isn't what I really want to know."

"What's that?" I asked, intrigued, leaning toward her so that our heads were nearly touching. "Is Carlisle a good place for finding a man?" she asked, her eyes big and searching mine.

I nearly fell back in my chair—at least I did in my mind. I was a hell of a person to ask that question. I was still wearing a nursing bra, and I had burp stains on my own blouse, and my eyelids were perpetually weighed down with lack of sleep. I had no idea if Carlisle was a good place to find a man. I doubted it. I told her that I guessed she could go to Fast Eddie's, and I thought there was this other place called Blondie's, but really I didn't know.

And therein was born a great and unlikely friendship. When Stephanie arrived the next fall, I suspected we wouldn't have much in common. I wouldn't be going on any man-hunts with her.

But then she started attending women's studies meetings and I began to see her many facets. There was the same audacity and willingness to ask any question. But there was also a person who always showed up to meetings having read the memos ahead of time, and who paid sufficient attention that when I had questions she gave reasonable responses. In summer study groups, she read the material meticulously. Her annotations in the margins fascinated me, as they nearly constituted an additional book unto themselves. She was really fun to argue with (if you had done the reading—but if you hadn't, you might as well just forget it). She was the quintessential *critical* thinker.

In a few years I moved out of the basement and we had offices on the same floor of Denny. We were an odd pair of friends, but that didn't stop us. In the late afternoons, the window between when I finished my teaching day and Stephanie was just starting, we would often drop by one another's offices to talk. We would talk about everything—from ideas for video clips we would show to our media classes, to problems we were having with students, to difficult situations we were having with colleagues. She was one of those rare people who could be simultaneously loyal to the core and look you in eye and tell you that you were probably wrong. And that search for a man? I soon learned not to dismiss that, as it was a profound wish for a life partner. That life partner she would eventually meet in David not only loved Stephanie dearly when she was healthy, when they were having fun and making plans, but also when Stephanie became sick. When Stephanie found her man, she found a wonderful one.

As I write this, it has almost been two years since my friend and colleague Stephanie Larson died. Almost exactly two years ago I sat in her living room with her talking about her illness and the most recent surgical fiasco she had endured when she asked me if I would see to it that her memoir was published. After she died, my early attempts to do just that didn't go very far. David and I worked with a consultant who warned that there was no market for such negative life stories. For me, it was unfamiliar territory outside of university presses, few of which took memoirs. Probably most difficult, I kept experiencing the "magical thinking" that Joan Didion described in her memoir about her husband's death—I kept thinking that Stephanie would step into my room and tell me she was going to manage the editing of her memoir. Instead, there wasn't anyone there, just my own depression at her death compounded whenever I tried to pull out the manuscript and work on it.

Thankfully, Stephanie's husband, David, and her very good friend and the department coordinator, Vickie Kuhn, kept pressing even when lack of direction seemed to overwhelm the project. They found Meghan Allen, one of Stephanie's former students, who did a simply beautiful job editing the manuscript, an absolute tribute to professor who meant so much to her.

As readers turn to the memoir, I think they will disagree with the consultant who said that no one wants to hear a negative story. I think, instead, that they will find a story that is alternatingly funny, blunt, analytic, unflinching, honest, and, above all, fully human. I think it will come as a relief to those of us who feel suffocated by all the positive thinking and pink teddy bears. I am so very grateful for Stephanie's stamina in finishing this memoir, and of the gift of her "complaint"—of her own keenly observed and challenging vision of the medical system and of her experience with it.

—*Amy Farrell*

Chapter 1: Introduction

"Stephie! I gained a pound! I'm coming back!" That's what my father said the last time I talked to him on the phone. He wasn't coming back; he was dying. But that wasn't something he talked about with me: he probably didn't discuss it with anyone. It is hard to imagine that he didn't believe he was at the end, given how emaciated he had become. The doctors had stopped the chemotherapy for his lymphoma. His heart was damaged. His lungs were shot.

My weight fluctuates a lot. It drops dramatically after surgeries and during the first week to ten days after I get chemotherapy. It creeps back up the week before treatment and then spikes when I take breaks from these poisons. Most of the time I am heavy enough to look normal, but that's probably because for most women, normal is diet-induced. My weight doesn't reveal the fact that I am terminally ill. It doesn't have to, because I'll readily tell you that I'm dying.

My father had a deep respect for doctors, especially those who spoke decisively and optimistically to him, leading him to believe that he was on their team. He believed in their skills, education, and expertise. He particularly adored his oncologist whom he saw as an expert *among* experts. It was no surprise that Dad believed in his oncologist's casual dismissal of his chest pains on the night that he died. All he had was indigestion—nothing to worry about. Even if my father had lived through the heart attack that followed a few hours later, I doubt he would have changed his opinion of his doctor. "Anyone can make a mistake," he would have said. Dad died a true believer in the American medical system and its personnel.

I can't say that I believe in my doctors, nor do I think that replacing them with others will make a difference. They say they want to "take a look inside" to see "what's really going on." I don't think they will understand what I say or what is happening to my body. I don't think they were trained to listen to me, observe me or consider complex interactions. They know how to order tests and see the results. They know how to operate and seem to enjoy the challenge of it. To them, I am at my most interesting when I am silent, unconscious, and physically opened. They have been trained to treat bodies as machines. Doesn't that make them mechanics? No wonder they'd rather look at my engine than listen to me ping.

I find it hard to trust their diagnoses even when I want them to be true—they have been wrong too often. It seems the more time I spent with doctors the less I believe in them, but I may just be accumulating additional evidence to support the distrust I have felt for decades. The distrust initially came from my fear of being mistreated by doctors whom my mother referred to as "bad eggs." However, after decades of medical experiences with over fifty different doctors and an education in social sciences, I've come to recognize medicine as a social institution of control with routines and norms that monitor, define, ignore, judge, and punish me when my physical responses are unexpected or when my attitudes challenge authority. The dehumanization that I experience at their hands is more disheartening to me than the failure to be healed.

Despite my lack of faith in the church of medicine, I find myself constantly forced to genuflect at its altar. I don't have much of a choice when I become seriously ill or injured. I don't have a choice when routine examinations and tests constitute preventative medicine; and *when* these examinations and tests are no longer the ones that are determined by my sex and age, I am told they are necessary because of my chronic conditions. Traditional medicine might not be the only game in town, but it's the only one with a stamp of legitimacy in America.

I don't believe that medicine, willpower, or optimism can heal me. My father was a believer: a hard worker. He was the son of an Italian immigrant laborer. He didn't go to college. But he worked his way up a corporate ladder from distributing papers, eventually becoming Vice President of a large, daily newspaper. Despite his success, he never felt accepted or appreciated by those he called "the Dartmouth crowd." He knew that they considered him uncouth and impulsive, whereas he thought of himself as practical, intuitive, and no-nonsense. Yet, he still believed that determination paid off and that a strong will could overcome obstacles.

My father was the master of positive thinking and believing that "anything is possible if you . . . ." Fill in the blank: try hard, believe strongly, or follow the rules. He called himself a motivator. His pep talks were the soundtrack of my upbringing. To listen to him you would think that my sister was going to be a brain surgeon. My brother was going to be a track star. I would win a Pulitzer Prize.

I wasn't a cynic at the start. In some capacities, I inherited my father's optimism. When I was thirteen, I had a huge crush on a cute boy in my summer school typing class. The constant tap-tap-tapping in the class made it nearly impossible for me to introduce myself. He was going to high school in a few months and I was going back to junior high. Of course, I talked this problem over with my father: we talked about all of my problems. He suggested a plan—it was big, it was bold, it might work. We'd have a party with a bus to take us to the beach. It would include my friends and my sister's, since the cute boy had been in her math class. While they'd never been friends, he knew her. So while it was a bit of a stretch that she'd invite him (and he might see right through it), having a big guest list would make it plausible. Sure enough, with an entire day at the beach and two hour-long bus rides there and back, I had plenty of time to talk to him. He was the last to leave our house. As we sat talking in the backyard, I remember telling myself to memorize the moment because it was perfect and it was fleeting. It was the only day I spent with this boy, whom I believed was my destiny. I was convinced that we would end up together, until I read his obituary in the newspaper five years later.

Not everything was possible, and yet, my father believed that he could work, will, and endure his way back to good health. He was not alone in this ideology. American culture told him: "Keep fighting! Don't give up! You can do it!" During the four years between his cancer diagnosis and his death, my father wore a surgical mask whenever he was around people. He thought that he was protecting himself from their germs. He hoped it would keep him safe. Feeling like he had some power was worth the silent stares and the occasional questions ("Are you a doctor?" "Are you contagious?" "Are you going to rob me?"). To a man who defined himself by what he could do, the stigma of looking strange was not as great as the stigma of being sick. Being sick kept him from doing the things that he loved to do.

I am a hard worker too, and was raised with the middle-class privileges that my father's success provided. He could afford to send me to college and I never doubted that that was what I would do. My friends, teachers, counselors, and popular culture told me I should. I attended the University of Central Florida (called Florida Technological University when I enrolled) because it was in my home town. It was cheap. It was familiar. It was close.

After getting my B.S., I went upstate to Florida State University to earn a Ph.D. in political science. I was hired as an assistant professor at George Washington University in Washington, D.C. before moving on to Dickinson College. It was at this liberal arts college in rural Pennsylvania that I made my career advancing from assistant professor to full professor. Despite having gone only to public schools, which my colleagues believed suggested bad pedigree, I have only taught at private schools. I specialized in topics (media, popular culture, public opinion) that are often considered frivolous in the macho discipline of political science. (Others look at weapons, wars, constitutions, laws, and budgets.) Despite some obstacles, hard work and determination got me far professionally, just as my father told me it would.

My successes as a student and eventually as a professor were empowering, but my confidence in these arenas has never transferred to my role as a medical patient. Unlike my father, I do not believe that anything I do, anything that I will to happen, or anything that I endure, can physically save me. (Though trying to save myself has long been my priority.) I had a good diet, exercised, and avoided unhealthy habits, but I wasn't convinced that doing so would protect me from diseases. I was careful, but I knew that wouldn't prevent me from getting hurt. I did not think that persistently seeking medical *attention* would result in me getting medical *care*. My body's fate—how long it would last, what shape it would be in, how much pain it would experience, how it would be treated by doctors—was largely beyond my control. My body's fate, and my father's fate, eluded the controlling influence of optimism.

My father never talked about death. He didn't speculate about what he thought, hoped or feared came next. We were not a church-going family. I remember asking Dad what his faith was and him describing himself as a "fallen Catholic" whose religion was "humanitarianism." He believed in the Golden Rule, fairness, and equality. These ideas were too vague to get him into heaven according to my Born-Again-Christian friends (a group he thought I hung out with because it included cute boys). Once he was ill, he became too preoccupied with treatments and trying to keep working to have religious discussions.

My father didn't cry in front of us or tell us about his pain even when I could see it taking over. There were also no, here's-something-you-probably-didn't-know-about-your-old-man stories, or I-want-you-to-remember-that declarations. He didn't pass along any mementoes with special, personal meanings. Maybe he didn't have anything that he needed to say. Maybe he did, but thought that saying something would destroy the illusion that everything would be all right or jinx the chance that it might be. I can't say for sure if he believed this illusion, or if he just wanted us to.

He didn't seem to be taking stock of his life, but I was in my mid-twenties and had already moved away from central Florida by the time that he got sick. When he couldn't sleep at night, he would pace the floors or sit on the couch downstairs with the television tuned to old movies that he wasn't really watching. He would call me sometimes and not say much and then hang up abruptly. Was he giving me chances to say something? Was he bored? Did he just want to remind me (and himself) that he was still alive?

While my father didn't talk much about cancer, I can't stop talking about it. I long to be understood, so I go on and on about what is happening, how I feel and what I think. I say, "I am dying," even though most people seem to equate that statement with giving up. I fluctuate between trying to make sense of things that make no sense and trying to resist looking for meaning from an illness that essentially means I will suffer and then cease. I express the emotions that I am feeling while I feel them and talk about them again after they pass. I talk. I cry. I yell. I laugh. I whine. I apologize for whining. I write. I am relentlessly honest about everything that is happening to my body, to my life, my thoughts, and my dreams.

I am a detective trying to solve the mystery of my body. I enumerate the clues. I rate the pains and compare their locations to yesterday's, this morning's and the one five minutes ago. I am a lawyer trying to convict the medical system for its crimes against me. I have a lot of evidence, but I can only cross-examine the witnesses in my mind. I am an essayist trying to find the right words when no words are sufficient.

I don't know what my father needed in his final months but I do know that my father didn't want to die. He was only fifty-eight years old. He wasn't ready to give up the life that he loved and tried so hard to build. He struggled to do the things that he did before he was sick. He'd go to work even though he couldn't accomplish much. He'd start conversations that he would become too distracted to finish. He hoped that he could beat cancer with the force of his personality and his strong will to live.

I don't want to die either. I am only fifty.[1] There's a lot more I'd like to do, but that doesn't change how I think about this disease. I believe the medical research that shows how deadly this cancer is. I know how sick I feel from the chemotherapy. I know that treatments have no long-term effect and that their short-term utility is questionable. Denying these things won't change them.

---

[1] Editor's Note: Stephanie Larson wrote and edited this memoir between her diagnosis in 2006 and her death in 2011. She was fifty-one years old when she died.

Pretending I am all right or that I will be again won't distract me from my disease, or persuade me that everything will be fine. It won't honor who I was and who I am now. My goal is to be honest and authentic with myself and everyone else.

When people ask me how I'm doing, they seem rattled when I fail to say "fine." I might say "hanging in there," or "better than I was last month" or "not great." None of these answers satisfy what they want from me. None of the responses celebrate the fact that I am still here and the idea that surviving at any cost is good news. I don't know what to call my bluntly-honest approach—is it brave or cowardly? Is it self-centered or useful for others? Is it a gift to my family and friends or a gift from them to me? Maybe it is all of these things. I know it is not polite. But it's never polite to challenge conventions or say things that make people uncomfortable. That's what I am doing.

In my profession we call this "resisting the dominant ideology."

We use a lot of fancy terms in academia. When we can't find the right words we make them up. We "construct" arguments and "deconstruct" images, commercials, entertainment, and rhetoric. We critique everything, including each other. It's a whiny profession when you think about it. But these skills help us *see* ideologies—systems of thought about how the world should work—rather than see *through* them. Ideology privileges certain ideas, behaviors, and even types of people, groups, or countries. Ideology normalizes inequality. It makes the inequality invisible. It reassures us that the world is working the way it should even when we see something that seems wrong. Once you look *at* the ideology instead of *through it*, you notice lots of inequality. It can make you angry and frustrated when other people don't see it.

Once I became chronically and terminally ill, I started to see an ideology of health, modern medicine, and cancer. I saw how the ideology, and the actions and words that went along with it, oppressed me (and other patients, whether or not they recognized it). I see how the positive-thinking mantra and the fighting-a-battle analogies that permeate discussions about cancer encourage those of us who are dying from cancer to view our deaths as *our* failure to heal.

Now that I have terminal cancer, the foreground of my life story seems to have become the background. It feels disorienting because my medical experiences are only part of my life story. They have been the saddest parts—some of them longer than others. The rest of my life has been pretty wonderful. I came from a loving, stable family. I have always had great friends. My professional life has been fulfilling and enjoyable. I have been financially secure. I have never stopped learning. I know, and like, myself. Finding a life-partner wasn't easy, but the search has had some highlights, and I ended up finding a wonderful mate.

I wish that my medical life experiences were a smaller part of my life story. One way that could have happened is if I hadn't gotten sick or injured so often. I don't spend much time thinking about that. It would lead to me blaming my body for its fragility when I can accept that this is simply the way bodies are. I remind myself how resilient and strong my body has been, too. It has done the best that it could. I think that no matter what we do, things happen to our bodies. So, I spend more time appreciating my body than blaming it. Some people are luckier than others. I marvel that my husband has never had an IV and that a friend in her sixties was only hospitalized when she gave birth to her daughter. I lament the students who died not long after I taught them—of AIDS, car accidents, and in Iraq.

Another way that my injuries or illnesses could have been a smaller part of my life is if the healthcare system had treated me differently. I have been repeatedly victimized by the medical profession, and it has led me to anticipate the worst from medicine. Many of my physical problems have been caused or exacerbated by medical treatment. My life has been risked as often as it has been saved by what doctors have done. Despite my vigilance and assertiveness (perhaps, in part, because of it), I continue to get hurt. It is my long-term abusive relationship with doctors that haunts my life story.

Chapter 2: "Don't Sweat, You'll Die": Feeling Unsafe Before Any Major Physical Problems

When people say things like "young people think they will live forever" or "when I was young and fearless . . . ," I can't relate. I have always been afraid of pain and tried to avoid it. My childhood was full of choices made with the goal of protecting my body from harm. This was true before anything dire happened to me. It was reinforced by how I interpreted what I saw and experienced, and initially, by my maternal grandmother's sardonic worldview. Armchair-bound later in life, my grandmother—a sharp and occasionally cantankerous woman—regaled me with her stories of a difficult childhood, unfulfilled hopes, and frustrations with people whom she considered "damned fools." Her heart and vascular problems had reduced her mobility, but she was still able to read, watch television, do her crossword puzzles, smoke her cigarettes, converse, and eat what she wanted. I loved to listen to her.

My grandmother used to say that it was a man's world and that she wished she had been born a man. I couldn't believe it. It seemed harder to be a boy: they had to be tough. "What about wars and fights? Girls can't get drafted. Men punch each other," I told her, predictably focusing my argument on safety concerns.

"You have no idea how much pain women have to endure," she replied. I assumed that she was talking about childbirth. My mother had claimed childbirth was easy. (She had been "knocked out" for most of it.) But Grandmother claimed it "tore her up." The stories she told of her life indicated that childbirth was only part of the trauma. Grandma didn't just warn me to hold scissors pointing outward and never run with them. Instead, she described a childhood accident that dramatically illustrated her point. I cannot remember the details of the story, but I would never forget the image of scissor blades lodged in a small foot. When she was diagnosed with tuberculosis as an adolescent, the doctor told her father, "You treat your horses better than your daughter." My great-grandfather had ignored her claims of exhaustion, and beat her when he caught her in the barn reading instead of working.

Her stories weren't limited to her childhood. She would describe how difficult it had been sewing in a sweatshop. They paid seamstresses by the piece, so speed was essential and accidents common. Sometimes her fingers got caught under the needle. She would mime the process, demonstrating with her invisible sewing machine how other women had gotten their fingers ripped apart. "I had to resist the instinct to pull the finger back while it was being repeatedly stabbed. I had to stop the machine," she would say instructively, removing her foot from an invisible pedal, "and lift the needle first." Somehow she was surprised that I didn't want her to teach me how to sew. "Just like your mother," she muttered, shaking her head with disappointment.

My grandmother would describe her current health problems and treatments in dreadful detail. She had hardening of the arteries, a weak heart, and a mysterious scar that ran from her thigh to the center of her chest from a grueling surgery. She also had the accompanying stories. The most memorable was about the excruciating test that had to be done twice because the nurse had failed to press a button at the right time and how loudly the doctor had yelled at her. She also described the bruises on her arms and hands where the "vampires" had stuck needles in her. I remember an odd, yet vivid, story about how she took a razor blade from her purse and used it to cut off a wart before feeling returned to her leg. Once, she lamented, "Nothing more can happen to me now that would make things any worse."

"You could die," I said. She replied,

"I'm not afraid to die. That would be fine."

"You could go blind," I offered. She apparently hadn't realized that she was dealing with an expert on awful things that could happen.

"You've got me there," she conceded. "Going blind would be worse."

It must have been around this time period that she told me, "If you ever want to kill yourself, don't put a gun to your temple; you could miss and be a vegetable. Put it in your mouth and angle it upward." She demonstrated—her forefinger the barrel of the gun. Thanks, Grandma. Good to know.

I spent less time talking to my father's mother, but that didn't stop her from purveying her neuroses upon me as well.

While watching my younger cousins play, she would yell, "Slow down! Don't sweat, you'll die!" and proceed to frantically fan and wipe little faces with dishtowels. I don't know where she got the idea that sweating killed people, but she was steadfast in her belief. Not convinced, my mother would shake her head and tsk about Grandmother's "crazy Old World thinking." It seemed that my father had not resisted the warnings. He'd mow the lawn with a towel around his neck or sometimes on top of his head, pausing frequently to wipe off sweat (and imaginary sweat) with it. Aside from occasionally taking an at-bat at his company's picnic game or joining my mother for a walk on the beach, I don't recall him physically exerting himself much. To him "playing football with the kids" involved throwing a Nerf® ball back and forth in the air-conditioned family room or walking us through elaborate "Wishbone-T" formations in the front yard.

Some of my caution seemed innate, but it was sharpened, early on, by experience. I don't remember being an unhappy baby, but according to my mother, I cried all the time. I was not soothed by milk, rocking, or lullabies. My memories begin in North Miami where I lived between the ages of three and six. I remember picking up a feather in the backyard and my grandmother yelled "Drop that! Birds are dirty. That will make you sick." I dropped it immediately and have not voluntarily touched a feather since. Yet my grandmother and my grandfather would take my sister and me to a local pond and give us bread to feed the ducks. In the home movie, I'm staggering around in my diapers and big clumsy shoes, holding bread, and staring at the ducks with a distressed look on my face. A duck more than half my size comes over and lurches to grab bread out my hand. I throw the bread at him and try to run away. But my grandfather holds one of my hands and insistently thrusts more bread into the other.

On every one of my young birthdays, my mother would recount the story of what had happened on my second. We were in the grocery store and when she turned her back on the cart, I would ask strangers for pennies. Some man had obliged. "What was he thinking?" she would rhetorically ask at this point in the story. In the car on the way home, I swallowed the penny, and stopped breathing. When my sister nonchalantly reported,

"Stephie's turning blue," my mother pulled the car over and somehow retrieved the penny.

"You would have died if I hadn't gotten that penny out, but I did. I scraped your throat with my wedding ring and you were spitting up blood, but you were alive!"

There was another oft-recounted story of my sister and me playing in the back seat of the car. This was during the reckless days before child car seat laws, so we were unrestrained and the car door was not properly shut. A stranger was signaling frantically to my mother as they drove next to each other on a freeway. She eventually figured out what he was trying to tell her and she pulled over. The story would always end with mom saying, "There I was thinking he was some kind of nut and the whole time you could have fallen out of the car and died." The message was clear: the world was a dangerous place for me.

It was during those years that I remember getting ringworm from making mud pies in the backyard and deciding never to touch mud or dirt, sit on the ground, or go barefoot outside again. Even when I was older, no amount of peer pressure would convince me to take my shoes off. For me, the reported pleasures of the cool grass between my toes did not overcome the risk of stepping on something sharp.

I began to weigh pleasure against risk many times in a day. My dad used to wrestle with my sister and me on the living room floor. Our job was to try to pin him down. My mother would watch, so I know it never got too rough. My sister would giggle and screech. But just as soon as I would enter the fray, I would panic. I'd think I was going to get hurt or have to go to the bathroom and not be able to get there in time. So I'd yell, "I've got to pee! I've got to pee!" The game would stop, and I'd be allowed to leave. Once I was free and realized that I didn't have to pee, my ambivalence about the game would return. I didn't want to be left out; I didn't want to be included.

When I was seven, I got a splinter in my finger from the sliding glass door. It was a big metal splinter, and there was lots of bleeding. I remember sobbing and pleading with my mother not to touch it. She said, "We can't leave it in there," and "It will feel better once it is out." But I still thought that as much as it hurt, I could and would rather endure the pain than have her touch the splinter. Of course, she insisted on taking it out and did so without a lot of difficulty. Even though it did feel better, I didn't revise my opinion. I became vigilant about not touching things that I

31

determined had "splinter potential." When I did have splinters I kept them to myself—soaking my finger in warm water, digging at the splinter with a needle, and hoping my body would push it out by morning. I still thought that pain was more endurable when I kept it to myself. I associated help with hurt.

That same year was the first time I had to spend any substantial time with doctors and nurses. I needed to get my tonsils out. I had spent months battling sore throats and what my mother called "whooping cough." The coughs would come at night and I wouldn't be able to catch my breath. If I couldn't breathe, I reasoned, I would die. So I'd panic, cough more, and gasp. My mother introduced a ritual to calm me. She'd make hot tea and put honey in it. I would hold it and blow on it until it was cool enough to drink and then drink it slowly.

When I was finally well enough for a tonsillectomy, I had to get a chest x-ray. They insisted that I take off my shirt. I was so embarrassed and upset that I stood at the x-ray machine sticking out my tongue in protest.

The next day I was admitted to the hospital and put in a room with two other children, one in a crib. I remember bringing a shiny little purse with LifeSavers® in it. They were my grandfather's solution to everything. He always had a few rolls lined up on the top of the highboy. I had dressed up for the trip to the hospital, so that must have meant that I'd bought into the hype about the "big event": an experience promoted in the book that I had been given to read about a little boy who got his tonsils out. The book showed

32

him getting a lot of attention, eating ice cream, and listening to his heartbeat through the doctor's stethoscope.

The nurse made me put my purse on the window sill, and change into the shabby hospital gown. She took me to get a blood test. I had been warned about this. My father had told me how much he hated it when they got blood out of his fingertip. My mother disagreed, saying it wasn't as bad as getting it out of the arm. The nurse went for the finger and she had to hold it firmly so that I wouldn't jerk away. I remember thinking, *This will hurt, but it will be over quickly.* However, after she got the blood sample my finger continued to bleed. I remember the concerned look on her face, her eyebrows furrowing. I wasn't even being operated on yet and something was wrong. She said, "This shouldn't still be bleeding; I don't understand this." Then she saw the little bracelet on my wrist. It had an elastic band. She said, "Oh this is the problem. You shouldn't be wearing this!" No one had told me not to wear the bracelet. *It isn't my fault*, I thought, but I still knew I was in trouble.

I remember being wheeled into the operating room and having a mask put on my face to breath in ether. That's how they did it back then. So I was spared the pain of feeling them put an IV into my arm. When I awoke in my hospital room, I didn't know where I was. I was still groggy and I couldn't see anything because my long brown hair was across my face. When I pulled my hair away from my eyes to see where I was, I felt my lip rip open, and I tasted blood. *What had they done to my face?* I tried to scream, but my throat hurt, and I only made a squeaky sound. My mother reassured me. "You're okay. Your hair was just stuck to your lip with blood and you ripped it open again." She explained that I had originally torn it during an adverse reaction to the anesthesia. She told me that she had thought it was the baby returning from her operation until she saw that it was me who was flailing and screaming. I didn't wonder then why they hadn't bothered to clean me up, or why my mother hadn't insisted that they do so. I think she probably assumed that they knew what they were doing. She didn't want to interfere and possibly do something wrong. Her belief in the infallibility of doctors and nurses had not yet been shaken. Eventually I did want my Life Savers®, but by then, ants had gotten to them. They were crawling all over my little purse. Nothing was safe here.

* * *

Even as a child, I craved my autonomy. My sister was born in December, 1958, and I was born in February, 1960. She was two grades ahead of me, yet I had always done whatever it took to keep up with her. The when-you-were-little stories my parents told us bore this out: I pounded away at wooden puzzles that were for children her age. When Connie got a "big-girl bed," I wanted one.

"You have to stay in a crib as long as you have a bottle," my dad explained. So I handed over the bottle, and I got a bed that day.

I played school with my grandmother, learning how to read, and do elementary math while my sister went to first grade. My brother's birth made attending kindergarten (not mandatory at that time) too difficult. So I had to wait until first grade. I loved everything about it except recess: I would hang back waiting until we could go back inside. The games didn't look like any fun to me. Tag: what was the point? Why would I want to be chased? Jump rope looked risky. Girls would trip and fall and invariably knees were skinned. Red Rover: terrifying. (And I was right about that one! The game was prohibited after all the broken arms caused by the person "sent over" crashing through the other team's arms.)

School was a window into a world of risk. In the first grade, I developed a fly phobia. We were shown a film in class warning us of the dangers of the housefly. The film was old: in black and white, with a *Leave-It-to-Beaver*-type kitchen, and a Mrs. Cleaver-like mother. But its obvious age did not negate the film's power for me. In one scene, it showed the fly eating out of dirty trash cans in an alley, and in another, how the fly ate by throwing up on the food before ingesting it. In the next scene, it was in the suburban kitchen while the mother made a cake. When she wasn't looking, the fly went in the cake batter.

I am not sure why my first grade teacher thought that we should watch this. I can't imagine that any of us were friendly with flies before learning how horrible they were. But for me, the bug went from being an annoyance to being a terrorist. If I saw a fly in the house, I would obsess about it. What diseases were they passing on to us from the dirty places that they had been? Would those diseases make me throw up? I would think about it throwing up on my food or on my hair. This was gross to me, and it precipitated my wearing a bathing cap on my head during days when there were flies in our house. It wasn't until I was an adult that I would eat food at a picnic.

Like all families with children, we did our share of vomiting. The first stomach flu I remember getting was the night I watched *The Wizard of Oz* on television. I was probably four years old and had Sloppy Joes for dinner. To this day I don't like the movie or the meal. But I doubt that I was more traumatized by the illness than any other child would have been.

The second family flu that I remember was when my brother was a newborn and I was five years old. It hit everyone in the family, including my grandmother, who had come to help take care of my brother. After the worst of it was over for me (I was weak but no longer in the puking stage) I went from room to room with my little chalkboard asking everyone how many times they had thrown up that day. This behavior foreshadowed fixation on throwing up as well as my career studying public opinion polls.

The third flu was only about a year later, but when I saw my sister throw up in her Jell-O® at the kitchen table, I started to obsess about whether I would get sick too, and when and where and how I could avoid it. I fought the bile down and sobbed while my mother tried to reassure me that "You'll feel better once you've got this up." I became increasingly fearful of vomiting.

By the time we moved from North Miami to Orlando, my preoccupation had gotten worse. If I heard that anyone had thrown up at school or on our block, I would promptly begin fretting about whether I would hurl. I would worry so much that my stomach would hurt and that feeling would frighten me more.

My big sister and I were still sharing a bedroom then. She never seemed to worry about anything and she was smart and knowledgeable. So when she would exclaim definitively, "You are *not* going to throw up. I *know* it!" I felt better. She was usually right. I had just worried myself into a stomachache.

One day when I was in junior high school and had my own bedroom, my little brother came home from school and vomited. I decided that to maximize my chances of not throwing up, I would do three things. First, I would avoid his germs. Second, I would not eat. And, third, I would ask for God's help. So, I barricaded myself in my bedroom, refusing to eat anything or allow anyone to come in. I read the Bible and prayed. I even put a towel under the door to keep the germs out. I didn't come out until I had to run to the bathroom to dry heave sixteen hours later. My efforts had failed. Hunched over the toilet, I wondered if there was a God. If there was, I wasn't sure he cared about me. I was powerless.

My sister didn't react the way that I did to our upbringing. These are not the stories that she tells about growing up—partially because she seems to remember little about her pre-adulthood and therefore rarely tells any stories. Nothing seemed to have made an impression on her, whereas too many things left too big of an impression on me. I don't know if she wasn't listening or she had a loud internal voice that refuted (or at least calibrated) the warnings that were amplified in my mind. She didn't see the world the way that I did even though we shared the same family, house and bedroom. Rather than worrying and trying to protect herself from the chance that she'd get sick or hurt, she had a whatever-happens-

happens mindset. "It's not worth worrying about now," she would say.

I envied her approach, but I couldn't emulate it, and I can't say that I was entirely convinced of its wisdom. How could she be ready when what was *going* to happen *did* happen? I sometimes found relief in her confident assurances and the evidence that she used to convince me that I would be safe. She had an answer for my mundane health worries (like my fear of throwing up), my acute ones ("You don't have a brain tumor; your headache is probably caused by having your bed covers up over your head. I've read about this. It's called a 'turtle headache.'"), and other concerns that I hadn't yet voiced ("If a shark comes near you in the ocean—pee. They don't like the acidity, so they'll go away"). She gave me a history lesson that helped me stop worrying about getting leprosy and a geography lecture that minimized my obsession with dying in quicksand.

I admit having experienced some satisfaction when her carefree approach didn't protect her during a camping trip that she took with her high school ecology club. I was shocked that she'd even gone. My brain flipped continuously through a litany of hazardous hypotheticals: *What about bugs carrying diseases? What about wild animals looking for food? What about rapists and murderers? You can't lock a tent!* Miraculously, I hadn't thought of alligators sharing the lake that she and her friends would swim in. But they did. This became apparent when one dove at my sister's feet and its tail hit her in the face. "Weren't there signs warning you?" I asked incredulously.

"Yeah, I guess so. But the sign wasn't *exactly* where we went swimming," she complained. "It didn't hurt me, anyway. No biggy. Everything's okay."

Everything wasn't okay. She had a tick in her abdomen. No one in my family had ever seen a tick. My parents were from New York City and they didn't enjoy the outdoors. They called friends for advice that varied: "Take her to the hospital"; "Light a match and blow it out. Then, put the match to the tick's end and it will pull out"; "Put Vaseline® on it, and it will suffocate"; "Put gasoline on the area and it will exit"; and "Pull it out with tweezers." I watched as my parent first tried to pull it out with tweezers. They seemed to get some of it, but not all. Next, they put Vaseline® on it. When nothing happened they tried applying gasoline. Right before my parents put a smoking match to the tick, it occurred to one of them that this probably wasn't a smart move. They didn't need to be nature experts to know that gasoline and fire weren't a good combination, so maybe, a blown-out match and gasoline wouldn't be either. They ended up taking her to the hospital.

* * *

As a child who was so afraid of getting hurt, I did not get involved in athletics. My parents didn't see the usefulness in organized sports. While my friends were going to ballet and tap lessons, gymnastics, and YMCA swim teams, I was at home reading a book and feeling left out. During the summers, my mother would allow us to "take something"—one thing, that she would drive us to and from. Usually we took art lessons, since that was the only activity she suggested.

The summer after fourth grade, I told my mother I wanted to join the YMCA girls' softball league. My best friend thought it would be fun to do together. We both joined, but we didn't get to play together. We were assigned to different teams. My team lost every game it played, most of them by huge margins. If there hadn't been a run-limit rule, we'd probably still be playing. I couldn't run fast or throw far and I was afraid of the ball. I actually hit the ball most of the time, but my running was so slow that even a chunky, uncoordinated girl in the outfield could throw me out at first. My mother said that it looked like I was trying to move through invisible Jell-O®. The tough girls on my team would yell, "Get the lead out of your ass, Greco!" It was mortifying and scary. These were the same little girls who would curse and punch each other in practice.

At first, I was regulated to the outfield. But, if a ball came my way, I would either close my eyes or back away from it. I remember praying that balls wouldn't come my way. Eventually, I was moved to second base by a replacement coach who thought I had potential. There, I could successfully throw to all the bases, catch routine pop flies, and allow the outfield to get the line drives. There was more action in the infield—less time for prayer, but enough time for fear.

Although my mother said that there was nothing wrong with changing my mind and no one would blame me for quitting before the season was over, I stuck it out. She wasn't thrilled with all the chauffeuring responsibilities, didn't like to see me so unhappy, and was leery of the coach. Our coach sometimes missed practices, hadn't instructed me on how to play the game, and used unsavory language with her daughter. All of this was troubling, but she tolerated my incompetence without threatening or belittling me, so I was more relieved than bothered by her.

Mom took me to the end-of-season banquet where the winning teams got their trophies and everyone else got their certificates of participation. It was in a school cafeteria and the entertainment was a film of the Orioles' 1966 World Series victory. It was my first banquet experience and I enjoyed it. There was no physical activity, so I felt like I could be myself. Even though I hadn't made any friends on the team, I liked the pretty, blonde pitcher and our tiny catcher. The others weren't nearly as threatening in their ugly dresses. Our coach was dressed in a low-cut, black shirt, leopard-print, furry miniskirt, and high heels. Her banquet appearance convinced my mother that she was a prostitute (something my mother had suspected all summer). When the coach gave me my certificate, she said, "No matter how many of these you get, you'll always be a lady." I wasn't sure what to make of that, but she said it kindly and I recall being pleased. Being a lady sounded less dangerous and more fun—more consistent with my feeling that I needed to protect myself.

It might seem like I was immobilized by my fears and grew up in a self-imposed quarantine. That wasn't the case. I had a good childhood. I did many of the same fun things that other children did. I rode my bike around the neighborhood even after I had fallen a few times. I played house and school with my sister, and grocery store and library by myself (because no one else seemed to think that these were any fun). Like most girls my age, I also played Barbie®, paper dolls, board games, and card games. I watched *The Brady Bunch*, *The Partridge Family*, and *Room 222*. I went miniature golfing, rode go karts, and went to movies. I went trick-or-treating.

I channeled my competitive instincts into making good grades, essay writing, and speech contests. In those arenas, I could be a winner. In sixth grade, our teacher assigned a paper on a topic of our choice. I remember my classmates chose sharks and space travel. Mine was: "Will the world end in war?" I included illustrations. The centerfold was of picture taken from *LOOK*® magazine of a Vietnamese man, bent over, and dying from a bullet wound to his midsection. I drew a cartoon of the world as a ticking time bomb with the USA and USSR colored in. I wasn't paralyzed by fear. I was just cautious.

Certainly some of my activities were constrained by my (or my father's) concerns about safety, but they were still enjoyable. I went to birthday parties, but once was forbidden from eating anything because the birthday girl's older brother had been arrested for smoking pot. I could go to slumber parties, but I was not allowed to spend the whole night. My father would pick me up when the girls were about to go to sleep and return me in the morning for breakfast so I didn't miss any fun. Why go to this trouble? He was worried about things happening to me that he didn't want to talk about. I swam a lot, but usually only in pools because they were chlorinated and didn't have marine life or algae in them. I was shore-bound at the beach, but not alone after my friends watched *Jaws*.

I also tried to minimize my worrying by avoiding stimuli that would give me more to fret about. No horror movies for me: when my grandparents watched *The Birds* on television, I left the room. The sounds coming through the closed door were bad enough. A few episodes of *Marcus Welby, MD* and I had learned about new diseases I could catch. No more medical television shows. Crime shows were out: rapes, murders, and stabbings were too frightening to be entertaining. News was tricky. I didn't want to see crime and war coverage, but I liked political scandals and elections. As a result, I watched the news selectively: some of the *Watergate Hearings*, all political conventions and election nights, but not the nightly news. I was drawn to comedies; their only vices seemed to be silliness and chauvinism. I could tolerate the former and wasn't sophisticated enough to recognize the latter.

I couldn't entirely restrict my reading materials because I was a good student. I had to read *Death Be Not Proud* (about a young man who died of a brain tumor), *The Diary of Anne Frank* (which began my nightmares about Nazis), and *Johnny Got His Gun* (about the thoughts and memories of a soldier who has all of his limbs and face blown off (he communicates by bumping out Morse code messages with his head against the headboard of his bed). When I could choose what I read, I chose wisely. Haikus were safe. I liked to read plays; they had lots of talking, not a lot of action, and were rarely graphic. I was too naive to understand violent subtexts that weren't explicitly played out on the stage. For example, I didn't figure out until I was eighteen that Blanche had been raped by Stanley in *A Streetcar Named Desire*.

What I couldn't protect myself from was going to the doctor for routine examinations and shots. I knew doctors and nurses could inflict pain and humiliation. Vaccinations hurt. Kidney infections hurt, and peeing into a cup was gross. Getting undressed for a strange man was distressing. I didn't limit myself to fear of the expected—the uncertainty of what was going to happen in the doctor's office also filled me with dread. One time, my mother brought me to a doctor because I had strange-looking blisters and scabs around my mouth. He peeled off one of the scabs and looked at it. "This is impetigo," he said.

"What's that?" my mother asked.

"It's a form of leprosy," was his horrifying response. Before he could explain that it was a fairly common bacterial infection that simply required I use a special soap and ointment, I pictured myself at a leper colony being thrown rotting vegetables to eat until my nose fell off (thank you, *Ben-Hur*).

Oddly enough, I never had anxiety about going to the dentist. Maybe it was because nothing horrible happened there. Maybe it was because most of my time was spent with a hygienist who didn't seem like a nurse. She was there the whole time chatting with me reassuringly. She'd tell me what she was doing. When I occasionally had to have cavities treated, I would know when they were going to give me the shot of Novocain®. I could prepare for it. When they put the gloppy fluoride treatment in my mouth, they left the timer where I could see it. I knew when the disgusting process would end.

There were always compliments included in the visit to the dentist, which went far toward buying my good will. One of the rituals of the dentist visit was when he would pop into the cubicle and ask me to "bite down." Then he'd look at my teeth. Enthusiastically, he would say "Perfect!" and leave. My sister and brother did not have perfect bites. They were both referred to the orthodontist for tooth-pulling and braces. Although my siblings took it in stride, the metal and rubber bands seemed awful to me. I had lucked out with my perfect bite.

Then, one time after the dentist looked in my mouth, he turned to my mother and said, "She has an under bite; she needs braces." I was shocked. I didn't want braces, especially now that I was in junior high. Just six months before, he pronounced his usual "Perfect!" Nothing dramatic had changed. Everything looked fine and worked well. Without hesitation or fear, I said, "No you don't. You got my brother and sister, but you're not going to get me." I looked at my mother to see if she'd overrule this disrespectful response. She just said,

"You heard her, she doesn't want braces." Apparently I looked fine to her too. The dentist didn't argue the point and never mentioned it again. From then on, when he looked at my teeth he would flatly note that they were "fine." I do have a slight underbite, but I found out years later that it wouldn't have been corrected with braces. The solution was major jaw surgery that would remove the back of my jaw, reposition it, and wire it into place. I would have had to eat through a straw during weeks of recovery. I never had braces or jaw surgery and I have never regretted those decisions.

* * *

When I was eleven, my albumin level registered as higher than normal on a routine yearly urine test. The doctor said that it could be a sign of something serious, so he wanted to take a closer look. This would entail some kind of scan that would look at my kidneys and bladder. It required that I clean out my bowels the night before so that during the scan they could fill my bladder with some sort of glowing substance.[2] The night before the scan I took the laxatives as the doctor required. I must have been told that they would make me go to the bathroom, but I had no idea what kind of night I was in for. Perhaps it was because I was a child or because I hadn't been told to eat lightly the day before the test, or maybe it was just the harshness of the adult laxatives on my body, but I remember the cramps and the purging as more violent than the ones that accompanied the abdominal surgery preps I would go through as an adult.

I don't remember drinking the glowing substance on the day of the test, although I do remember worrying about peeing while on the scan (a feeling they said was normal). It's possible that they administered the substance through a vein, though I don't recall getting an IV. I do vividly remember worrying about what

---

[2] Editor's Note: I preserved drug names, medical terminology, descriptions of medical procedures, etc. as remembered and reported by Larson. As a result, technical inaccuracies may exist.

might be wrong with me and what they might do to me if I were sick. I was scared and confused. The doctor was talking to my mother, not me, and she wasn't asking any questions: if he wanted a test, then I would have the test. If there was something wrong, he would fix it.

I also clearly recall the blood test that preceded the scan. This was the first time I would have a needle put into my arm to extract blood. When I saw the needle coming, I became upset. This was going to hurt. The nurse was annoyed that I was upset. I needed to calm down. "This is nothing," she quipped. "I do this all the time." But I had never done it, and her side of the needle seemed so much better than mine. She missed the vein. Oops . . . she was going to have to try the other arm. She missed again. I started crying. Then she successfully drew blood out of the top of my hand with a full-sized needle. I sobbed. She said that it hadn't been that bad and I needed to stop being a baby. Years later, when I was introduced to a butterfly needle (designed for inaccessible veins), the relative comfort of the butterfly needle made it clear that I *hadn't* cried unnecessarily that day. After I encountered the butterfly needle, I begged for it by name any time my veins failed.

The scan itself was awkward and uncomfortable, but not as bad as the effects of the laxatives. The results of the scan showed that I was fine. A urine sample a few months later confirmed this. I never again had a urinalysis that indicated high albumin. Yet, for the next two decades, I would conscientiously report this aberrant test when asked for my medical history. Nurses would always say that high albumin levels were "a fairly regular occurrence in children—nothing worth noting." To the nurses, this incident was irrelevant to my medical history. To me, it was an important part of my story. It was one of the ways that I learned that I didn't have to feel sick for something to be wrong with my body, that my veins didn't work very well, that medical tests weren't reliable and that doctors and nurses could (and would) inflict pain on me. I also learned that there was nothing I could do about any of this.

I wonder now why that doctor didn't spare me the ordeal of that scan. Why didn't he consider how hard it would be on an anxious eleven-year-old? Why didn't he order another non-intrusive urine sample first? Should my mother have insisted on that? Was this the same woman who scoffed at my paternal grandmother's warnings about overexertion? Is it even possible to wonder about these things without assuming that my middle-class parents, with their working-class upbringing, were able to treat doctors and their diagnoses with level of caution that didn't exist in the early 1970s?

My mother and most of her contemporaries didn't know (or have access to) the medical information available on the Internet. We can read, in graphic detail, about medical tests and protocols. We can comb through patients' recommendations and regrets. We know how much money doctors make from ordering tests and, unsurprisingly, how many unnecessary tests are ordered. We know how much radiation is given off by scans and how dangerous that radiation can be. It took a world-weary soothsayer such as my maternal grandmother to meet any man face-to-face and call him a "fool." By contrast, my mother remembers thinking "Doctors were gods." The lesson she remembers from my urinalysis was the relief that the test indicated nothing was wrong with me. She did not second-guess me having the procedure because she thought it was better to be safe than sorry. I was safe. But I didn't *feel* safe and I *was* sorry. I had gotten a glimpse into a world I didn't want anything to do with.

Chapter 3: "You Should See How Much Blood I'm Getting Out": My Knee Nightmare Begins

I started high school in the fall of 1975, eager to compete in speech tournaments, act in plays, and meet new boys. I wanted these boys to be like the Osmond brothers, Wally Cleaver and the guy in Beverly Cleary's book, *Fifteen*, who takes the girl to a Chinese restaurant for their first date. I wanted long conversations, hand-holding and kisses on the front porch. Dancing and free meals in restaurants sounded good too. The country might have been going through a sexual revolution, but I was longing for the 1950s. I never found those kinds of boys; maybe they never existed. High school became another disappointment in my quest to find love.

I had a boyfriend, Chuck, for a few months in ninth grade and it took three times as long to get over him. I hadn't even liked him. In fact, I told him from the start that I was destined to be with Tom (that boy in my sister's grade who I'd had a crush on since we'd spent that one perfect day on the beach together). I remember calling Tom "a Cadillac" among men. "How about hanging around with a Volkswagen with shiny hubcaps until the Cadillac comes around?" Chuck asked. He was clever and persistent. After the first kiss, I was hooked.

I soon had our lives together planned. After high school we would go to college in Orlando. After we graduated, we'd get married and move to St. Petersburg, Florida where I would work as a reporter and he would get a medical degree at the University of South Florida in Tampa. I thought that having a doctor as a husband would be ideal. If he told me not to worry about an ache, pain, or lump, I wouldn't have to. He would know when something was really wrong and know how to fix it. I wanted Chuck to be an anesthesiologist. Anesthesiologists didn't have to see their patients naked. They were the doctors who came in for scheduled operations—an ideal schedule for when we had children. Anesthesiologists made sure that the patients could sleep through pain (How kind!) and keep breathing (How important!). This plan had my father's fingerprints all over it. I remember him saying that choosing an anesthesiologist was the key to a successful operation.

I can see now why all of my future plans for us (coupled with my practically-militant vow of chastity) might have been overwhelming for a fifteen-year-old boy. But when he broke up with me to date my best friend—a large-breasted girl who lived on the lake, had access to a motor boat and lacked a curfew—I was shattered and confused.

Long before I would realize that high school boys were just as disappointing as junior high boys (except generally bigger, hairier, and pushier), I was confronted with my first major physical challenge. It was not the kind of challenge they celebrated in physical education classes. But that's where it started. It was my last year of gym and I had no regrets. No more smelly locker rooms, inadequate showers with other modest girls in their underwear and bras, ugly gym suits or threats to my grade point average. No more having to play games that I wasn't good at. No more walking the line between trying not to sweat, and trying not to be singled out as a slacker. No more being picked last for teams or, even worse, being considered a wasted pick by the team captain who let my height deceive her into thinking I could shoot a basketball. No more worrying about getting hurt when I inevitably lost my balance on a beam, had the wind knocked out of me by a kicked soccer ball, or got spiked by a volleyball. No more failing the President's Physical Fitness Test. *Thank God.*

I had cursed John F. Kennedy every year since seventh grade for the abomination of the President's Physical Fitness Test. The test had been his idea to promote fitness among adolescents by assessing them on various physical challenges and comparing their scores to a national, recommended level of performance. For me, it inspired anxiety and humiliation: I never came close to passing. I don't know what students got if they met or exceeded the standards. It might have been a pat on the back, a certificate or a medal. There was no bribe big enough to get me to meet the national standards because the problem wasn't motivation.

My mother's generation had to climb a rope hanging from the gym ceiling. My peers and I were tested on seven tasks: how far we could throw a softball; how far we could jump from a standing position; how long we could hang from a bar; how many sit-ups we could do; how fast we could run fifty yards; run/walk five-hundred yards; and complete the "shuttle run." I did well on the sit-ups and the broad jump because I practiced at home. I could do one hundred sit-ups (although I think our goal was only fifty). One year, after months of practice in my parents' bedroom, I jumped farther than anyone in my class (crushing the requirement). Thump, thump, thump—watch awkward Stephie hurl herself across the floor and measure the length with a yard stick.

The events I dreaded the most were the running ones. I still had the "running through Jell-O®" problem that my mother observed years earlier, so my fifty-yard dashes were dreadful. If I recall correctly it would take me 8.5 seconds of legs and arms flailing to complete the run. I remember one of my gym teachers asking me if I was serious, or just kidding around. I was no better at the shuttle run, which entailed ferrying two erasers, one at a time, from one place to another, at a dead sprint. The quick turns and bending for erasers did nothing to improve my speed and I usually wheezed my way through the final thirty yards. The 500-yard run/walk was always the last event. One year when I decided to walk it, keeping pace with the pale girl who had asthma, the teacher made me do it again. Running it made my side hurt, and I felt a little nauseous, but crossing the finish line signified the end of the unit. I would have another year before having to do this again. I suppose the standards went up as we aged, but I was so far from meeting them, I didn't notice.

Since most of my junior high attended a different high school than I did, I didn't know anyone in my tenth-grade gym class. Before I could demonstrate my lack of physical prowess on a field or court, we started the fitness test. *I might as well get this degradation over with*, I thought, as I ran my pitifully slow shuttle run. Unfortunately, the teacher had pushed the wrong button on the stopwatch, so she didn't have a score for me. I remember telling her that she could put down the lowest score in the class since I never did very well on the test. She said that I needed to run it again once everyone else had finished. It was the last class period of the day, so the dirt that we had been running on was badly torn up by the time I did the run again. That might explain why at one point my foot twisted and my leg kept going.

As I fell, it felt like I was moving in slow motion and then I was on the ground screaming from the pain in my leg and knee. Classmates rushed over to where I lay. The students surrounding me looked horrified. My leg didn't look like a leg anymore: the knee was pushed over to the right. Ingrid, a girl from one of my other classes, held my hand. Her friend, Teresa, chattered to distract me. I heard sirens and an ambulance arrived. The EMTs put an inflatable cast on my leg to immobilize it for the ride. I remember the agony of the paramedics taking off my shoe to put the cast on. They rushed me to the hospital. I cried and nervously asked questions. All they told me was that I'd be fine; the doctors would fix it.

I was quickly wheeled into an emergency room cubicle. Then the breakneck speed of events, which had both frightened me (*This must be serious*) and reassured me (*They're on top of the problem and seem so competent*), stopped. I waited and waited, aching and moaning on the gurney. No one told me what was going on or what was going to happen next. They simply asked me for my name and phone number, saying that they needed to call my mother before they could do anything. It was long before the days of cell phones and my mother was at another hospital visiting her father. My grandmother was home, but she couldn't drive and didn't think to give them my father's work number.

As time went on, my tendons and ligaments stayed stretched out, blood filled my knee socket, and I was in misery. When my mother finally arrived, she came into my cubicle and gasped. She told me later that my leg "looked like a pork chop—misshapen and discolored." She signed the forms that allowed the doctors to attend to a fifteen-year-old minor. They popped my knee back into place. Of course this hurt, but not as much as the dislocation and the waiting. Immediately afterward it felt better than it had for the two hours it had been out of place. They put me in an immobilizer, gave me crutches and sent me home.

Three days later, I went to an orthopedic doctor who my father insisted came highly recommended. Diligently following directions—no pressure on the leg, lots of ice, and aspirin—I had been uncomfortable all weekend. My knee swelled to the size of a volleyball and throbbed, but I assumed it would get better. I mentally prepared for a cast, focusing on how diminished the pain was since the relocation. Perhaps the worst was behind me.

All I remember about Dr. Mean's[3] looks is that he was a big guy. His manner is more memorable. He was exactly like the

---

[3] Editor's Note: To protect the privacy of individuals, Larson intentionally assigned pseudonyms to all medical personnel. In keeping with her intentions, I have preserved the pseudonyms and in cases when Larson had yet to assign pseudonyms I have created them in the style she defined.

high school boys that I was starting to be unimpressed by—bulky and aggressive. He was in a hurry and seemed irritated that we were there. He briefly looked me over and said, "This is a lateral dislocation. It needs to be drained. Then we'll put a cast on it. Nurse, prepare her." I started to ask a question, but he was already out the door. Flustered, the nurse followed him out. I started asking my mother the questions I wanted to ask the doctor: "What does that mean?"; "How do they drain it?"; "How long will it take?"; and of course the most important question, "Will it hurt?" I wanted to prepare myself.

"I don't know. I'm sure he'll come back and tell us more," she said. Then the nurse came in and started to clean my knee. She was annoyed, distracted, and called away before I could interrogate her. Then we heard blood-curdling screams from down the hall. A boy was screaming, gasping, and begging for mercy. It was chilling. A few minutes after he stopped, the doctor was back in my room.

"She hasn't prepared you yet?" he bellowed angrily, turning to leave.

"Wait," I called. "What do you mean by 'draining'? What are you going to do?" He looked at me with a grimace of annoyance.

"It's nothing! I just take the blood out. I just did it to a kid down the hall."

"The one who was screaming bloody murder?" I asked, feeling my eyes widen.

"Oh, yeah. So you heard him?" Then he was gone.

My mother and I looked at each other in shock. I started to whimper and hyperventilate. She knew she couldn't reassure me. What could she say? We could hear the doctor yelling at the nurse, who came in fuming. She briskly finished cleaning my knee and gave me a shot on the side of the knee. The idea of a shot in the knee freaked me out and hurt, but I knew that this was supposed to be what helped with the pain from the needle used for draining. What must *that* needle be like?

The doctor joined us. He pinched my knee: "Can you feel this?" he asked. I could. "Can you feel *this*?" Yes. "Well, I don't have time to wait for that to take effect," he said glaring at the nurse. "So let's get started. Get up on the table."

I should have refused. I should have said, "You need to find the time." But I was fifteen-years-old and he was the doctor so I lay down on the table. He came at me with a bigger needle than I had imagined was used on a human. He inserted it under my knee cap and started to extract blood. I alternated between screaming and gasping as he dug the needle in. It had hurt going in, but it was unbearable as he moved it around. At one point he pushed down on my knee cap with his left hand while guiding the needle under my knee with his right. My whole body jerked involuntarily in response to the pain. He growled, "Stop moving, or I'll stick it in again." I think I started begging him to stop or trying to tell him how much it hurt, as if he didn't know. I thought, *Is it supposed to hurt this much? Something must be wrong.* "You think *this* feels bad," he gloated, "you should *see* all the blood I'm sucking out of you." *Are those the words of a doctor?* I pondered, incredulously. *Maybe he said*

57

"getting out?" Either way, I remember thinking—no, *knowing*—that he was enjoying himself. His nurse hated him. The little boy down the hall hated him. My mother hated him and I hated him. But it didn't make any difference; he could hurt me as much as he wanted. He had the authority and the needle. My only defense was to change doctors. And we did.

For months I wore the ankle-to-thigh cast that Dr. Mean put on me that day. I got it signed by my new friends. I successfully used it in my campaign for student government, plastering my posters with, "Cast your vote for the girl in the cast!" as my slogan. I dragged it around at football games, clomping up the bleachers. I learned how to sleep perfectly still on my right side with my heavy straight right leg anchored to the bed and my left leg bent (a position I used exclusively for over a decade). I was transferred to a physical education class we affectionately called "Misfit PE" where we played board games and ping pong. I religiously completed the leg lifts and knee flexes that my new doctor recommended. I worried about having my knee drained again.

I had been told that the knee could fill with blood or water and might need to be drained again. I wasn't sure how much of the pain that I had experienced was due to the procedure and how much was due to Dr. Mean's traumatic technique. I needed a plan. Maybe I could talk my new doctor out of draining? Dr. Mellow seemed like a kind, laid-back man. Maybe he would be receptive to another approach? I practiced persuasive arguments in my head. Maybe I could get that kid in my English class to sell me some marijuana? I had never been tempted to take drugs before (I'd never even smoked a cigarette), but surely having my knee drained would be more tolerable if I were high.

I didn't have to get my knee drained again. The cast was taken off, and I was sent to a physical therapist. I was shown exercises to do at home. Most of these were types of leg lifts with weights on my ankles. I had packets of birdshot that would be placed in the pockets of a saddlebag-like thing that would be placed across my foot. We'd add more pellets as the weeks went by. Lift and hold, count to five, over and over again: it was difficult and monotonous.

When I returned to Dr. Mellow, he examined my knee. I sat on the end of the examination table. He had me extend my knee from bent to straight, while he held my ankle for resistance. I had regained all of my motion, but not my strength. He had me repeat the move. "You're not doing your exercises," he scolded sternly.

"Yes, I am," I said. I *had* been doing the exercises. My mother agreed, noting,

"She does seem to do a lot of exercises." He admonished me to do more. I was to increase the number of repetitions before our next visit. So, I did more exercises.

At the next visit, he again had me bend and straighten my leg. Again, he said, "You're not doing your exercises. You are not going to get better if you don't do them. You have to take this seriously."

I hated being in trouble. I was Little Miss Obedient. I had to defend myself so I truthfully reported how much weight I was lifting in my little foot satchel and how many repetitions I did each day. He said, "Show me." I think he thought that he was calling my bluff and I wouldn't be able to do the exercises that I said I could do. So I demonstrated defiantly. "Those are the wrong exercises," he said, stopping me mid-demonstration. "They are building up the wrong muscle. You need to strengthen the muscle that holds your knee cap in, not the one that pulls it out." He pointed out how my knee cap pulled toward the right trying to escape the socket every time I bent my knee. My biggest problem wasn't strength; it was stability.

"You need to exercise your knee the way the physical therapist told you to," he objected, "not this way." Once again he was blaming me.

"This *is* the way the physical therapist told me to do my exercises," I insisted. My mother backed me up:

"Stephie does what she's told."

Finally, Dr. Mellow called the physical therapist. She confirmed that she had trained me to do the exercises I was doing. The script he had written for her office was hard to read. This is what she thought he wanted me to do. For weeks, my leg muscles had shriveled in my heavy, plaster cast (a remedy for dislocations that is no longer used), and now key muscles had continued to atrophy while I dutifully exercised muscles that weren't injured. The doctor concluded that the solution to my problem—a chronic-subluxing patella (for the uninitiated: continually-dislocating kneecap)—would be surgical. He recommended that he perform a "lateral release" where they cut the ligaments that pull the knee cap outward, "clean up" the damaged cartilage under the knee, and move the muscle from the inner part of the leg over the top of the knee to help "hold it in." Since I was walking comfortably, I was surprised by this recommendation. So was my mother. She took me to another doctor for a second opinion. That doctor confirmed that my knee cap wasn't resting comfortably in the knee socket; it was pulling to the right. The operation Dr. Mellow had recommended was the conventional surgical approach to try and correct it.

That summer, I had the surgery. I was in the hospital for a week. It took me days to lift my leg off of the bed without using the toes of my left foot to help. Perhaps because my pain was in a limb instead of my core, I could distract myself from most of it. My knee ached, but that was similar to the weekend after the dislocation. Since the pain was familiar and within the realm of what the nurses were telling me I would feel I wasn't afraid. I was uncomfortable. The scar looked (and felt) nasty—crusted with dried blood and oozing with sticky puss. Physical therapy in the hospital taught me how to walk again: to roll off of my toe instead of protectively lifting my leg. The pain from that motion was more intense, but similar to what I'd felt after the cast came off. It didn't alarm me. There weren't big surprises, except perhaps the terrible constipation. I had willed my body not to create excrement until I could hobble to the bathroom on my own. No gross bedpans for me! I must have had at least one IV, but I don't remember it, so it must have gone smoothly. I remember getting flowers, daily presents from my mother and lots of visits and phone calls from friends. One of them introduced me to Kurt Vonnegut books, which kept me busy the rest of the summer.

The incision was six inches long, thick, and red. Though faded slightly, it is still visible today, thirty-four years later. *Not attractive*, I thought, with concern. The scar was something of a disappointment because I had considered my legs my finest feature, next to my eyes. I had wanted to attract a "legs man," whom I suspected would be more mature than those who were attracted to more sexually-defined body parts. Admittedly, this was a strange way to look at things, but that's how I felt at the time. I felt like one of my most marketable features was now marred, and there wasn't anything I could do about it.

Maybe it was better this way, because my grandmother had always said that beauty was a curse. She hadn't elaborated, but I think she meant that you couldn't trust the men that beauty attracted. She had a failed first marriage and an unhappy second one to my grandfather. My mother said, "Beauty hurts," and when I started plucking my eyebrows, I had to agree. In retrospect it seemed like she raised me to believe that beauty wasn't worth the trouble because the only makeup my mother routinely wore was lipstick. It was hard to tell, in the black-and-white photographs from her pre-marriage years if that had always been the case. There she was, posing with her hand on her hip next to her roadster with a slightly suggestive smile. Maybe the lesson was that you only needed to work at beauty until you got married? When I asked her why she didn't wear makeup more often, she said, "then people would expect it. Better to have them get used to the unadorned face and be pleasantly surprised sometimes, than get them used to seeing makeup and disappointed when they see how you look without it." It made sense to me. Not shaving your legs didn't make sense. That seemed to be taking it too far. Yet my mother resisted the convention. Even though, like me, her legs were her outstanding feature. So having an ugly scar seemed like a problem to me mostly because I had not yet found Mr. Right.

After getting out of the hospital, I spent the summer recovering. There was more time on crutches, a walking brace, more knee exercises, and lots of visits to the doctor. Unfortunately, my knee continued to slide to the right when I straightened it, just like it had before surgery. The doctor admitted that the operation hadn't worked. He said there was another surgery that we could try, which would attempt to fix the problem by moving bone instead of muscle. He talked about cutting bones, using screws, and full-leg and hip casts. It sounded awful. "What's the chance that that operation will work?" my mother asked.

"Well, it doesn't have as good a track record as the one we tried," he admitted.

"What if this doesn't get fixed?" she asked.

The doctor explained it was likely that I would develop arthritis in my knee at a fairly young age. His exact words were: "She'll have an eighty-year-old knee by the time she's thirty."

He also said that the knee joint would never be very strong. My chances of having another dislocation were high. Therefore, I should limit my physical activity. Specifically, I should never ski, water ski, roller skate, ice skate, run, jump, or kneel. And, I should avoid walking up or down stairs.

"For how long?" I asked.

"For the rest of your life," he replied.

I knew that I wouldn't have the second operation. I had learned that doctors would operate even when they were unsure of a positive outcome. Just because they could do another operation didn't mean I had to let them. I had already wasted a summer trying the operation that he originally said had the best chance of working and it had been irritating, uncomfortable, and disappointing. I could always have the second operation later if things got worse. Eleventh grade was starting soon and I wanted to experience it on two legs. So I left Dr. Mellow with his bad handwriting and bleak predictions behind—knowing that despite his daunting list of activities to avoid, I could still do the things that I wanted to do.

I would act in plays, compete in speech tournaments, go to football games and watch movies with my friends. I would excel in classes. So what if I needed to be careful with my knee? I had always been careful with my body. I now had license to stop people from trying to get me to be less careful. "Sorry, I can't go do that, I have a bad knee," I could (and would) say. If anyone challenged me, I could cup their hand over my knee while I straightened my leg and they could feel the abrupt, powerful slide of my knee cap as it pulled to the outside. It was persuasive (and creepy). I chose to think of it as a party trick or a conversation starter, rather than a deformity. The scar was a mark of what I had endured and visual evidence of my uniqueness. Therefore, I was never embarrassed by it. I decided to embrace a life that didn't need two good knees and tried not to think too much about that life's limitations. I would continue to prioritize thoughts and words over motion. I didn't think that I was hiding in books and conversations; I was living the life I was given. It was a life that I would enjoy and be good at.

Chapter 4: "I'm the Doctor; You're the Patient": My Appendix and Complications from Its Ruin

I went to college at a state school in Orlando; it was the only place that I applied to, since my parents agreed to foot the bill. The plan had been to live at home and commute to school. However, my father changed jobs and went into business for himself a few hours away. So, I ended up living in the dorms and university apartments. I worked part-time jobs throughout school—as a phone sales representative, a typist, a cashier, and an office assistant—spending money on pizzas, gin and tonics, and transmissions for my twenty-year-old Toyota Corona. My parents paid my tuition as well as my room and board. Careful to live within my means, I never had a credit card or a checkbook and I managed to save money for graduate school. I graduated in three years with a double major in communications and political science in addition to a minor in speech.

Some of my friends would probably have said that I worked hard and played hard in college, but that would be a misrepresentation, considering how seriously I took everything. My play was every bit as goal-directed as my schoolwork, but playing felt far more difficult to succeed at than working. I was determined to find Mr. Right while following the rules that would keep my body safe. I might have been out at the fraternity parties, local clubs, and basketball games, but I never had a carefree attitude about being at those places. Because I was outgoing and quick to kiss boys, I had a lot of first dates. Because I was serious, intense, and didn't believe in sex before marriage, I had few second dates. Each disappointment led me to wonder what was wrong with me. Why couldn't I find *him*?

One of my theories was that I *had* found Mr. Right; he just didn't realize it yet. His name was Kris, a tall, dark, and handsome Radio-and-Television major who loved an audience and a laugh. We took classes together and like most college students, hung out at my dorm. But we also went to movies, dinners, and dancing. He wasn't dating anyone and seemed to spend all of his free time with me, which led me to believe that we were building a relationship. He would act annoyed and competitive whenever I'd have a date, and so after a year of pseudo-dating, I told him how I felt. He said that he considered me a close friend, and emphasized this point by giving me a Valentine's Day card with the word "friend" underlined. He explained that he only dated blondes. Despite this explanation, we continued as before—I, a brunette, and he, not dating one. It never occurred to me to dye my hair. If I had, it might have forced him to reveal the real reasons he wouldn't date me.

By the spring of my sophomore year, Kris started a long-distance relationship with a girl at his best friend's college. In retaliation, I went on a few dates with his best friend, Mark, when he came to town. The three of us would go out dancing and drinking, and they would make spectacles out of themselves.

Maybe we all did, but their antics seemed to come naturally while mine were more derivative. Kris played "My Best Friend's Girlfriend, She Used Be Mine" by The Cars on his college radio show and dedicated it to me. I hoped that this was all a part of the dance that would lead to an interesting how-your-grandfather-and-I-fell-in-love story. But I feared that it wasn't.

That spring break, I stayed in Orlando to work extra hours at the mall, get an early start on term papers, and see some high school friends. Lots of my college friends left campus and went home for the week. Some of them went to local beaches, but none of them flew off to Cancun or Europe for the week like the students I would eventually teach. That wasn't our world. My spring break extravagance was Sunday brunch with my best friend and my gay debate partner from high school. We went to the restaurant on top of the Contemporary Hotel at Walt Disney World, where it was all-you-can-eat with unlimited champagne. We ate and drank our money's worth. I overheard the waiters talking about us when I went, again, to refill my plate. One said, "I wouldn't have believed it, if I hadn't seen it myself."

A few days later, I had abdominal pains. I had been experiencing cramps and exhaustion the week before, even missing a few classes because of it, but it was nothing like this. As much as I didn't want to go to the doctor, on the third day of pain I decided it was worth a try. It was difficult to walk from my apartment to my car in the parking lot. I was bent over, clutching my abdomen, and walking slowly: my face contorted. This walk became the origin of a rumor that spread through the apartment complex that I

68

had had a miscarriage or better still, a botched abortion. The rumor about the abortion came later, but seemed to persist longer.

I went to my family doctor's office, but saw a partner whom I had never met. He observed me, asked me to describe my symptoms, pressed on my abdomen, and listened to it with a stethoscope. He asked me about my periods—I said that I was at the end of one, but that I had always been irregular. I also said, "I think my appendix is bursting." He was sure that I was wrong because he could hear bowel sounds and the pain wasn't centralized on one side. He concluded that I had a "female problem" that was likely to resolve itself, neither prescribing me anything nor asking if I had a gynecologist. I remember thinking that being examined by the doctor should calm my mind, but the uneasiness in my body didn't allow it.

That evening I was exhausted, aching, and not hungry. I tried to distract myself by watching television, but I couldn't concentrate on it. I went to bed on the little mattress I had in the small bedroom in the apartment and slept fitfully. When I woke up, I could barely stand. My roommate, whom I had just recently met and moved in with, had the master bedroom with a bedroom set. She was away for the week, so I decided to sleep in her bed. It was an out-of-character intrusion for me, but the pain had increased, and I couldn't imagine sleeping on my floor mattress any longer. The pain intensified that day, so I called the doctor's office. The voice on the other end of the phone dismissed me with a curt, "Mylanta® should help."

But the next day the pain was even worse, which seemed unimaginable. I called the doctor's office again in the morning. I was told by the nurse to put a hot water bottle on my abdomen. I tried to rest that day and managed to sleep a little. It was like passing out momentarily only to be awakened again. A friend called, and I said that I was too sick to get out of bed. She said that she'd bring something for me to eat; I don't remember eating any of it, but I did sip the lemonade she brought. She asked if I had seen a doctor yet and I told her that I had: he had promised that I would get better. She must have told me to call the doctor again. When I did, I was reprimanded by the nurse: I needed to remember that I was not the doctor's only patient. He had told me what to do, and now I needed to stop calling them. If the nurse had asked me when I had last urinated, I wouldn't have been able to tell her (it had been at least twenty-four hours), but I didn't know that this was an important thing to report. Peeing didn't seem like much of a problem compared to the pain.

My suffering continued, and I kept thinking that there must be something that could be done. Afraid to be rebuked again, I called the office at night hoping to get a different nurse. This time I was told by another doctor that I could go to the hospital and get a shot for the pain. However, it was the only shot I would get, so I needed to make sure it was, as he put it, "the right time." It's hard to believe that he told me that, but I remember it clearly. I thought that the pain couldn't get any worse, but I had thought the same thing the day before. I didn't want to use my shot before the pain reached its peak, so I stayed put.

I might have been nodding off the next day—or I might have been passing out and coming to. I heard heavy footsteps followed by the rattle of the front door knob. Unable to move, I realized how vulnerable I was to an attacker. (It was probably an apartment exterminator who had keys to the building.) I started yelling and heard him run away. The boys who lived above me and those from across the walkway decided to try to synchronize their music. They played Willie Nelson's "Mamas, Don't Let Your Babies Grow Up to Be Cowboys" repeatedly on full blast, but never quite at the same time intensifying my private hell. I started yelling, "Stop it! Stop it! Stop it!" before drifting off again. When I came to, the music had stopped, and I heard a voice in my head say, "If you stay in this bed another night, you will be dead." It was a calm, clear, male voice that I attributed to God. I called my father and said, "I am sick and I don't want to stay here alone anymore. Could you come get me and bring me home?" Probably because I had never called and interrupted him at work before, he knew something was wrong. He arrived ninety minutes later.

He didn't expect to find me pale and writhing in pain, with an abdomen so distended that I looked about six months pregnant. He drove me to the hospital. Every bump along the road made me scream. I do not remember how long it took before they operated on me. I know I told my story to at least three healthcare professionals. I know that they had time to do a sonogram, two pelvic exams, a blood test—all while wheeling me back and forth in corridors, carelessly pushing me into doorways, and riding me up and down elevators as I screamed. Everyone told me angrily that what they were doing didn't hurt. They didn't know why I was moaning, gasping, crying, and involuntarily jerking when they pressed down on my abdomen. Day turned to night, and I was asked to sign a form that would permit them to give me a hysterectomy. I was ready to sign anything for some relief.

It felt like only seconds had elapsed between the time I was wheeled into surgery and the moment I woke up in recovery. The now familiar pain inside my gut persisted, and added to it was a new one. There was a burning, aching, torn feeling on the outside of my abdomen that connected to the horror on the inside. For the first twenty-four hours or so, adrift on swells of relentless pain, I floated between waking and sleeping. When I occasionally surfaced, the pain was so extreme that it left room for nothing else. I knew that I might die but I was too tortured to value the life I had, or had planned to have, over death. Death would free me from my body and, I believed, put me in the hands of a loving God.

My purported recovery period was interrupted occasionally by bizarre and horrifying moments with medical professionals and fellow patients. The first was when a nurse came into my private room at the end of the hall to yell at me for moaning too loudly. She told me that I was disruptive and selfish. I needed to be more considerate. It took me a few moments to decipher what she was saying because I had been deep inside of myself—unaware that I was making any sounds.

The second strange moment was when I awoke to find a feeble, old man looking down at me. He had pulled up his hospital gown, and his hand was on his penis. I tried to scream, but only muffled, throaty growls seemed to come out. I had no idea what he was intending to do, but I knew that I couldn't stop him. I was entangled in tubes and wires, and anchored to the bed by my embattled midsection. Thankfully, the nurse, who had yelled at me earlier, came in and interrupted him. As I thrashed about on the bed, panicking, I expected another chastising; instead, she led the man away, telling him that this was not his room. She said nothing to me as she did this, and once she was gone she didn't return.

A third intrusion (that I remember) came from a doctor who inserted a subclavian artery line. This was a bedside surgery, he explained—necessary to try to revive my kidneys, which still weren't working. I assumed that surgery would include anesthesia and was unpleasantly surprised that it didn't. As he cut a small hole in my chest and shoved a tube into the subclavian artery, I felt a new type of pain in a part of my body that had previously been spared. The tube flushed fluid through my system to jump-start my kidneys. He said that the flush required that I remain flat and still despite the additional pain that it would cause me. If I was not perfectly still, I could suffer internal organ damage as the fluid rushed through my body. I steeled myself, determined not to cause further injury.

A carpenter's level was used to make sure that I was flat. I had never seen a level before. I used it as my focal point to help will any physical reaction to the pain away. I watched the air bubbles in the level as the top part of my bed was lowered. Every adjustment of the bed intensified my pain. *Don't move or you will hurt yourself more*, I kept repeating in my head until the procedure was over. The experience taught me that no matter how horrible pain was, it could always get worse. It was a lesson I would recall throughout my life.

* * *

The next day my parents updated me on what had happened. Before the doctors could perform the hysterectomy, my appendix had ruptured. The doctor admitted that it had probably been leaking for a while. My abdomen was full of poison—poison that could not be surgically removed without the surgeon's scalpel spreading it. Instead, antibiotics were being used to kill the infection. The kidney flush had worked and saved me from a lifetime of dialysis. My father's go-get-'em demeanor could not conceal his continuing concern. I knew I had almost died. And, I knew that I could still die.

It was then that I saw my abdomen for the first time since the surgery. There was a vertical incision from my pelvic bone to my belly button. This incision was about a quarter of an inch thick, held together (and yet open) with seven, big, red, plastic bands that were anchored on each side of the line in holes half-inches apart. There were two, soft drainage tubes coming out of my lower abdomen, one on either side of the incision. Pus and blood were matted to my surgical dressing, which needed to be pulled off before the nurses cleaned my incision. It was awful to look at and worse to have touched.

My room was quarantined because of my open wound. Visitors and medical personnel were supposed to wear protective clothing and gloves, but that was observed erratically at best. Mercifully, the quarantine sign kept the traffic through my room at a minimum. The insufferably cheerful candy stripers routinely mistook the warning to mean that they could catch whatever I had.

The last night of my supposed recovery stage at the hospital was the only time that my sister and brother joined my parents in my room. Even though I looked and felt better than I had earlier, my fourteen-year-old brother looked scared and sat far away from me. The rest of the family was enthusiastic about my recovery, and they were there for the first meal that I was allowed to eat. My father paid for the upgraded food tray—it was within his power to do that, so he did, hoping to help me. I didn't want to seem ungrateful, so even though I had no interest in food, I ate a little of the chocolate silk pie. It was the first time that I thought that my nightmare might be ending. The pain inside my abdomen had eased. The surgical-recovery pain was manageable and I knew from experience that this type of pain would get better with time. As long as things were better on the inside, things on the outside would improve.

My hopes were short-lived.

* * *

The next day it was clear to me that things were not better on the inside; the nightmare was not over, and something had gone seriously wrong. The pain was severe and different in a way that I couldn't specifically explain or describe to the nurses. They assured me that it was trapped gas, and that gas pains could be extreme. I knew the gas pains could be terrible, but this was something else.

One nurse offered me Tums®, which I accepted, but I was still in enough pain by noon that I begged the nurse who took over to do something. When the nurse left the room, my mother—upset from having watched me suffer all day—followed her. When she implored the nurse to help me, the nurse offered my mother a sedative. "I don't need drugs, my daughter does!" my mother protested. The nurse explained that the surgeon had written "no pain medication" on my chart because pain medication slowed down recovery.

I was not recovering. I was getting worse. I told every medical staff person who visited that day that something had changed, and I needed help. One nurse looked concerned, but told me that she didn't want to call the doctor—it was Sunday and he didn't like to have his weekends disturbed. But as the day continued, she must have changed her mind because he arrived later that afternoon.

As soon as he entered my room, I could see that he was angry. His jaw was clenched, his eyes cold, and he was moving quickly. He asked my mother to leave the room. I tried to explain how the pain had changed, thinking that he might be able to make sense of the subtle difference in quality and intensity. I could see that he wasn't listening. He gruffly examined my incision, pressing on my abdomen. "There's nothing new wrong with you," he said. "I know because I'm the doctor and you're the patient. You are a selfish, whiny baby. You want something to cry about? I'll give you something to cry about." Then he grabbed the two drainage tubes from the side of my lower abdomen and yanked them out of my body. I screamed and sobbed. He left the room.

* * *

Pain is a terrible thing. It distorts time. It reminds you of your own susceptibility to illness and injury. But people remind you of your helplessness. I learned later that the doctor had gone directly to my mother who was weeping in the hallway and said, "There's nothing wrong with your daughter except that you baby her." Then he stormed off the floor. I stopped asking for help because I knew that I wouldn't get any. I also knew now that angering the medical staff meant that they could hurt me. Dr. Evil had power, and I was his victim. All I could do was to hate him, and I did. Later that evening a nurse came in to my room saying,

"If anyone asks, I didn't give this to you." She added something to my IV. Soon all the pain washed away. It was the first relief I felt since my initial cramping. I wanted to hold on to it, but it was like smelling perfume—sweet, intoxicating and gone as soon as it fills your senses. I fell into a peaceful, sound sleep.

The next morning another nurse came in to take my vitals and check my IV. As soon as the thermometer was in my mouth she started to lecture me. She had heard all about the scene that I had caused the day before and encouraged me to remember that doctors and nurses were experts. They knew more about what was going on than I did. Her final words to me that day, "Trust us; we know what we're doing," were delivered as she sauntered confidently out of my room, leaving the thermometer in my mouth.

Not long afterward, Dr. Evil returned. This time he didn't make eye contact. He said that the morning's blood tests had indicated that my white blood cell count was soaring. The infection was out of control, and he needed to operate on me again. A nurse would soon be in to prep me. I wanted him to say that he should have taken my pain more seriously. I wanted him to apologize for treating me so badly, to say that he would listen to me in the future when I said there was a problem. Of course, he didn't say any of these things. But I had been right. *He* had been wrong. We both knew it. I thought that maybe without acknowledging it this experience would change things between us. It didn't. He remained an arrogant, nasty, insensitive ass. He was like the pain: something I couldn't alter, but had to endure.

* * *

The second surgery left me more incapacitated than the first. I had more uncomfortable tubes and was attached to even more apparatuses. I had a catheter as well as bags for nutrition, hydration, and antibiotics. Apparently they had difficulty finding a vein for my surgery IV because my entire arm was puffy and red. It soon became black and blue. On the right side of my bed was a large machine that intermittently sucked green bile out of my abdomen through a gastrointestinal (GI) tube, depositing it into a clear jar. A tube was taped into my right nostril and ran down my dry, scraped throat into my gut. I never adjusted to that hard, plastic tube and how it felt in my nose and throat. It caused me to gag when I swallowed and dry heave without warning.

I thought I was getting better when they took the GI tube out, but was horrified when they had to put it back in. A nurse shoved it up my nose and asked me to help her push it down my throat by swallowing hard. Something went wrong and it ended up coming out of my mouth. She had to pull it out and try again. Everything about the process was awful— hearing and feeling the crack of cartilage in my nose, feeling the scraping of the tube down my throat, not being able to breathe while it happened and knowing that it wouldn't even feel fine when it was done. It was an assault that made me feel like I was being suffocated. I now wonder if the panic it induced in me might feel something akin to waterboarding.

As I recovered from my second surgery, I noticed that the day nurses seemed to dislike me. My mother thought it was because people dislike those whom they wrong, and they had all wronged me. I thought it might have been because they were the most flirtatious with Dr. Evil. I always knew when they were with him because of all the giggling in the halls. (Once, my mother saw him pinch one of them on the ass.) The day nurses ignored my complaint that the IV didn't feel like it was in the right place. It was up to the next shift to find that my collapsed vein had allowed the medication to swell my soft tissue. If they could help it, the day nurses simply avoided me. The senior day nurses routinely sent one of the nurses-in-training to clean the incision from the second surgery, which was in the same place as the first incision but longer, sorer, and more open. The nurse-in-training was never supervised and she wasn't very careful either. When I suggested that dabbing the open wound with the gauze hurt less than rubbing it, she told me that she knew what she was doing. It was a familiar and unconvincing line.

This phase of my hospital stay lasted for weeks. It included a constant, cramping, burning pain and a poking, sharp pain in my abdomen. A day after surgery, they started me on walks. I couldn't stand up straight, but as long as two other people were available to push my carts and medicine, I could press a pillow to my abdomen and shuffle along in a bent position. These walks were supposed to help my bowels recover, move trapped gas around, and keep me from developing bed sores. Apparently a lot of patients complained about walks because nurses would tell me it was time for a walk as though I had already given them a hard time. I never did. I was diligent about the walks regardless of how difficult they were.

The dry heaving increased during a period of time when I observed that the bile-sucking machine wasn't working correctly. Of course, I reported it to the nurses, but that didn't help. I remember telling one that the machine "wasn't sucking anymore" and I was feeling sicker. She didn't even look at the machine. She just looked at me like I was an idiot and asked, "Do you know what 'intermittent' means?" I said,

"Yes, it means that starts and stops and starts again!"

Since the nurses wouldn't take my concerns seriously, I tried to get the hospital front desk to connect me to the people who distributed and maintained the machines. When I tracked them down, they said that they couldn't check the machine on a patient's request; they needed to be called by a nurse. I said that the nurses were ignoring me and maybe they could act like it was their own idea and just come by? They wouldn't.

Eventually the buildup of bile allowed the infection to strengthen causing my white blood cell count to climb even higher. Dr. Evil was on vacation, but his associate told my father that he would need to operate a third time. My father asked him if the bile drainage problem that I had complained about could have something to do with the infection. I think he was trying to placate my father by looking into my concerns because the doctor brought me to radiology where the position of my GI tube was examined. It revealed that the tube was not in the right place. It needed to be pushed further down into my abdomen to reach the fluid that it was supposed to drain. The trip to radiology was uncomfortable. Lying flat made me dry heave; having the tube pulled and pushed again though my nose and throat was awful, but at least I avoided another operation. Dr. Evil's associate even told my father, "Your daughter was right," which was nice, but I would rather he have told me directly. He had already aligned himself with Dr. Evil, and that had been clear the first time I met him.

There had been so many problems with my veins and IVs that they wanted to have another direct line put in. The doctor who had put in my original subclavian arterial line came to put in another one on the other side of my chest. Before I could even think about what I was saying, I protested, "No. Don't do that. My body is telling me that that's not a good idea."

"You're just saying that because you know it hurts," he explained, dismissively. But that wasn't the reason I was rejecting the second line. I didn't understand it myself, but I *knew* that it was a bad idea and it shouldn't be done. But it didn't matter what I thought. He was going to do it anyway. Once again, the bed was leveled, my chest was cut, and a long needle was stuck in it. Then the doctor said, "Well, that didn't work. Sometimes they don't. Still, I needed to try." Then he was gone.

The next doctor to try to get a tube into one of my arteries was Dr. Evil's sidekick. He came in with two of my least favorite day nurses at his side. "I've heard all about you," he said sternly as he moved rapidly about the room preparing . . . *for what?* "I'm not going to put up with any of your complaining," he continued. "I need to do a cutdown. It's going to hurt a lot, but I don't want to hear one peep out of you." Then, he put a light on his head and a nurse held down my arm. He cut a two-inch incision at the crux of my arm and started shoving a small tube through it. Silently, I endured what would be one of the top five, most painful things that I ever experienced. I stared at him, mentally chanting, *I hate you. I hate you. I hate you.* When he was done, he looked at me and saw the angry determination in my eyes as I stared at him. I had done what he asked, no—demanded of me, and *still* silently conveyed my objection to the procedure and my disdain for his insensitivity. I wasn't the problem patient he'd been led to believe I was, and he knew it. He looked uncomfortable and didn't seem to know what to say next. I could see that he wasn't evil. I didn't need to hate him anymore. After all, he was just the sidekick.

I started to feel more exhausted. I had trouble taking deep breaths. I reported this problem to an afternoon nurse. She said that I was probably hyperventilating because I was upset. If I could calm myself down, I would feel better. I was too weak to finish my walk through the hallways that day. The nurse who was assisting me told me she would allow me to "cut the walk short *this* time," as if I were pulling a scam on her. Another nurse said that my breathing problem was in my head. It sure felt like it was in my body. Nevertheless, I mentally instructed myself to, *calm down*, breathing in when I thought, *calm* and out as I thought, *down*.

I didn't realize how much time elapsed as I concentrated, but I knew it was late when I saw Dr. Ghost. He was a tall, thin, pale man with hair like Gene Wilder. He was soft-spoken, and never seemed to be in a rush. I had rarely seen him during the day, but occasionally he would turn up by my bedside at night. He wasn't a surgeon, but I knew that in some way he was working on my case.

Dr. Ghost asked me what I was doing up so late. I could barely assemble enough breath to explain, "I'm trying to breathe." He asked me what the problem with my breathing was, and I said the nurses believed I was too emotional and needed to calm down. He said that a chest x-ray might tell a different story and promptly ordered one. It was another uncomfortable trip to radiology because standing up straight was as difficult as lying flat, but at least this time no one touched the nose tube.

In the morning, Dr. Evil came trotting into my room with his day-nurse entourage. Referencing the prior night's chest x-ray as though he'd ordered it himself, he said, "An x-ray revealed that you have a punctured lung. Since it happened days ago when they tried to insert the subclavian arterial line, there is no time to waste." I was immediately turned onto my right side and asked to put my arm behind my head. Then he cut me on the side of my breast and shoved a large tube through the incision into my lung. (A friend of mine whose lung collapsed from a gunshot wound also had this procedure done. When I spoke to her, she insisted that the gunshot wound was less painful. She imagined that the procedure resembled the feeling of being impaled.) Dr. Evil finished the procedure and swept out of the room. It was then that I realized that I could breathe again. But each breath rekindled the pain.

I kept hoping that the pain would ease, but it didn't. I looked at my mother with a panic that she had become familiar with and I said, "It feels like they're still cutting!" For hours, a cutting sensation accompanied my every breath. I thought I would go insane from re-experiencing this trauma over and over again. So, I once again went into my self-hypnotic, trance-like chanting. This time the mantra was: *It feels like they're still cutting. It feels like they're still cutting.* . . . I remember that my father was there that day, so it must have been a weekend. He practically crawled under the bed with the telephone receiver so that I could receive a call from Mark, Kris's best friend. This was the only phone call I took during my time in the hospital. I don't remember what Mark said, but I recall finding his voice soothing. He would later become a minister, and I think his reassuring calmness probably helps him with that job.

Late that night, in the same position, feeling the same pain, focusing on the same words, I didn't notice Dr. Ghost enter the room. "Why aren't you asleep tonight?" he asked kindly.

"It feels like they're still cutting," was all I could say, unwilling (or perhaps unable) to break the focus that kept me from whatever madness was in this seemingly bottomless anguish. He turned on the lights to look at the wound, then left and returned with a night nurse. Dr. Evil and his minions had not taped the tube into the hole or bandaged the wound correctly; therefore, it had been constantly shifting position, resulting in the continuous-cutting sensation. Before they started, Dr. Ghost had the nurse add a pain medication to my IV. The second night of peaceful sleep of my hospital stay followed. It no longer felt like they were cutting. Dr. Ghost talked to my parents the next day. He told them that he had ignored Dr. Evil's order regarding painkillers because I was close to going into shock, which would have slowed my recovery even more. He expressed surprise that I hadn't gone into shock. He thought that most people in my circumstances and condition would have.

"Don't let them tell you that your daughter isn't tough," he said.

The collapsed lung brought the respiratory team to my room to prescribe exercises. They were encouraging so I worked hard for them, blowing in and out of a little plastic apparatus, trying to keep the ball inside airborne. The addition of a big respiration machine with a tube running into my side made walks even trickier. It also provided me with one more machine that could malfunction.

I was still savoring Dr. Ghost's praise when I first smelled smoke. *Was there a fire or electrical short in the respirator machine? Or was it in the bile-sucking machine again?* I called a nurse but it wasn't until black smoke started pouring out the air vent that she or my mother smelled anything. The nurse made a call, and the floor started evacuating. There was no way I was going to be able to move fast enough to get out of the room, so the nurse called for assistance in getting me out. Her request was misunderstood, so a Code Blue went out over the public address system, broadcasting that I had flat-lined. Men with defibrillator pads ran in to revive me. Fortunately, the nurse was able to stop them before they sent an electrical current through my chest. The nurse and my mother maneuvered my bed out into the hallway, but we stopped at the elevator doors, which had been disabled by the firemen who came running up the stairs in full gear. There was no way I could escape the floor, so I hoped they could take care of the problem. I remember my mother and a doctor waiting with me.

"I can't believe this," the doctor said. I could. I was beyond surprise.

How could I be surprised by a system that allowed the doctor who originally misdiagnosed me and ignored my calls to be my admitting doctor? How could I be surprised by a system that then permitted him to charge me for daily visits during which he did nothing? Every time I saw him, my blood would boil. It didn't help that he was always so cheerful and said inane things like, "You're spending so much time here, you could be a nurse." How could I be surprised after Dr. Evil ordered a rectal tube to release trapped gas? It was an uncomfortable and humiliating experience to have a nurse stick a tube (with a plastic balloon on the other end) up my ass. When I told him that this wasn't effective and that I wanted it discontinued, he laughed and said, "I don't think it ever actually works, but it is a great way for nurses to get back at patients." Get back at us for what? Is it for being sick, being in pain or not responding well to their treatments? What had I ever done to these people besides try to help them help me?

* * *

All told, the hospital stay lasted seven weeks. It wasn't clear until the final few days of the stay that I would live. I was finally cured because Dr. Ghost went to a medical conference and shared my case with other doctors. He asked them for suggestions for antibiotic combinations that might successfully fight my peritonitis. One of those suggestions worked. Years later, I was sad to learn that Dr. Ghost no longer practiced medicine. "There was something in the newspaper about a malpractice suit," my uncle said. That was hard to believe. Maybe he was a scapegoat, or disillusioned by having to work in such a heartless profession. Or maybe he just made a mistake.

The hospital seemed like an entirely different place when I was recovering. I began writing letters to my friends, explaining what had happened to me and why I had been unreachable for nearly two months. Many of them didn't know I had been in the hospital because my new roommate had simply told them, "She's not here. I'll have her call you back when she returns." Maybe this was her way of getting back at me for sleeping in her bed. My friend Robin eventually tired of this refrain and demanded,

"Why isn't she ever home anymore?" That's how she finally learned that I was in the hospital. She came with my favorite lemonade, not knowing that I couldn't take anything by mouth.

A friend from work had known because I had my father notify my employer. I remember waking up after surgery and seeing her sitting in my room holding a single rose. She looked petrified. I was also visited during the final week by my friend Jeff. I don't know how he found out, but he was upset that he hadn't known sooner. He said that he could have been helped me by praying. I remember how surprised my mother was when he dropped to his knees, raised a hand in the air, and called on Jesus to heal me.

Kris had come to visit me once, on Mother's Day, telling me about all the fun I was missing. He had a new friend whom he said I'd like. Since I wasn't around, they were hanging out all the time. She was funny, fun and smart, and as an added bonus—also short and blonde. Before he left, he asked if he could take some of my flowers home to his mother. I'd like to say that his visit gave me a new perspective on him and cured me of my longings, but it didn't. It just made me sad. His friend Mark sent me a love letter in German (which he spoke, but I didn't). Another friend came to read and translate it for me. He was in town for a visit the last week of my hospital stay and came dressed in a huge bozo shirt long enough to look like a dress. I remember how he made the afternoon nurses laugh. Too bad laughter filled such a small part of the time I spent there.

There were still challenges when I was released from the hospital. My first meal at home made me so sick I was almost readmitted. After that I developed a daily routine that helped me readjust to food and gain strength. I slept ten hours a night, and took about two hours trying to go to the bathroom and shower, while resting in between. Then I'd go downstairs for my half-a-banana breakfast, after which I'd read for a while, write letters to friends, and walk laps around the living room while playing the best side of the *London Calling* album by The Clash. Next came lunch—the other half of the banana. Later my brother would come home from school and bring in the mail. He'd usually pretend that nothing had arrived for me and then giggle when he revealed at least one card or letter in his back pocket. We'd watch *General Hospital* together and have some vanilla ice cream. Then I'd write or read until my parents came home from work. Each day, I'd try to eat a little more for dinner than I had the day before.

My friend Frank visited when I was home from the hospital. We had been on the speech team together in high school. He was one of the quirky, nerdy boys who quoted *Star Trek* dialogue and played a lot of *Risk*®. I remember how angry he was about what had happened to me. He paced, clenching and unclenching his fists as I told him about it. These doctors would be punished when he ruled the world, he reassured me. I appreciated the sentiments, but didn't put much stock in his plans. I had heard him talk about building an empire before but never took it very seriously. Years later, I would learn that he was in federal prison for embezzling millions of dollars. In his defense, he said he needed to because "Taking over the world is expensive."

My mother often said that I already had more than my share of pain, and should be healthy from then on. Wouldn't it be nice if there were a finite and fair amount of pain for each individual to experience in his or her lifetime? I would never have chosen to endure so much of mine all at once. But if that was how it worked, I was glad to have mine behind me. It was a nice thought, but I had been through too much to believe that anything about health was fair.

Despite my parents' belief in fairness, they discouraged me from trying to sue the doctors or hospital for what had happened. My father said that if I wanted to pursue it, then he'd contact a lawyer, but I needed to go to the meeting alone. I did, but the lawyer didn't think I had a case that could be won. First, it would be difficult to get a doctor to testify against other doctors, but juries needed to hear their testimony to find challenges credible. Second, appendicitis was difficult to diagnose, though he thought a simple blood test would have secured me a hospital bed right away. Third, he didn't *see* any permanent harm. He said a jury would look at me and see a healthy girl who had been healed. He didn't think they could be convinced that I had been wronged. I thanked him for his opinion and didn't give a lawsuit another thought. I knew that I had been damaged but that my trauma wouldn't be evident to a jury. The important thing was to put this behind me and get on with my life.

Before I could do that, I needed to see Dr. Evil one more time so that he could remove my stitches. I suspected that he'd make this as uncomfortable as possible, but it didn't end up hurting very much. Perhaps that is why he had to find some other way to try and hurt me. As he clipped each stitch, he looked at my scar and said, "That's probably the most hideous scar I've ever given anyone." I almost laughed in his face. I knew the scar was ugly, but why would I care about that when I was alive, pain-free, and beyond his sadistic reach? Did he actually think he could hurt my ego? Or was he just trying to remind me that the ugliness he had brought to my life would be with me forever? He continued,

"I think you should consider plastic surgery." I said,

"No way. I would never go through surgery for cosmetic reasons, especially after what I've been through." He looked surprised.

"Well, I take a lot of pride in my work and that scar doesn't represent me as a surgeon. So don't tell anyone that's mine." So, Dr. Evil wanted something from me now. He wasn't going to get it. As I looked at him for the last time, I knew that there was no scar horrendous enough to represent him.

Chapter 5: "Not My Body Part": My Knee Problems Continue

By the time the second session of summer school began in 1980, I felt like myself again. Actually, I felt better. I was enjoying the euphoria of having escaped death. Just like the clichés say: I didn't sweat the small stuff; I appreciated every day; and I saw every day as a miracle. As much as I tried to hold onto them, these feelings faded, enduring just long enough to help me adjust to Kris graduating and moving away, and to Mark dating someone else. Neither would be my Mr. Right. Those same feelings of euphoria might also have drawn Scott to me. He was looking for Ms. Right and had assumed she'd be a cheerful, joyful girl like Marie Osmond or Debbie Boone. I did not fit that mold, though my recently-eluded death glow might have made it seem like I did.

Scott was a trustworthy, straight-laced romantic who wooed me enthusiastically. He planned elaborate dates and created Barry Manilow-infused soundtracks to accompany them. He sent me lots of flowers commemorating anniversaries that I didn't remember, like our first phone call or the day he told me he loved me. He would drive me to my parents' house for the weekend. He got his father to fix my junkie old car; he gave me half of the money he won playing Jai-Alai on our date, because he "wouldn't have been here to win it without you." When I had the flu, he showed up at my work with a bag of remedies, dramatically pulling each out of the bag like a magician and his hat. Once he picked me up from a dance club late at night because he didn't trust that the person I was with would be sober enough to safely drive me home. He didn't dance, he didn't drink, but he didn't want to stop me from enjoying myself.

My knee limitations and puffy abdomen (with scars so pronounced that my bathing suit clung to their outlines) didn't discourage Scott. He played softball and tennis with his friends; he didn't need a girlfriend for that. He focused on smile and my eyes. The post-surgery limitations on my diet weren't problems either since his palate was extremely narrow and conventional. He wasn't horrified by my story because he had heard plenty of gruesome tales from his mother—an emergency medical technician. So it seemed like my medical baggage wouldn't be a problem in our relationship.

During a yearly examination, I was told I would need a mammogram because there were suspicious lumps in my breasts—not something that I expected dealing with in my twenties. I wanted to be reassured, but when I told Scott, he seemed more alarmed than I was. He inundated me with increasingly confrontational and almost angry questions: "What does this mean? What's going to happen? What am *I* supposed to do?" And finally, "I don't know what you want from me!" Ironically, *I* ended up reassuring *him*:

"It's probably nothing," I predicted. "You don't have to worry about it. I'll take care of it. Let's talk about something else." It turned out that the lumps were normal, but the scare had reminded me that being loved didn't make me any less alone when it came to health problems. Another person could worry about me and commiserate with me, but he would not feel what I would feel. He couldn't completely understand my nearly-debilitating fear of pain. He would not share my distrust of doctors and nurses. If I became seriously injured or ill again, I would be on my own in a body that didn't work, squaring off against a medical system that might hurt me more than help me. Fortunately, I was blessed with many years of good health, and I didn't have to deal with this.

Scott and I got married after my first year in graduate school at Florida State University, where I was working towards a Ph.D. in Political Science. Our lives in Tallahassee were quiet and laid-back. We put our energy into school and work. Scott and I didn't go dancing as I had throughout college—refusing to let my bad knee get in the way of a good time, I would resolutely planted my right leg away from the crowd and focus on my upper body movements. Scott and I spent our evenings watching movies and eating pizza. Sometimes we'd go to a friend's house for *Trivial Pursuit®* and junk food. It wasn't a life that should have taxed my knee and yet my knee got worse. My knee's slide had become a painful pop and jerk that made it difficult to walk. My usual remedies of ice at night, limited activity for a few days, and aspirin weren't helping with the pain. Every step became difficult. Every night I would go to bed with a swollen knee, and each morning it would look better. I would try to not to aggravate it, but that required not bending my right knee. When I tried to walk straight-legged I got back pains. I suspected that a wheelchair was in my future, but I couldn't bring myself to admit defeat yet, and so I went to an orthopedist.

The doctor took my history, examined my knee, and ordered some x-rays. *Would he recommend the bone-moving operation with the screws?* I wondered, shuddering at the thought. No, the operations for this problem were notorious for not working well, he assessed. He determined it'd be better to solve it with physical therapy—building the muscle up to hold my knee in place. I objected, explaining that I tried that, but he replied that physical therapy had made lots of advancements in the ten years since my surgery. There was something called "biofeedback" that could help. He also said that by taking aspirin every day, I could easily toughen up what little cartilage was left under my knee. I forget exactly how many aspirins he recommended, but I recall that the number seemed excessive.

"For how long?" I asked.

"Indefinitely," he replied, clarifying, "your problem is not going away."

"But won't that be hard on my stomach? Won't it cause ulcers?"

"I don't know," he admitted. "That's not my body part." I wondered if he was so steeped in his specialized training that he could not understand what I was saying, or if he was just startled by being challenged (even indirectly). He didn't try to explain, qualify, or justify what he had said. Apparently he did not find anything odd about admitting that he cared only for my bones and joints and had no concern for the rest of me. He was simply living up to his medical training—to be a specialist. He wasn't going to take any responsibility for the consequences his recommendation might have on my digestive system.

"They're all my body parts," I said before ending the appointment.

* * *

Years later, I had a lump in my jaw that didn't go away for a few weeks. I went to see my primary care physician and told him that I was concerned about a growth on my jaw that felt like a marble. I reported when I had noticed it, how it moved without discomfort, and that it became sore if I touched it for too long. He was reading some papers while I talked and continued to read as I pointed to the location of the growth. When he finally looked up, he said, "It's probably swollen glands. That's a common problem." He put his hands along the sides of my upper neck and felt for them. "No, you don't have swollen glands. I don't feel any lump. You're fine," he said nonchalantly.

"That's not where the lump is," I explained, guiding his hand to the ball on my jaw. "That's where," I told him, demonstrating how the lump slid across the bone.

"Oh, yes, I feel it," he said. He started walking toward the door as he admitted, "I don't know what that is, but I'm not worried about it." Before he could slip out, I interjected,

"If it was on your jaw would you be worried about it, especially if you didn't know what it was?" He stopped and made eye contact with me for the first time during the appointment. Smiling sheepishly, he acknowledged,

"Yes, I suppose I would be worried." He came back, spent more time feeling the lump and asked me several questions about it. Some of the answers he would have known if he had listened to my initial report. But I didn't care if I had to repeat myself. He explained that because the lump was neither attached to bone nor soft, he felt confident that it was not a serious problem. He said that if it changed in the next few weeks I should contact him again, and he would give me a referral to a specialist.

Maybe I hadn't needed to ask him to put himself in my shoes in order for him to take the problem seriously. Maybe he simply didn't realize that I was a patient who needed more of an explanation to accept his diagnosis. Maybe I should have gained confidence in primary care physicians from this experience because ultimately, he was right and the lump was nothing to worry about. (In a few weeks, it disappeared.) But instead, I interpreted this experience as additional evidence that I couldn't trust doctors to automatically take me, or my symptoms, seriously.

* * *

I didn't take the aspirin as prescribed by my doctor, but I did go to the physical therapist, where I received an all-too-familiar knee exercise regime. After a few weeks the biofeedback indicated that I was getting the most out of my muscle, but it wasn't enough to hold the kneecap in place. The therapist recommended a knee brace. It was a foot-long, elastic sleeve with a circular hole for the kneecap. I would slide it on and then tighten it with a rubber device attached to the brace with Velcro®. At the spot where my kneecap came out of the hole in the brace, the rubber device contained a metal object that held the kneecap in place when I bent my leg. I put it on when I would get out of the shower in the morning and take it off before I went to sleep at night. It felt like a miracle, allowing me to walk without pain. I was to wear versions of this brace for the next ten years.

The brace drew attention. Strangers assumed that I was an injured athlete and talked to me about sports. I marveled that people could be so intrusive, wondering whether they would ask people in wheelchairs what had happened to them. Did they ask blind people, "When are you going to see again?" I doubted it. Yet, the idea that I would always wear a knee brace seemed to vex people. It jarred with their overall impression of me—a healthy-looking, quick-walking, young woman—and challenged their beliefs about the American medical system. Some strangers would insist that doctors could "do something" and that I had "given up too soon." I remember one woman telling me that she would rather be dead than wear something so ugly. I didn't think the brace was ugly. It was beautiful because I could walk without pain. The brace saved me from playing "surgery roulette," a gamble that many weak-kneed people were invariably lured into by the hope that *this* would be the surgery that solved their pain.

I eventually had a second knee surgery after graduate school when I was working my first professional job as an Assistant Professor in Washington, D.C. I gave in to the common wisdom that medicine had made many advances since my first operation. It was foolish *not* to do something, especially now that I was in a metropolitan area with presumably better doctors than

Florida. I went to an orthopedist who talked me into having arthroscopic surgery. He said it was outpatient surgery, ("nothing to it," were his words) and it *should* take care of my problem.

It didn't. Instead, it took three tries to get an IV in and I developed back problems from the physical therapy that followed the surgery. They had positioned me incorrectly on one of the machines and so instead of building my leg muscles, I pulled something in my back. My knee kept sliding out of position. After an unsuccessful attempt to use all of his body weight to hold my knee in place while I bent it, the physical therapist conceded, "Don't let any doctor talk you into thinking that you can get that muscle to hold that kneecap in." After the surgery and physical therapy, I was back in the brace.

I was still wearing the brace when I started my second teaching job, this time in Carlisle, Pennsylvania. After my divorce from Scott in 1990, when I was thirty, I accepted a job at Dickinson College. I had been living there a few years when my knee brace days finally ended. I had known for some time that I should replace the brace; it was old and worn, but my Pennsylvania orthopedist was unfamiliar with the device and where to get it. I never found out if he had managed to track a supplier down, because I was literally forced out of the old brace when I dislocated my knee while wearing it.

This dislocation was no less memorable than the first. I was in New Orleans for a political science conference. I had joined four male colleagues for dinner and we had just arrived at the Old Absinthe House, a famous bar/restaurant on Bourbon Street. I had gone to the upstairs restroom and simply lost my footing coming down the marble spiral staircase. I knew that I had dislocated my knee as soon as I hit the floor. The manager ran over when he heard me scream. Concerned, he questioned, "Are you okay?"

"No!" I cried. "I dislocated my knee."

"Are you alone?"

"No, I'm with the men at the end of the bar." The manager brought them over. They looked a little pale, and one held my hand while an ambulance came. The EMT drew my blood, (probably to see what my blood alcohol level was), mercifully finding a vein without a problem. One of the EMTs said lightheartedly,

"I think you're the first sober person I've ever picked up on Bourbon Street." They took me to Tulane University Hospital. Its emergency room was deserted, so I got a lot of attention. After an x-ray and a confirmation of my diagnosis, they gave me crutches, a prescription for some painkillers, and told me to go to my orthopedist when I got home. They gave me the x-rays, but I left them in the cab.

My colleague got me to my room, put me to bed, and promised to call my friend Lydia to fill her in on what happened. Lydia came through. The next day she brought me painkillers and some food. I slept a lot. The following day she brought Chinese takeout. With a lot of help from her and some from the sky cabs, I flew home. My friends Kelly and Wendy picked me up at the airport. They had both been field hockey players and were currently coaches, so I knew they had seen their share of knee

injuries. They agreed that I had the biggest swollen knee they'd
ever seen.

Being on crutches after my first surgery at sixteen had not
been easy, but at least I had my mother to take care of me. She
drove me to doctor's appointments, cooked my meals, and helped
me get around the house. Being on crutches in my mid-thirties, in
the midst of a semester of teaching and living alone, was much
more difficult. I wasn't dating anyone at the time, so there was no
default helper. Maneuvering around my home wasn't a problem (I
had purposely bought a one-story house in anticipation of being
wheelchair-bound), but just about everything else was. How could
I eat if I couldn't carry something and move at the same time? I
would toss bottled water onto a chair and then hobble over to the
chair with my crutches to drink it, but I couldn't do that with food.
The immobilizer around my leg meant I drove with my left foot on
the pedals and my right leg on the front seat. This was effective,
but probably illegal.

Fortunately, friends rallied to help me. Surprisingly, the
ones who offered me rides, brought me food, and listened to me
whine did not include a few of the people I thought were my
closest friends. The woman who I considered my best friend
actually said, "Give me a call when you're up and running again,
and we'll go to a movie." There was no knee bending in my
immediate future and it would be months before I was able to sit in
a theater.

As I struggled to fulfill my professional and personal
responsibilities, all the time worrying about what possible solution

(if any) would be offered by the doctor this time, I had to deal with acquaintances joking about my being on crutches. Since I had to find a way to ascend two flights of stairs to teach a class, I wasn't in any shape to be teased about the elevator being broken. Sitting on the first step, I used my arms to lift myself to the next. Then, I doggedly dragged my book bag and crutches after me. I repeated this process until I reached the landing, used the stair rail to drag myself to my feet, propped myself up with my crutches and swung into class. When I was trying to balance myself on crutches with books hanging in a book bag from my neck, I didn't want to hear any clever comments. When I was sitting in the grass trying to locate the screw that had come out of the crutch and caused me to fall on my face, I needed help more than I needed a joke.

I had reached my limit of insensitive remarks when one day I was wobbling back to my office after teaching an "Introduction to Women's Studies" class. I was trying to talk to a student when a male colleague passed with a mischievous look in his eye. "There's nothing sexier than a woman on crutches," he quipped.

"Right, that's why I dislocated my knee," I said sarcastically. Maybe he thought I was playing along, but I wasn't. I was trying to leave without looking like he'd upset me. I wanted to say, "I'm at work and we're not friends. Don't comment about my sexual appeal," but I didn't have the energy to stand on one foot, book bag around my neck, any longer.

When we got to my office, I could see that my student was rattled. "How could he say that?" she asked. I tried to make it a teaching moment, to help her see how this was an example of the patriarchy that she had been reading about in class. He had probably been unaware that he was exercising his male privilege, saying whatever he wanted to say to a girl. Still looking puzzled, she replied, "Yeah, I see that, but do you *really* think he thinks that women on crutches are *sexy*?" I couldn't tell if she thought it was impossible for a woman on crutches to be sexy or if she was troubled by the idea that he would find a wounded women sexy *because* of her limitations. (Probably the former.) I agreed that it was troubling to think that men might find women who couldn't run away sexier than those who could stand on their own two feet. *If being around a woman who needed help made this man feel more masculine, then why hadn't he ever helped me open doors, carry books or move around obstacles in the hallways? Why was I even trying to figure this out? I shouldn't have to deal with this, too,* I thought. I knew I should have just put it out of my mind, but he had gotten to me, and I resented it.

Only after I went to talk to the chair of his department did I feel better. I acknowledged that my colleague hadn't been hitting on me, but argued that the inappropriate, insensitive and discomforting nature of his comment constituted sexual harassment. The chair begrudgingly agreed to talk to my colleague. I never got an apology, but I did get ignored by the colleague for years.

During this time on crutches, I tried to fulfill all of my obligations. One was to give a speech a few hours away at a YWCA, which was part of my work with the Pennsylvania Humanities Council. I leaned on a table so that the audience could see me. It helped make my leg more comfortable, but I noticed that I was dizzy. This got worse that night, so the next day, I went to my primary care physician. He said that I had an ear infection that should easily be taken care of with drugs. I took the drugs and that night had an allergic reaction. Huge, itchy, red, puffy, blotches erupted all over my skin. I called the doctor's office. They said to stop taking the drug and take Benadryl®. They would see me the following week.

Hobbling, still a little dizzy, blotchy, and itchy, I went to a lunch meeting at work. "Look at you, you shouldn't be here! You should be at the doctor's," chided an Associate Dean. I told her that I had called them, and they didn't have an opening until the next week. I was waiting my turn. But the Dean didn't sanction my compliance: "You need to see them now. Either call them and say that you are having shortness of breath or show up and once they get one look at you they'll fit you in," she advised. Demanding attention from a doctor was a novel idea to me. I was good at taking no for an answer. I had certainly never thought of lying about my symptoms to get medical attention. "Go," she urged gently. "The Benadryl® isn't working. You need something stronger. You shouldn't have to suffer for a week. You don't have to. The doctors work for you, not the other way around. You're paying them to do a job."

I took a moment and tried to think of myself as a healthcare consumer. It was a novel idea. I couldn't say that I was sold on it, but I went to the doctor's office anyway. The receptionist was alarmed enough to let me see a nurse, who got me some drugs that eventually helped. I felt relieved until I talked to a friend who had the same reaction to the same drug. Her doctor had given her a shot that made the problem disappear in hours instead of days. My small victory didn't entirely change my assumptions about the medical system. Even *if* I was a consumer, instead of a victim, I still wasn't all-powerful. If a plumber said he wasn't available that week, my faucet would keep dripping. Healthcare wasn't like buying a dress, either. I couldn't say, "You need my business more than I need your product." If I couldn't fix something, I was at the mercy of those who could.

* * *

Eventually, my knee injury healed enough for me to go to physical therapy, since my Pennsylvania doctor said there weren't any new surgical solutions to my problem. I remember liking the physical therapist. She was animated, energetic, and a good listener. When she asked me to tell her about my knee, I started with "twenty years ago . . . ," and she said, "Uh oh, that's bad news." When she heard that I had a chronic-subluxing patella, she grimaced: "Those are the hardest to fix. I'd rather see a blown out ACL." She didn't minimize my injury; she didn't say that I was going to be fine, but she did think she could help. She had strong professional opinions and wasn't reluctant to share them when I asked. Her approach made me feel understood, worthwhile, and hopeful.

The operation I had in 1976 had never worked on any patient she had seen. Despite the fact that surgeons like to operate and patients wanted to believe in surgical solutions, she recommended that I stay away from surgery as long as I could. The surgery that *would* fix my problem was a knee replacement, but they didn't last long enough for me to get one yet. I was too young. She joked, "Try to figure out when you're likely to die, subtract ten years, and get a new knee then." Apparently knee replacements only lasted about a decade. Finally, I had something definite to say to the old men who badgered me about getting a knee replacement like they had.

As for solutions, the physical therapist had some new ones. She believed that exercises would help, but she didn't stick to the same ones that I had been given by previous physical therapists. She was convinced that I needed to work on my balance and my hip. She noted that I walked with my toe pointed inward because I was subconsciously trying to protect my knee—to hold it in so that it wouldn't slide out. But this was the worst position for it. She showed me how this angled my leg in a way that actually made the knee slide out more. Being careful and trying to protect myself had actually jeopardized me. I couldn't help but wonder if this message had a universal application for my life.

She put me on a stationary bike, lowering the seat to cut down the motion of my knee. She showed me how I could adjust all kinds of exercises so that I worked important muscles without risking damage to the joint. She said, "Don't believe the motto: no pain, no gain. Especially when it comes to your knee. Stop whatever you're doing when you feel pain. Whatever you're doing will be causing more damage than good." This was reassuring advice.

Eventually the physical therapist used the McConnell Taping technique, which entailed realigning my patella so it tracked correctly and then taping it into place. The first time she tried this, she asked me to try to walk with the tape on. These were the first steps that I took bending my knee after my second dislocation. She asked me how it felt. I said, "Odd, like I am walking on a pillow." She laughed.

"That's called cartilage. It is supposed to feel that way when you walk." There wasn't any popping, sliding, or pain. It was amazing. Then, she taught me how to put the tape on myself. I could start walking again without the immobilizer and without a knee brace. It felt like a miracle.

Having a little tape across my knee was hardly noticeable, yet it gave me more support than the brace. I looked normal and I felt great. The tape liberated me; so much so that soon after, I agreed to take an active vacation with a quirky, attractive man I met at a wedding. We sailed up the East Coast on a thirty-two-foot sailboat. It had sounded romantic, but turned out to be more adventure than vacation. A few days into the trip, Cameron told me that the boat had been deemed *almost* seaworthy. There were problems with the engine, so we spent a lot of time bobbing, waiting for a breeze. The toilet didn't work, so I wouldn't eat or drink much until we docked for the night. The sail got torn in a storm that even he admitted had been dangerous.

Cameron was frustrated with my lack of sailing experience and was fastidious about his defective boat. After passing too close to a garbage barge, the boat became infested with flies. He insisted that I only kill flies on the mast pole because he didn't want fly guts on the boat's wood or upholstery. Sailing was a lot more like camping than I expected and Cameron reminded me of Felix Unger from *The Odd Couple* comedy I had watched as a kid. Nevertheless, it was a bold journey for a woman who had always chosen the safe route. I felt liberated from more than just a knee brace. I had *needed* an adventure more than a vacation.

The story of my knee does not officially end here. A few years later, I started having some more pain in my knees. The same Pennsylvania doctor who sent me to therapy to get out of the brace thought it was time I go back to wearing one. He thought physical therapy wouldn't help this time because he could see the kneecap sliding when I straightened my leg on the end of the examination table; the muscle wouldn't have a chance against that pull. Nevertheless, he agreed to refer me to therapy since I wanted to give it a try.

I showed my new physical therapist the knee slide. He asked me if I spent a lot of time sitting on the end of tables straightening my leg. I laughed: "Not outside of the doctor's office, I don't."

"That's what I thought," he said. "So let's not worry about that. Let's try to get you to walk without pain and swelling." It was like a twist on the old joke about the patient who says, "Doctor it hurts when I do this"; and the doctor replies, "Stop doing that."

This physical therapist thought that much of my problem was with the position of my foot and the fact that my right leg was a half-inch shorter than my left. Why had it taken someone in the medical profession over twenty years to notice that? He fit me with an orthotic, a special sole to put in my shoe. He trained me to put pressure on the outside of my foot when I walked. That took care of the problem and I didn't need to return to a brace. That was over ten years ago, and every time I feel a pull in my knee I consciously shift my weight to the outside of my foot and marvel at how much better it feels. Once again, a physical therapist was my hero.

Most of the people I know now don't remember that I had a knee problem. They can't recall the brace. But for twenty-five years, my right knee was like walking around with an egg in my pocket: I watched it, worried about it, contorted myself to keep it safe, and still ended up watching it crack and break more than once. That's not easy to forget.

My knee problems and how they were treated by doctors have taught me a few things that resonate with my other health experiences. First, no matter how hard I tried, I couldn't protect myself from harm. I tried to be careful with my body and not ask too much of it. Second, even though most people did not know what I'd been through or what was wrong with my body, it did not stop them from telling me what I should be doing differently. They interpreted my acceptance of my physical limitations as a mistake, perhaps even a character flaw. They thought I lacked persistence and faith in doctors who could heal me. Third, no matter what anyone said or thought, doctors didn't have solutions to my knee problem, and some of them couldn't admit that. There was always something else that they could try if I would let them. They'd get paid for trying, regardless of their success or failure. Once I realized that this was how it worked, I could better protect myself from them. Some of them hurt me more than they helped me; others just couldn't help. Like my appendix nightmare, my knee problems had exposed an unhealthy healthcare system. I concluded that the only way to save myself from doctors was to stay well enough to avoid them.

Chapter 6: "You're Fine": Hit by a Dodge Ram Van

In my late thirties, my life (finally) felt balanced. My body felt good and I felt good about it. I was out of the brace, exercising regularly, and unencumbered by any physical challenges. The confidence and zeal I had for being a professor were both at their highest. I was publishing more often and in better journals and I had a new book out. I began to travel, enjoying some of the money that I had cautiously squirreled away. I had become more discerning about whom I spent time with and as a result my circle of friends was strong and full of interesting, caring people. When necessary, I was secure choosing work or solitude over socializing, yet there were still a lot of dinners out and conversations over beers. All that was missing was a significant other. At thirty-nine, I decided to make finding him a priority. Fortunately, there was a relatively new social networking site that would allow me to take the initiative: the *Yahoo! Personals Web Page*®.

In the late 1990s, using the Internet to find love seemed foolish at best and dangerous at worst. But I decided that if I followed a careful protocol and kept my sense of humor, it would be worth trying. Living in small town, rural Pennsylvania meant that available (and suitable) men were precious rarities. Too often, I had tried to make relationships work that should have been rejected quickly. With the advent of Internet dating, I didn't have to use that approach. I had a virtual supermarket of men!

I called it "Yahoo dating" for more reasons than the website's name. Many of the men who posted ads that I answered were "Yahoos," Jonathan Swift's satirical rendering of mankind's worst traits. I would read the ads looking for evidence of intelligence, humor, and self-awareness. I'd email the men who seemed to have these qualities, asking, "What do you do for a living and what do you like the most and least about it?" One man delivered mail at a community college. He liked that he didn't usually have to talk to people and disliked how stressful it was when he did have to talk. He didn't make it to the next stage of Yahoo dating—the telephone call.

A few men made it through this second stage but shouldn't have. Some misrepresented themselves to me; others seemed to misrepresent themselves to both of us. One asked if I had any physical deal breakers. He thought it would save us some time and a date if we were unlikely to have chemistry. I confessed that I wasn't attracted to fat men who were fat all over (rather than just a bit heavy or carrying a beer gut). He laughed reassuringly. When we met at a restaurant, he had fingers the sizes of sausages and was too large to fit into a booth.

I had a wonderful phone conversation with another man insisted on sending me the address to his web page so that I could see what he looked like. I was relieved to see how cute he was, a little leery of the pet snake he was posing with, but disheartened when I read that he never dated women taller than he was. He was only five-foot-eight. I called him back to explain it wouldn't work out. I was taller than his height limit, but he still wanted to meet me; in preparation for our date, he would draw a mark on his office wall to represent my height and practice standing next to it. *Was he charmingly quirky or just plain odd?* I wondered. After a pleasant dinner out, we met at his house for our second date. He had a pet ferret that had its very own messy, little bedroom, *The Book of Satan* on his mantel and he looked horrified when I gave him a homemade lemon square. He disclosed that he was afraid of dessert: the look on his face when he tasted it confirmed that. "It's like a little pie—crunchy and sour at the same time. I don't understand how anyone can swallow that," he pronounced. It was our final date.

Many first dates were also the last dates. One man was extremely late in meeting me for our first drink. Eventually he arrived, red-faced and wet. I considered disqualifying him for rudeness on the spot, but decided to hear his excuse or better still, his apology. He said he had been on time but hadn't thought to enter the bar to look for me. He had been standing outside in the rain . . . *for an hour*. I disqualified him for stupidity.

There was something about the way that another man looked around the bar that caused me to ask, "Are you married or just living with someone? You shouldn't be here because some of us are *serious* about this dating thing." He was shocked, insisting that he, too, was serious . . . about figuring out if he should leave the woman he was living with. Another first date asked if I wanted to hear a joke. Frankly, I didn't, because jokes tend to be racist, sexist, homophobic, gross, or too stupid to be funny. It was unlikely that I would laugh, which would be awkward for both of us. No offense. But he insisted that his joke didn't fit into these categories and proceeded to tell me a joke in which the punch line was about a woman's vagina smelling like tuna fish. I think it was a black woman, but I can't swear to it. In any case, that was our last date. I suspect that his friends heard about the humorless feminist who answered his *Yahoo* ® advertisement. I know that my friends enjoyed hearing my entertaining dating stories. Their favorite was my evening with George.

George seemed to need a lot of reassurance and affirmation during our phone conversation. "Were there any red flags in my ad?" he asked. I responded frankly,

"It did lead me to believe that you weren't very tall, but I can't put my finger on why." Then, he asked the question tall men don't ask:

"What do you consider tall?" I replied,

"Well, I'm six feet tall."

"Oh, I'm a little shorter than that, but it doesn't bother me," he said, with an edge of nervousness. "I like dating tall girls. I think of it as improving my gene pool."

"Not on a first date," I told him flippantly. We agreed to meet for a drink at a bar closer to my house than to his. He lived about twenty miles away, across the Susquehanna River near Three Mile Island. Three Mile Island is home to a nuclear power plant that had suffered a partial meltdown in March of 1979. Another red flag, especially when he said that living where he did was worth the risk because rent was cheap. I thought he was using the wrong currency to decide what was cost-beneficial.

I sat at the bar while snow started to accumulate outside. He was late. Then an attractive guy who looked about the right age sat next to me. I was pleasantly surprised. He smiled, said hello, and waited for the bartender. "You *are* pretty tall," I told him. He seemed a little surprised, but replied,

"I guess so. I'm five-ten." There was an awkward silence. As soon as I had formed my next question in my head, I knew the answer.

"You're not George, are you?" He shook his head.

"No. Are you meeting someone you don't know?" A man opened the front door and loudly dropped his umbrella. He was chubby, short, with carrot-colored hair, ruddy skin, and thick glasses. George had arrived. We both stared at George as he gave me a little wave. The attractive man said, "Well . . . good luck with that," and walked away.

The conversation with George was no better than the first impression he had made. He was a snob who thought he deserved a better life than the one he had. I drank my beers and tried to be cheerful. He kept complimenting me: "You're so pretty"; "It sounds like you have a great job"; "I love the way you talk"; and "You're so funny." He was running out of things to compliment. Since I couldn't honestly reciprocate, I would just thank him. Then he said, "You have a big bladder! You haven't had to pee once tonight." I joked that he probably shouldn't say that anything on a six-foot woman was big.

And then he started apologizing. I told him that we should probably get the check since the snow was getting worse. Then I said that although I knew this was awkward, we wouldn't be going out again. His face fell, and I took my big bladder to the bathroom to give him some time alone. He later sent me an email informing me that his car had broken down on the bridge going home. While he didn't blame me for his having to walk two miles in the snow or for having to buy a new car, he did think I should have given him more of a chance.

As my year of using the Internet to find love was coming to an end, my enthusiasm for the process was waning. A few weeks before turning forty, I decided to reply to one more advertisement. That's how I found James—one of the nicest men I've ever known. For almost three and a half years, we were in a committed relationship.

After a decade of post-divorce dating, I was exhausted from trying to remake the wrong man into the right one. I was able to relax with James. He could take care of himself, and I soon found out that he could take care of me, even though I had never made that a criterion for a mate. I was financially stable. I had a low-interest loan on an affordable house and a car that was paid off. I didn't use credit cards, and I had a healthy savings account. I had tenure at a college that supported my teaching and research interests. I had lots of friends with whom I could spend time. I hired people to do the things that seemed daunting to me— maintaining the air conditioner, mowing the lawn, and fixing my car.

Despite how full my life was, I considered a man frosting on the cake. The cake was already pretty tasty, but it didn't look quite right, and it wasn't as sweet as I wanted. I wasn't sure that James would be the man who added that sweetness. He didn't give me a sugar high or the crash that would typically follow. I was the one who was more eager to go out, see people, and have fun. He was bored with the superficiality of most social occasions. So I went out with friends during the week and had a quiet, cozy time with James on the weekends. We had fun, but it was quiet fun after he'd accomplished what he needed to get done.

Although we were different, I always felt that James appreciated me for who I was. One of his favorite things about me was how I argued. I stayed focused on the issue at hand, making my case and listening to the other person's points, looking for a resolution rather than a fight. I was prone to crying but tears never kept me from articulating a cogent five-point argument with supporting evidence and a conclusion. James was an engineer by profession and by temperament. He wanted to solve problems in a deliberate, unemotional way. In his words, he liked to "observe, organize data, assess, strategize, enact the plan, test it, observe, and retest it." It was similar to my social-scientific approach, except he fixed things while I analyzed culture.

James and I understood one another, but I was never completely convinced that we were right for each other. I often wondered whether the problem was that we were not spending enough time together—we lived and worked ninety minutes away from each other. On weekends, we alternated between staying at his house and mine. I always thought that on weekends at my house, things went better. We had more fun in our work/play ratio and enjoyed each other more. It was easier to sleep. I was in a better mood. For a while, I wondered if the solution to our relationship turmoil was that we just needed to escape his house.

In contrast to my modern, Florida-style ranch house with its white furniture, beige walls and carpet, and gas-burning fireplace, James's house was an A-frame made entirely of wood. The walls, floors, ceiling, and furniture were wood. It was even heated by a wood-burning stove. I wasn't comfortable on his waterbed or his wooden couch. There wasn't enough light. I told a friend that when I was there I sometimes felt like I was in a coffin—wood was all around me. But James couldn't understand why I didn't love the place like he did. It was on a huge piece of property out in the country and he loved the privacy. The neighbors were so far away they couldn't even see the house—a trait I thought would appeal to robbers and rapists. James loved seeing the families of deer move through his backyard and found shooting groundhogs invigorating. I was afraid of animals and guns.

Things were constantly breaking at his house, and so there was always work to be done. He was frequently hurting himself trying to make repairs; his ex-wife had injured her back while living there, as did the girlfriend who lived there with him after we broke up. I joked that the house was cursed. He surprised me by saying, "Not the house, the land." Apparently he had found a book in the local library about a witch coven that had lived in the area long ago.

They had been run out of town, but not before they had put a curse on the land and all those who dwelled on it. It included his lot.

I'm not sure that I believe in curses, but I did feel like we had bad fortune together. I had never felt very lucky, but James and his family seemed even less so. James was raised outside of Johnstown, where a dam had broken in 1889 and destroyed the town. I remember crying the first time we visited there—driving down into the beautiful valley, but feeling the heaviness of the historic loss and the bleakness that remained there. I was speechless when his grandmother, battling dementia in the small house in which she had raised her children, lucidly recalled her days in an orphanage where she stayed for years when her family was too poor to care for her. She said she could still smell the soup and remembered how they had smacked her hand when she stole a taste of it in the kitchen. I heard the death of his grandfather's death, a blind, ex-coal miner who fell off the roof while shoveling snow. I wanted to bring James lightness and joy. Although I could sometimes make him smile or laugh, it was fleeting and never seemed to reach his core. Our first summer together, the darkness of my own life moved from the background to sit beside us. The health problems and the fears returned when I least expected them, when I was trying to escape our serious work-focused lives for a weekend of foolishness.

* * *

James couldn't understand why I would want to spend a long weekend on a road trip with my friend Cameron and two other wacky guys since its only purpose was to have silly fun. The guys had chosen a snack food theme and itinerary. They enjoyed planning and researching road trips like "Mound-Mania," when we went to eastern Ohio to see a Native American burial ground in a Hardee's parking lot. Or "Loser-Mania," when we saw the minor-league hockey team with the worst record and attended a regional *Star Trek* convention. My companions were quick-witted fellows who usually amused me.

Cameron was my companion from the sailing adventure. It would be a stretch to call him an ex-boyfriend, but I had been swept away by the fantasy of him. He was smart, handsome, adventurous, rebellious, funny, and outgoing. We had the same mental pace and energy. He could draw me outside of my comfort zone, and for the first time in my life, it felt appealing. Dating him for a few weeks and maintaining a flirtatious friendship afterward had kept me on an emotional hook for longer than I would like to admit. This odd limbo was probably sustained in part because we had not dated for six weeks.

My six-week rule for dating was simple but surprising to most of the people I shared it with. After my divorce at thirty, I knew it didn't make much sense to become a (born-again) virgin until (a second) marriage. I was aware that my eagerness to find love made me vulnerable and so I wanted a boundary that was clear and reasonable. After some early trial and error, it became clear to me that it was reasonable to refuse sex under any circumstance during the first six weeks of dating. It didn't matter how long the dates lasted or how wonderful they were. The rule weeded out users, players, and cheaters. They weren't patient enough to last. It also allowed enough time for a man (and me) to reveal who we really were, not just who we wanted the other person to see. Most of the men I dated in my thirties didn't make it through the six weeks.

It was the end of the six weeks when I joined Cameron on his sailboat. That's when he told me how much he appreciated the rule. He had always had sex early in his relationships, and they rarely lasted long or were very meaningful. He said he didn't want our relationship to end. (That sounded *good* to me). I was more important to him than the others had been. (That sounded *great*.) He said that he knew now that once he had sex with someone he didn't want to be with them anymore, so we should never have sex (which did *not* sound good). He continued to be affectionate, complimentary, and tease me about when we would get married, but we were no longer dating. Of course, by then, I thought I had fallen in love with him. He couldn't commit, but we couldn't entirely let one another go.

Lots of mixed signals and two years later, we were still friends and going on a road trip to eastern Pennsylvania to tour snack food factories. I hadn't given up on the idea that if he ever settled down and I hadn't found Mr. Right, we would end up together. It's hard to say what he thought. He said that he wasn't threatened by any of the other men I had dated but he did claim to be thrown off when he met James. "You seem serious about this one," he noted.

Something was off about "Snack-tour" from the beginning. The rental car that we were supposed to get wasn't available and four of us (me, Cameron, Cameron's brother Charles, and Cameron's brother's friend Harvey) jammed into my Geo Prism. I had thought that Harvey was an odd, funny guy when we went on the Mound-Mania trip, but his creepy side was showing on this trip. He talked often and eagerly about scalping. We were all tired; alternatively trying too hard to have fun and not trying hard enough. The brothers baited each other. The mushroom museum was small and boring. The Franklin Mint, lamely included because of a pun, was commercial and self-important. Only at the Herr's potato chip factory did we have some kitschy fun. We sampled ketchup-flavored potato chips before they were widely distributed; the boys asked the tour guide stupid questions; and we posed in front of silly murals of the company's mascot. In one memorable shot, I feigned horror as a van full of potato chips driven by a squirrel barreled toward me.

Our next stop was supposed to be a hotel. Cameron was driving. I sat behind him, next to his brother. We all saw the large van run a stop sign on the cross street ahead of us. We had the right of way and were going a reasonable speed. There was no way we could avoid getting hit, so I turned my body toward the center of the car. The van slammed into the passenger-side door nearest to me, rolling the car onto its right side. When the rolling stopped, glass was everywhere. I dangled from my seatbelt. My chest hurt; my side hurt; my hip hurt; my face and arms were bleeding. As I screamed, Harvey and Cameron quickly pulled themselves out of

Cameron's window. The driver of the van came up to my window. "Oh my God, oh my God! Are you okay?" she cried.

"No!" I yelled. "Call 911! Call 911!"

The EMTs came quickly. I heard them strategizing. Did they need to call the helicopter to have me airlifted? Would they need the Jaws of Life™ to get Charles and me out? They ended up sawing the roof of the car off and pulled Charles out first. He had a sore neck and some small cuts. I had the most serious injuries. I kept insisting that my hip must be broken but the paramedics were reassuring and efficient. I remember that one kept asking me questions that seemed irrelevant: "Where were you all going?" and "Where are you from?" He also said some things that I found incredible, namely "You'll be fine," and "You'll be able to resume your trip tomorrow."

The boys turned down medical assistance at the hospital and retreated to the waiting room. I was left alone on a gurney. I wasn't supposed to move and was told to keep my head still in case there was a neck injury. This became increasingly hard as time went on. Eventually, Cameron came to check on me, letting me know that he would take care of everything. He was sure that the doctors would see me soon. I asked him to call James. Ironically, the delay in treating me was caused because the driver of the van was being treated. She was the only one who lost consciousness, fainting when she saw the disaster she caused.

Eventually a doctor arrived and looked me over. I told him that I thought my hip was broken. He ordered an x-ray and concluded that I was fine. I was lucky to have suffered no breaks—

only soft tissue damage and cuts. He prescribed painkillers, advised me to see my primary care physician the following week, and released me. By this time, Cameron had arranged a car and hotel. He had also gotten me a lawyer. I said that I didn't need a lawyer. My car was totaled, my body was bruised, and my weekend was ruined. But the boys all agreed that I would make big money if I sued. I remember saying, "That is not how my world works." They laughed and argued that since the night's expenses would be paid for by the lawsuit, it made the most sense for me to put the hotel rooms on my credit card. They were in the euphoric post-catastrophe stage, but I was not. They had already started to refer to the trip as "Snackscident." I was too tired to challenge them, and I was feeling sorer by the minute. I tried to walk to the hotel room, but each step shot currents of pain through my body. Leaning on Charles, I managed to get to the room where I showered off the blood and pulled shards of glass out of my ears and skin. Washcloth after washcloth filled with blood, skin, and glass. I took the painkillers and slept. I woke a few times that night, from pain and (once) the sound of my own screams. This was one hell of a way to be fine.

The next day was a long one. I had to borrow a wheelchair from another hotel guest to make it from my room to the car. We went to where my car was impounded to collect our belongings. The car was a mess. David and the guys took pictures: posing ghoulishly as I sat aching. They wanted to collect evidence for my lawsuit so they took pictures of my demolished car and of the van that hit us. (It had a small dent in its front fender.) The name of the other car (a "Dodge Ram") made me a little sick. They took pictures of the skid marks on the street. By the time we got to my house, I couldn't walk at all. The few painful steps I had taken the night before were impossible to repeat. *When had I become such a wimp?* I reflected. I had walked with worse injuries than this. Now I had to lean on two, grown men to get from the car to my couch.

I don't think that the guys understood how much pain I was in or they wouldn't have spent the night. They wouldn't have kept me up late with rented movies and joviality. I don't think I fully understood either, or I would have insisted that James come over as he had offered to do. When I tried to get down the hall to the bathroom, I got some indication of what I was facing. I had one hand on each wall to hold myself up, and I wobbled and gasped with each shuffling step. I eventually gave up and sank to my hands and knees. It was easier to drag myself across the floor.

The next day, James arrived. He facilitated getting my guests to leave and told me to stay in bed. He brought me food, water, my pills, and something to read. While I slept he cleaned the house, swept out the garage, went grocery shopping, and made dinner. He found the crutches that I had used after my knee dislocation and told me to start using them. I said, "If I needed crutches, wouldn't they have given them to me in the hospital? They said I was fine."

"You don't seem fine," he said. "You can use the crutches until you are." So I did.

If I had a primary care physician, it was in name only. I didn't have a relationship with any of the doctors there. The group that I had been going to was a large one. I had seen different doctors the few times I had been there for checkups, flu, and back pains. None of the office staff recognized me. I thought of it as the office-that-held-my-medical-records, or the place-with-the-phone-system-that-had-no-human-voice-option. It didn't seem like much of a problem that I hated my primary care physician office. The only doctors I had needed in my thirties were my gynecologist and my orthopedist.

The week after the car accident, I saw the most junior member of the group. I told her what happened and I gave her the hospital's discharge order. I showed her my bruises (massive black and blue marks that covered about a foot of my left side). I told her that I couldn't put any pressure on my left side, and that I was using an old pair of crutches to get around. I asked if it would be okay to use the crutches to attend a conference in California the following weekend. It was a business trip that I was looking forward to and needed as a condition of grant I had received. She advised me to stay home from work for a week. At the end of that time I should be off of the painkillers and finished with the crutches. I was fine, she parroted—just bruised.

I got a call from the lawyer Cameron had procured without my permission. I told him that I wasn't convinced legal action was for me. He persisted. There was no risk in pursuing the matter, he said. He worked on contingency: he only got paid if he won me money. He offered his assistance with the annoying hassles like insurance papers. I agreed. We would be in touch.

A week went by. I adapted well because the problem was similar to a knee injury. I had aches and if I moved the wrong way, sharp, fleeting pains, but I was still able to distract myself with work and reading. Feeding myself was tricky. I would go through the Wendy's drive-through, order a baked potato and iced tea, and eat in my garage. I would put my biggest purse around my neck, fill it with microwave popcorn and a bottle of water, and hobble to the couch for dinner. The bruising improved, but walking remained impossible. I knew I was supposed to be getting better and I wasn't.

I wasn't getting better, yet two doctors had told me that I was supposed to be fine. Both expected me to walk by the end of the week. So I decided one morning that I would. The pain was searing, and I fell. Then I started to panic. What was wrong with me? What if I was supposed to be doing something and I wasn't doing it? Would this be like the knee—I should have been doing different exercises and as a result the muscles atrophied? Was this like the appendix—I should have gotten a second opinion and I could die if I don't? What was the right thing to do? *Try to walk? Don't try to walk?* I decided that I needed to see a specialist. I called the office of the orthopedic doctor I had seen for my knee. They were the largest practice in the area.

I told the secretary how I had been injured, rehashing the accident and the troubling persistence of pain from my injuries. She asked whether I had a lawyer; I did. The secretary cut me off immediately: none of the doctors in the practice accepted patients with lawyers. I asked if it would it help that one of the doctors was my knee doctor or if I got a referral from my primary care physician. But it didn't matter. The secretary was ready with a retort: the doctors didn't like to testify, or do all the paperwork that litigation entailed.

I got the list of orthopedics who accepted my insurance, and I called another office on the list. They said the same thing. I called a third and heard the same story. I could hear the shrillness creep into my voice. I knew I was about to cry; the receptionist knew it, too.

"I can't walk! I'm supposed to be able to walk!" I exclaimed. In a hushed tone, as if she were telling me a secret code, she confided,

"You can go to the emergency room. If the doctor there refers you to the orthopedic on call, they can't refuse you." She hung up abruptly.

I knew that many people use the emergency room for primary medical care, but I had never been one of them. Victims of heart attacks, stabbings, and gunshot wounds went to the emergency room. *Was this an emergency?* If I calmed down and sat on my couch, I could return to reading journal articles and taking notes. I wasn't about to die. I had already been to an emergency room. I had already seen a doctor—two doctors! It seemed like cheating to go to *another* emergency room so that *despite* my status as a litigant, I could have access to a specialist. I was so worried about my condition that I went anyway.

The doctor on call appeared to be about the same age as the undergraduate students I teach. I hoped she wouldn't be so deferential and accept the judgment of the first hospital. I filled her in on the particulars of the accident, the first and second diagnoses, and how I'd been struggling ever since. I still couldn't walk. I asked her if she wanted to see me try. She didn't. She examined me and came up with a new diagnosis. My effort to avoid the impact of the collision and/or my efforts to try to walk since the accident had caused me to have a condition with a name I have since forgotten. It was a condition that she said is typically found among runners. *Runners?*—this didn't ring true. Her recommendation was to stay on the crutches for two more weeks and not to put any weight on my left side while I used them. "No toe touching the floor when I am standing?" I asked, knowing that the "toe touch" made a world of difference for crutching.

"No," she said.

"After the two weeks, should I go to an orthopedic specialist that you could refer?" I asked hopefully.

"No," she said. "I don't see any reason for you to go to a specialist. I really think that you will be fine."

Two exhausting, uncomfortable weeks later, I still couldn't walk. I called my lawyer to terminate our relationship so that I could see a specialist. He berated me for not calling him sooner. He could help me get a doctor. They weren't supposed to blacklist me. Unfortunately, the doctors he knew were in Philadelphia. He'd have to get back to me. In the meantime, he wanted to let me know that our chances of getting a settlement from the van driver's insurance were diminished because I had signed a limited tort agreement. He lectured me about how foolish I was to have given away full tort for a small reduction in premiums. I wasn't sure what he was talking about. My insurance agent had reassured me that limited tort simply "limited people who wanted to sue over a broken fingernail." I would still be able to sue if I were seriously injured. The lawyer scoffed,

"That's the kind of thing those agents say. They get bonuses for selling limited tort. Serious illness is defined as loss of life, dismemberment, or significant long-term impairment, like being in wheelchair or having brain damage." After we hung up, I wondered why he decided to keep my case. Perhaps, he was the only other person who thought that my inability to walk weeks after the injury was indicative of a major problem. The only difference was that I hoped it wasn't, and he probably hoped it was.

I finally got an appointment with the only orthopedist in the area who accepted litigants. I'll call him Dr. Bottom-Feeder. He had no partners. He was disheveled. A colleague had shared bad things about the care he received from him.

At my appointment, I told Dr. Bottom-Feeder about the accident and aftermath, closing my story by pointing out that I *still* couldn't walk. I asked if he wanted to see me try. He didn't. In his opinion, there was no reason that I couldn't walk. He believed that I was just afraid to walk because it would hurt, and that I needed to work through the pain. I should start by trying to walk in a pool and lead up to walking on land.

I tried to walk in James's pool. It hurt to walk in the water, but at least I couldn't fall. After taking baby steps in the pool for about twenty minutes, I was in such pain that I had to lie down on the little bed that James had brought up from the basement. A deep ache kept me awake most of the night. The pain consumed my left side and radiated down my leg. I was worse off the next day. I dreaded my pool sessions and the hours of agony that would follow. "You shouldn't do this anymore," James said.

"The doctor said I should," I replied.

"So what," James challenged, "He can't make you do it." I wondered if it was true that a doctor couldn't *make* me do something. It hadn't been true with my appendix, but that was twenty years earlier and I had been trapped in the hospital. But wasn't there some implicit agreement between a patient and a doctor? That to get better, the patient does what the doctor tells them? I was willing to endure a lot of pain to walk again. But I also felt like I was doing myself more harm than good by trying to walk in the pool. None of the doctors' opinions about this accident seemed valid to me: I wasn't fine; this wasn't a runner's injury; and this wasn't a normal level of pain to endure during a recovery. There was something wrong. They missed something.

Returning to Dr. Bottom-Feeder, I told him about my efforts to walk in the pool and the pain that I experienced. He did an x-ray of my thigh, which wasn't broken either. He ordered an MRI of my back and a test to see if I had nerve damage. Before his receptionist called to make the appointments, she shuddered as she read the order for the nerve damage test. She said, "That's a nasty one. I had that on my arm." That test had to be terrible for an employee in the healthcare profession to admit that something was painful. They typically used code words, like "pinch" and "uncomfortable."

The back MRI was uneventful because it didn't hurt, and I am not claustrophobic. I was slid into a long tube and listened to my own CD of relaxing music while they took magnetic images of my back. The nerve damage test was a different story. The doctor asked several short questions and listened patiently to my long answers. I told him I couldn't walk and I asked if he wanted to see me try. He said, "Sure." I took the step and folded in on myself the way I always did using my right leg to catch me so that I wouldn't fall.

"I don't think you have nerve damage. I think you need a bone scan," he offered.

"Can you order one for me?" I prodded, hopefully. He couldn't because he was not my doctor. He only did nerve damage testing. I needed to convince my doctor to order one for me. I liked this guy. He seemed to care, so I tried not to scream or cry as he ran electrical currents through me while hitting my nerves with large needles. It was a challenge because he started at the base of my backbone and went down to the soles of my feet. A friend of mine told me that his grandfather said that this nerve damage test had been worse than World War II, and he had seen action.

At my next appointment, Dr. Bottom-Feeder said that the tests indicated that there was nothing wrong with my nerves, but that I did have a bulging disc in my lower back. The symptoms that I was reporting weren't entirely consistent with the MRI. I asked what he meant. He said that most people with back problems are more comfortable standing and lying flat than they were sitting. They also found standing more painful than walking. Yet I was comfortable unless I tried to walk.

"So perhaps my problem isn't a bulging disk," I said. "Maybe I need to have a bone scan." He said,

"I'm not an expert on backs, but I know a doctor at Hershey Medical Center who is. He comes to this office every few weeks to help me out. I'd like to have him examine you."

"Okay, but could I have a bone scan, too . . . . *please*?" Maybe it was my pleading expression—or maybe it was the fact that doctors get extra money for every test they order—but he agreed to order a bone scan.

The lawyer was pleased to hear about the bulging disk. There was no evidence that it was there before the accident. Back injuries were hard to fix and could worsen over time. This could be the lifelong, serious damage that we needed to overcome the limited-tort problem. It wasn't hard for me to contain my enthusiasm. He told me that we might need to name Cameron in our suit since he was the one driving. If we won, Cameron's insurance company would pay so it wouldn't be as though I were financially devastating a friend. Cameron didn't see it this way. I reminded him that he had called the lawyer, I still didn't have a car, and I couldn't walk. Harvey sent me a nasty reply to the email in which I asked for his portion of the hotel bill. I told the lawyer not to cite Cameron.

The bone scan was scheduled for the same day that I would meet with the Hershey back specialist. I answered the specialist's questions; he examined the MRI and told me that he thought I had bursitis in my hip. He thought an injection in my hip would ease the pain and swelling, allowing me to walk. I said, "What about the bulging disk?" He mused,

"Well, that bulge isn't consistent with your symptoms. The bulge is on the right side and your pain is on the left." Somehow Dr. Bottom-Feeder had missed this. The needle was large, the injection unpleasant, but not memorably so. What stands out in my mind is that I took my first successful steps after it. They were not pain-free steps, but walking was possible for the first time in months. The recommendation for physical therapy made me even more hopeful.

Although I wondered if it was still necessary, I went through with the bone scan. For the scan, I was positioned on a table in ways that helped them see certain body parts. I remember being instructed to make "frog legs" while I was on my back. I could tell they were trying hard to hone in on something, but I knew that technicians weren't supposed to answer patients' questions, so I didn't ask any.

A few days later, Dr. Bottom-Feeder called me. "I have good news," he said. "The bone scan revealed that you have a cracked pelvis." *This was good news?* "There are multiple fractures in your hip that were too small to be seen on an x-ray." I asked about the bursitis diagnosis. "Well, you probably developed that because you were trying to walk on a broken hip. That might also lead to some arthritis later in life." *More good news!* "The locations of your fractures meant that this was not a weight-bearing injury." He was saying what I had said all along—it wasn't that I didn't *want* to walk because it hurt; it was that I *couldn't* walk. "Since it's been three months since the injury, you should be seeing a lot of improvement" he predicted, recommending "Just take it easy and don't push yourself." As we were about to hang up, Dr. Bottom-Feeder casually interjected, "Oh—the scan also revealed that you had broken ribs, but there was nothing that could be done about that either." Long after I hung up the phone, the words "nothing could be done," echoed in my mind.

I thought that everything would have worked out the same if I had never gone to a doctor and then I realized that things would have turned out *better*. If I had never seen a doctor, I wouldn't have tried so diligently to walk on a broken hip or have caused the long-term damage that would come from having followed that advice. The pain of trying to expedite my recovery before my body was ready was surely worse than if I had allowed myself the time for the natural healing process to occur. I had more evidence to support the thesis that I didn't want to believe: that the medical system did not work. Or at least it didn't work well for understanding and helping me.

It took a year to be able to sleep through the night on my left side and just as long to settle the lawsuit. The Dodge Ram driver's insurance company awarded me about 4,000 dollars. My medical file was subpoenaed for the lawsuit. In it I saw Dr. Bottom-Feeder's critical comments about me. He thought that I exaggerated my level of pain since it was "not consistent with the diagnosis of soft tissue damage." Nowhere did it say, "The patient was right all along. Five doctors and an EMT squad were wrong. She had broken her hip. She could not walk. She was not fine." But, of course, by this time, I hadn't expected it to.

Chapter 7: "This Is a Good Cancer": My Uterine

I've begun thinking of my experiences medical industry as a series of thunderstorms. In my forties, I would see a lot of rain. Some storms came out of nowhere, like the fractured hip from the car accident. Others built slowly. I could see them coming and hope they'd blow over. The first black cloud of my next storm took the form of an abnormal pap smear.

I always hated getting pap smears. No woman likes them, but I had probably struggled with them more than most. In fact, my Tallahassee gynecologist had sent me to a psychologist because he was unable to complete the test. He diagnosed me with a "mild case of vaginismus." Rather than allowing him to give me a routine pelvic exam, the muscles surrounding my vagina would spasm involuntarily and literally close up. Once again my body was trying to protect itself in a counterproductive way that ended up making things worse.

My first visits to the gynecologist were before my marriage. I had been trained too well by my father to keep my legs crossed with men. The fact that *this* man happened to be a doctor was not enough to make me feel normal about the experience. If a stranger did this to me outside of a medical office, wouldn't he be arrested? How could all these other women so easily adjust their thinking about what was happening to their bodies in these rooms, in these stirrups? How did they get their bodies to cooperate? Maybe it was because they trusted doctors and I no longer did. Or perhaps it was my inherent, hyper-vigilant phobic instinct that kept me from trusting?

The psychologist I was sent to in order to treat my fear of the gynecological exam was a pregnant woman who was also an RN. She was having low blood pressure problems and would periodically have to rush blood to her head so that she wouldn't pass out. "Excuse me," she would say politely, before abruptly putting her head down between her legs, below the seat of her chair.

She tried to demystify the process that I would be going through by explaining how the exam worked, why it was necessary, and by showing me the speculum. Since it was my early experiences with pap smears that likely caused my anxiety, it struck me as odd that she thought this information would help. The doctor who performed my first pap smear (before the appendix experience) seemed angry at me the whole time and grew angrier as I cried. Maybe my body was rebelling against his declaration that I "better get used to this"? It sounded like a threat from which I would rather run than acquiesce. The psychologist never asked me about this experience. I'm not sure what difference it would have made if she had. We were both focused on achieving a procedural goal, not in gaining a deeper understanding of my psyche.

In addition to the physiology lessons, she gave me homework that entailed practicing what would happen to me at the doctor's office. I was supposed to lay by myself on my bed with my legs in the appropriate position and imagine the process. I was supposed to use a tampon as the speculum while doing my stress-releasing breathing. Always the conscientious student, I did the assignment even though it seemed ridiculous. It felt like getting ready for war by holding a water pistol and saying, "This is a real gun."

The psychologist seemed eager for me to say that I was ready to try again. I knew the doctor would be reporting back to her. I didn't want to disappoint the psychologist or the gynecologist. They had tried to be compassionate by offering me help. The gynecologist even suggested that he'd forgo the rectal exam to make the process easier. I tried to look on the bright side—he had mercifully small hands. I willed myself not to remember the picture in his office of him in hunting gear with a dead deer over his shoulder. I reminded myself that I wanted a prescription for birth control pills before my wedding and I rescheduled the exam. I used the psychologist's techniques. I breathed. I visualized. I tried to relax. Mission accomplished.

I had many routine pap smears before the abnormal one in my early forties. I became calmer about the process, only allowing myself to fret about the procedure on the day it was scheduled. My anxiety centered on the procedure, not the diseases that the exam might reveal. When my doctor asked me to return for a follow-up pap smear, for the first time, my anxiety resettled on the possibilities an abnormal pap smear suggested. I returned for the follow-up and a few days later, I called for the results during a break in the three-hour research methods class I was teaching. A nurse said that I should talk to the doctor, but that she was gone for the day.

"Couldn't you tell me anything now?" I asked. She did.

"Well, you have HPV." It was hard to hear her on my primitive cell phone.

"What?" I asked, in horror. "Did you say I have HIV?"

"No, HPV. Human Papillomavirus."

"Oh, well, that's good." I was comparing it to HIV, the virus that can lead to AIDS and based upon what I knew about AIDS then, a few years of hell followed by death.

"Not really. It's a virus that leads to cervical cancer." She was comparing it to cancer.

"Oh my God, do I have cervical cancer, or am I going to get it?" I spluttered.

"You should talk to the doctor. All I know is that you have HPV. I really shouldn't be talking about this. Call back tomorrow." She hung up.

After teaching for another ninety minutes, I went to the office to look up HPV on the Internet. It was a fairly common virus that was usually sexually transmitted. Men could spread it but were unaffected by it. For women it could be silently present, result in genital warts, and/or lead to cervical cancer. There were over one hundred different types and about thirty were linked to cancer. I wrote down the names of the worst ones, and prepared to ask the doctor the next day what strain I had. I went to meet a friend for dinner and a drink to celebrate my forty-second birthday. It wasn't much of a celebration, but it was nice to have someone to talk to about my diagnosis. Like me, she'd never heard of the virus. She said, "How bad could it be if neither of us ever heard of it?" I wasn't reassured. To me, bodies were disasters waiting to happen. The things that could go wrong with them seemed random and endless.

I never got to talk to the doctor, but I did get a call from a nurse practitioner. She was sorry that the nurse had upset me with incomplete information. She confirmed that I had a dangerous type of HPV, but that it was also the most common. She said that most women my age contracted HPV in their "sexually-promiscuous twenties" and then the virus went dormant or just undetected. *One more way I didn't fit the norm*, I thought, remembering how I had spent my twenties—married to Scott, both of us previously virgins. She said that HPV didn't cause cervical cancer, but it had to be present for a woman to get the disease, explaining "Think of it as if you're on a ladder to cervical cancer and you just went up a step, but that doesn't mean that you are going to keep climbing." I certainly didn't want to climb that ladder.

"Should I get a hysterectomy?" I asked.

"Oh, no, we wouldn't recommend that. That would be too extreme. We'll just have more frequent pap smears and keep our eyes on it. If you get another abnormal result, we'll need to pursue it further." I didn't want to think about what hideous procedure that benign statement veiled. I was satisfied. She wasn't quite done.

"I do want to talk to you about your blood pressure. I see from your chart that it has been steadily creeping up. Considering that, your age, and the fact that you've been on the pill for so many years, it's time to consider some other kind of birth control."

I postponed getting off of the pill for a few months while I tried to bring down my blood pressure with a heart-smart diet. During that delay, I was at the University of Nebraska grading Advanced Placement (AP) tests for a week with other political-science professors and high school social-studies teachers. That is where I began bleeding. I bled and bled and bled. It was inconvenient. I was in a traditional dorm with the bathrooms at the end of the hall—little stalls and rows of sinks and showers where the water from three shared a single drain. It was embarrassing. Privacy was limited when you shared the same bathroom and the same schedule—everyone had to be at their grading tables from 8:00 a.m. to 5:30 p.m. Everyone took the same regimented fifteen-minute breaks and hour-long lunches. It was obvious why I was late to the table in the morning because it was clear that I was in the bathroom a lot. It wasn't a mystery why I left dinner with blood on my shorts. It wasn't easy to manage. I had no car and I needed lots of supplies—pads, tampons, detergent, and iron pills. I tried to call my gynecologist in Pennsylvania, but I didn't have a cell phone and the phones in the dorms didn't allow for long-distance calls. When I did reach her, I had trouble communicating the severity of the situation. It was scary—much worse than any period I'd ever had. My blood clots were larger than ping pong balls; I was eventually overflowing two supers and a pad in forty-five minutes while lying down.

My friends at the grading offered lots of opinions: "It is nothing to worry about—you're at that pre-menopausal age when periods change. Mine did. It was hell"; "Maybe you are losing a baby you didn't know you were carrying. Birth control pills fail, you know"; "You should fly home to your doctor"; "You should be at the emergency room"; and, "You should try to get your mind off it. Have a beer." None of these comments were convincing. I knew something was wrong, but instead of worrying about what was actually wrong with me, I worried about getting my doctors to take my condition seriously. I didn't want to endure the consequences of another undetected illness or injury.

On the advice of a nurse at the gynecology office, I doubled my birth control pills and the bleeding slowed down. She suspected that I was on the wrong birth control pills and that taking me off them would solve the problem. I went into the office when I returned from Nebraska, trying calmly and specifically to report the extent of the bleeding and how unprecedented it was for me. Thankfully, the nurse practitioner didn't need much convincing to order a sonogram.

The sonogram was odd, but not painful. Even people who haven't had sonograms are probably familiar with the process—or at least part of it. They'd know from all the television coverage of expectant mothers that a gel is put on the abdomen and a hand-sized device is run over the outside of it to reveal what's going on inside. What's not so obvious is that a microphone-sized device is inserted through the vagina into the uterus. It is moved around to get a better view of what's going on. This looks (and feels) like someone driving a stick-shift in your privates. Odd, but not painful and since no one needed to find a vein to do it, I took it well.

The results revealed that I had bleeding polyps in my uterus. I was told that this was a fairly common problem and easily taken care of. I would need a dilation and curettage (D&C), which would scrape the lining of my uterus in order to remove the polyps embedded in that lining. It was a minor out-patient surgery. The recovery period would only be a week. Of course, I needed to have some pre-op tests—an electrocardiogram (EKG), a chest x-ray, and a blood test. The day before the surgery, I would meet with the doctor. This, in itself, was unusual. My office visits had always been with the nurse practitioners. I'd never been sick enough to earn the privilege of meeting with the doctor.

When I told James what was going to happen, I burst into tears. I could see him struggle between his pragmatic, reasonable side and his sweet, sympathetic side. I knew what he was thinking as he held me in his arms and watched me cry: Was I just being neurotic and dramatic? Was this the usual, pre-surgery stress? Was there something I wasn't telling him? All I could say as I sobbed was, "They've got me again," as I panicked that my healthy period was over. The medical world that I functioned so ineffectively in had tracked me down. It was a world in which I remembered having no rights, no autonomy, no authority, and no options. It was a world in which everything hurt, and the hurt isolated me.

A few days later I had my tests. The EKG and chest x-ray were uneventful. The blood-drawing was not. For weeks, I had been looking at my own blood—in the toilet, in the shower, on the tampons, and on my clothes. It seemed like I had lost gallons of it. Now I needed to have a tiny vial of blood drawn out of my arm and experience told me it would not be easy to get. I was told by various nurses and phlebotomists that my veins were deep, small, and rolled. I knew to drink lots of water the night before a blood test and direct the nurse away from the promising-looking vein on my right, inner arm. When I went to the hospital, I hoped for the best, but I was anxious as always. The nurse looked at the scar on my left arm (the cutdown from my appendix nightmare) and whined, "Oh no, when I see that scar I know I'm going to have trouble."

I was angry—*how dare she say that to me?* I worried that hitting a vein in my arm with a confident nurse was hard enough, and this one had already admitted defeat. I had never agreed to the cutdown, which remained one of the most excruciating memories of my life. It felt like she was blaming *me* for having the cutdown because it would inconvenience *her.* How much trouble could she really experience on her side of the needle? Although she anticipated her inability to find a vein, she wouldn't listen to me when I explained that the vein on my right, inner arm never worked out. She tried it anyway and missed. Next, she tried the backside of my arm—a place that I'd never seen anyone try before—and failed again. I started to cry and she said harshly, "What's the matter with you? It can't be what I'm doing. This doesn't hurt." I asked for another nurse. The second nurse found a vein in my hand as the other nurse complained about how much trouble I had been.

The next day I went for my pre-op meeting at my doctor's office. It started with the nurse practitioner reviewing what would happen the next day. When she got to the part about my getting an IV, I burst into tears. By then, my arms and hand had big black and blue marks on them from the day before. I knew that it was even harder to find suitable veins for and three spots were already out of the running. I cried and cried, knowing that the reaction was not commensurate with the problem, but unable to stop myself. When I was sent to see the doctor who was going to perform the surgery, she talked to me calmly and quietly, like I was a child or a hysteric. She gave me my first prescription for Ativan® (a drug to calm anxiety) with instructions to take one the next morning on the way to the hospital. She explained again how minor the surgery was, how common bleeding polyps were, and told me to get a good night's sleep.

The following day I had surgery. James dropped me off at the hospital, but since it was a minor surgery and he had an important day at work, he didn't stay. The IV went into the first vein. I came through the operation fine and woke in a recovery room without incident. A friend picked me up and drove me home where I slept through most of the post-op aching.

A few days went by. The bleeding had stopped. I told myself that the dread I felt had come from fear instead of intuition. I berated myself for being so immature about the whole procedure. I hoped that the experience of having a doctor correctly diagnose and solve a manageable problem would help offset my other experiences in the medical system. I reassured myself that they didn't have me after all.

When I got a phone call from the doctor, I immediately started to report how I was feeling, assuming that she was interested in a post-op progress report. I'll admit that it was an odd assumption to make; I had never received such a call before. She waited for me to finish and then said, "That's fine. What I am calling about is the lab report. Of course, everything we take out of the human body is sent to a lab. This is routine. I was surprised to find that your lab report revealed that you have endometrial cancer cells in the material that I scraped from your uterus."

What?

The doctor continued: "Most patients don't hear much after I say that they have cancer, so I don't want to overwhelm you with information right now." She was right. Her voice rattled softly in the husk of the phone. I could barely hear her. "It is a good cancer to have. It is highly curable. It is at an early stage. I have referred you to Dr. Kind. He is very good. You need to call his office and set up an appointment. Do you have a pen?"

I felt dazed. I had cancer, but no pen. I located a pen. I still had cancer. I had a good cancer, but it didn't feel good knowing that. I asked, "What will they do?"

"You will need to ask Dr. Kind about that, but typically he would perform a hysterectomy. That's abdominal surgery." I knew all about abdominal surgery.

"Will I need chemotherapy?" I asked, thinking about my veins and how many veins must be needed for chemotherapy.

"Not necessarily. You need to talk to him." I hung up and a new friend, Julie, called saying that she'd be a little late for our lunch date.

I said, "I have cancer, but I still want to meet for lunch."

Julie was an academic, too. She specialized in women's health issues from a sociological perspective, but she still knew a lot about the science. She interviewed women about their bodies for her research and was a good listener. It was serendipitous that she was my lunch date and a relief that she offered to help me though the medical labyrinth. Our lunch was a long one, and I noticed at the end of the one-sided conversation that all I'd talked about was the appendix hospitalization. I remarked to her, "I have cancer, but I can't stop talking about my appendix. That happened twenty-two years ago, but it feels like yesterday." *And it feels like tomorrow*, I thought.

"That's because you were medically raped," was her reply, "and you're afraid it is going to happen again. It doesn't have to happen again. We can make sure that it doesn't."

I had never thought of what happened as a medical rape, but the experience and my emotional scars made it seem like an appropriate analogy. It was somehow liberating to think of what happened to me as a horrifying aberration rather than a routine abuse in a dehumanizing institution. If it was a trauma, it might not happen again. If it was a trauma, couldn't I get over it? Maybe a good experience in the same setting would help me do that. Maybe that would actually make this cancer "good."

First, I had to get an appointment to see Dr. Kind, the gynecological oncologist that my surgeon referred me to. I knew this call was too important to avoid, postpone, or botch. So I made it that afternoon, and it went smoothly. I was given an appointment for two days later.

The next afternoon I found a message on my answering machine from the doctor's office canceling the appointment and rescheduling it for a week later than the original appointment. I couldn't believe it. Didn't they know I had cancer? How much should I expect the cancer to grow in a week? I thought about finding a doctor who could see me sooner, but then I wondered if the better doctors just had fuller schedules. I contemplated calling back and trying to get an earlier appointment . . . but if they had an earlier appointment available, wouldn't they have given it to me already? Would asking for an earlier one mark me as a problem patient? Was I overreacting? I wasn't the only woman with cancer. I wasn't more important than the others who were waiting for appointments. Or was it essential to my health that I be assertive now? *Remember the appendix,* I instructed myself. *No,* I countered, *forget the appendix. This is different. I should call the doctors back. Yes, call. Don't call. Calm down.*

I decided to call the office with a carefully-constructed script that balanced assertiveness and deference. After I practiced reading it, I made the call and read it again. The person on the other end of the phone said, "This is the answering service. Would you like to leave a message?" Oh . . . I looked at the clock. It was

11:00 p.m. *Where did the day go? How did I miss the fact that it was long after business hours?*

"Oh, never mind, I'll call them tomorrow," I said, hanging up.

I tried to do other things, but I couldn't concentrate. Tomorrow seemed too far away. I tried to go to sleep. I couldn't stop thinking. Maybe I should have left a message? What if there was only one earlier appointment and someone else called in the morning and got it? Would they live and I die because I hadn't left a message? What message should I leave? The answering service operator wasn't going to write down my whole script. How would I know if the right tone was conveyed in the message? I called back without a script, and I tried to explain the situation to the operator.

"Hi. This is Stephanie Larson again. I called before and said I didn't want to leave a message, but I think I should leave a message because I have cancer, and I shouldn't have to wait two weeks to see a doctor. I mean it must be growing in there and I need to do something about that. Don't write that down. Write down that I need an earlier appointment . . . no, that sounds too demanding. Say that I want an earlier appointment . . . or does that sound too needy or like I have something more important to do on the day they gave me an appointment? Oh . . ." It was one in the morning and I was lost. *Where was that assertive professor I spent most of my time being?* "I'm sorry, I'm just overwhelmed. I have cancer and I am scared. I need these doctors' help."

"Honey," the service operator said, sympathetically, "you need to ask for God's help, but how about I say that you called and that they should call you back in the morning? Now, give me your name and number and go to bed." It sounded like a good plan. They called the next day and I got an earlier appointment.

Julie accompanied me to meet the doctor who would do my surgery. It was Dr. Kind's colleague, young Dr. Sure. Julie brought a tape recorder, and I was surprised by how at ease the doctor was with her request to tape our meeting. Dr. Sure initially controlled the pace and tone of the meeting, but between Julie's expertise on women's health and my experience with abdominal surgery, we were able to ask and receive answers to all of my questions. Dr. Sure reiterated that that this was a curable cancer and that 80 percent of uterine cancer patients did not have reoccurrences of the disease after the hysterectomy. I was glad to hear that most uterine cancer patients did not require chemotherapy. It would depend upon what he found during the operation, but the pathology report from my D & C was encouraging.

He described the operation and the recovery experience. He seemed perplexed when my questions focused on abdominal surgery and complications rather than cancer itself. I told him that I was worried that my prior abdominal surgeries and seven weeks of peritonitis would complicate the surgery. He was used to seeing adhesions from previous surgeries, and didn't think he would face anything new or unusual. He did not foresee that I would need a nose tube or drainage tubes. Medicine had "come a long way since 1980," he said, and the importance of managing a patient's pain was now seen as essential to recovery. During the examination that

151

followed, he saw my appendix scars for the first time. The look on his face was fleeting, but revealing. It seems that my body had made my point better than I could.

Julie advised me to get a second opinion, and found another doctor to give it. My mother had arrived in time to attend that appointment with us. My records were supposed to be sent to this doctor, but when we got there for the appointment, the receptionist said they didn't have them. She suggested rescheduling the appointment, running more blood tests, or having the meeting without records. All three options were problematic. There was not enough time to reschedule before my scheduled surgery, getting more blood drawn filled me with dread, and not having records would compromise the doctor's ability to make a recommendation.

Julie calmly told the receptionist that the best solution would be for her to call Dr. Sure's office and get the records faxed over. All I needed to do was sign a waiver and I did. After ten minutes, Julie went back up to the desk to receive an update. They hadn't called yet, but they would do it now. Ten minutes later, Julie checked again: they'd called, but hadn't received the record. They would call again to make sure they were being sent. Ten minutes later, she checked again. The records had arrived.

My mother and I marveled at Julie's cool effectiveness. We were both locked in assumptions born of, or reinforced by, the appendix drama. My mother assumed that patients and their families should quietly yield to medical professionals who knew what they were doing and had protocols that had to be followed. I assumed that patients were at the mercy of healthcare practitioners who would treat you worse if you challenged them. Watching Julie disprove these assumptions, even in a small way, was more eye-opening than anything the second doctor said about my condition. She, too, recommended a hysterectomy and thought my prospects were good.

Leaving the appointment, my mother turned to face Julie and said, "That was amazing. I remember when Stephanie was in the hospital for the appendix. Early on I went up to Dr. Evil, outside of her room to ask him a question. He snapped at me— 'Can't you see I'm talking to a nurse?' He was so rude. I decided then and there never to talk to him again." I was floored. How could she have given up so easily? I knew how hard it had been for my mother to watch me suffer. I also knew that her pride wasn't more important to her than I was. I could only conclude that Dr. Evil, as well as the system that sustained him, had made my mother feel just as powerless as I had felt. She had been at the foot of my bed for hours, but I was alone in my pain, and now it seemed that I had been alone in my unsuccessful efforts to receive responsive and compassionate medical attention.

This time I wouldn't be alone. I had emotional support from my mother and James, and advocacy from Julie. I was a 42-year-old patient who had been around the block (or in this case, the hospital) before. I wanted there to be a point to having cancer and more abdominal surgery. I wanted the world to make sense. Maybe it would, as long as this time we could all be more powerful versions of our past selves. This time would be different. It *had* to be different.

Since I didn't have any children at the age of forty-two, it seemed to reassure everyone that a hysterectomy was not going to be emotionally difficult for me. When Julie had asked Dr. Sure why the operation needed to include the ovaries, she made it clear that it wasn't because I wanted to keep them to have children. It was because of the hormonal changes that taking the ovaries would create. She and I never talked about whether I wanted children, but like most of my friends, she assumed I didn't. They had never seen me gush over their children or cry on their shoulders about the ticking of my biological clock. I tried to love the life I had, not demean it for what was missing. But that didn't mean that I didn't want to be a mother.

In fact, I chose my profession based on how well the schedule worked for raising children. When I was young and naïve enough to think that you could plan such things, I decided I would have two children. And I wanted another loving parent to offset the impact of my deficiencies. It was the one thing in my life I was convinced was best done by a team. Scott and I had wanted to get our careers and finances in order before having or adopting children, but by the time we were professionally and financially stable, our marriage was ending. One of my multi-year relationships with a Mr. Wrong had included weekends with his incredible six- (and then seven-) year-old son. It was as close as I ever came to mothering. I ended up having to say goodbye to the boy in a letter because of the ugly circumstances of the end of my relationship with his father. I still think about that boy and miss him in a way I can't explain. But I was resilient and still hopeful.

Being in my early forties was not necessarily too late to have that three-person family. Maybe after all of this was over, it would be with James and an adopted daughter.

After the hysterectomy, I was only in the hospital for a few days. Things went pretty smoothly. Finding a vein for an IV was difficult, but they called in the most experienced phlebotomist to start a new line when the one used for my surgery gave out. The five-inch, vertical surgical incision looked better than the one it replaced. It hurt, but I had a morphine pump, which I didn't need to use very much. When they wanted me to, I walked with ease. The amount of urine that I produced seemed to delight the nurses. I had a great room with a view of the Susquehanna River. My mom was there in the afternoons. James joined us in the early evenings. I received a lot of flowers.

We waited for me to produce stool. That was the condition under which I would earn a release. It became the focus of all our activities. I tried to stimulate my bowels by walking the halls. Nurses tried suppositories. Finally, after a few days I produced something stool-like, and the next phase of the exit plan began. They gave me a little food. When I didn't throw it up, they decided to release me. I wanted to escape the daily shots, IVs, constant intrusions, and plastic, pulsating knee socks. However, I wasn't impressed with what my intestines had accomplished. Dr. Kind was doing rounds the day I was released. He reassured me that it was time to go and that I would be fine. "Go home," he encouraged, "and eat whatever you want." I had pills for pain if I needed them. I would see Dr. Sure in a week. By then he'd have called me about the pathology report.

I went home to more flowers and my own bed. I wasn't hungry and I wasn't regular. My mother urged me to eat anyway. I ate a little. Nothing changed. The next day one of my favorite dishes arrived from a friend: chicken and rice with olives and Mexican spices. Mom urged me to eat. It did taste good, so I ate. I became more tired and still couldn't go to the bathroom. It felt like an anchor was on my abdomen, weighing me down to the bed. I wasn't peeing as much as usual. My abdomen started to hurt. It concerned me enough to call the doctor's office, but Dr. Sure wasn't worried. He said that it sometimes took a while for intestines to come back from a surgery. He told me to take stool softeners, stop taking painkillers, and eat lightly. I had already stopped taking the painkillers and had been on the softeners for two days so I decided to stop eating entirely and just drink water. The constipation continued. The abdominal pain intensified.

I called the doctor again and reported my lack of progress. I was calm and precise. He said to try an enema and drink more water. I tried to follow the directions on the enema box, but can't say for sure that I did it right. It didn't change anything except my mood. I chugged some water and promptly threw up. The pain was more intense. Finally, I started to panic. Something was wrong and the doctor didn't think so. I had been here before.

I decided to call my friend Cindy. She'd had Crohn's disease, which had led to colon cancer. She knew a lot about intestines. I told her what was going on. "I think you have an intestinal blockage," she said. "Don't eat anything. Only take small sips of water, but take them frequently. If you start throwing up again, go to the emergency room for an x-ray. They can tell easily if you're blocked. Since you're having constant abdominal pain and severe spasms, it seems like your intestine is trying to push your food through. If you manage to pass anything, look at it before you flush. If it looks like coffee grounds (dark and granular), then it is probably a small intestinal blockage." *If only Cindy could be my doctor*, I thought.

When I hung up with Cindy, I recounted her diagnosis to my mother, verbatim. My mother was aghast. "You can't possibly believe your friend over a doctor, can you?" she asked. Yes, I could.

That evening Dr. Sure called back. I was relieved. I thought he was taking me seriously and wanted to check on my condition. Instead, he was calling to tell me the pathology report. "Good news, Stephanie. The pathology report revealed that there was no cancer. I had them do it a second time to make sure. So it's likely that the only cancer was in the lining, which was removed by the D & C." It was hard to focus on anything but my abdomen, so all I said was,

"Okay."

"You should be happier" he chastised. "This is the best news we could have gotten." I was sorry to disappoint him, but I didn't have the energy to please. "Yeah, I will be happy when this abdominal pain goes away. Do you think I could have an intestinal blockage?" I asked.

"Probably not. Those are extremely painful; you would know if you had one of those. But why don't you come to the office tomorrow morning and I'll check you out?" I didn't care if he was pacifying me. I was glad to get the appointment. Later that night, I expelled a coffee-ground-like substance into the toilet. The pain continued and I couldn't sleep. I kept sipping water.

The next day, Dr. Sure examined me and said he thought everything was all right because he could hear bowel sounds. I had heard that one before. Maybe bowel sounds were my body's way of screaming for help. He ordered an x-ray anyway. Sure enough, I had a partial blockage of the small intestine. I needed to stop eating immediately (I hadn't eaten in thirty-six hours) and only drink water to take the steroids that he prescribed. His assistant was going to start looking for a bed at one of the area hospitals. I was assigned to a room with a young, bald woman who had apparently been there a long time. She spoke loudly to the nurses. She refused to eat. She said she was tired of throwing up. The television was loud.

A doctor came in to speak with my roommate. "You have to eat," the doctor said to the girl. "You have to sleep. You can't keep staying up all night watching television." I dreaded the long hours that were ahead of me. I would be a frustrated visitor in my own room. I would never be able to ask someone in such a bad situation to turn down a television. *How will I get any rest?* I fretted.

My mother and I waited for an IV team. My arms and hands were still black and blue from my previous hospital stay. A nurse told me that Dr. Sure had ordered a peripherally inserted central catheter (PICC line) instead of an IV because of the bad state of my veins. We had to wait for radiology to call. I was hot and thirsty. The nurse confirmed that I had a temperature and was dehydrated. But I was still not allowed to drink water. They would give me hydration as soon as they got the PICC line in. The plan was to continuously hydrate me and hope that this helped soften the intestine so the blockage would pass. Dr. Sure had instructed the nurses not to put in a nose tube unless I started vomiting.

I wasn't sure how to feel about a PICC line. Since it would keep me from having blood drawings and IVs, I was in favor of it. But getting a procedure done on my veins was worrisome. What if it was as bad as the procedures to access my veins during my appendix crisis? I wanted to ask questions about the procedure, but the nurses weren't around long enough, and their aides didn't know anything. I was wheeled down to radiology. They'd be putting in the PICC line on my left side since I was right-handed. According to the radiologist, this would make using my hands less awkward. *Less awkward for doing what?* I contemplated. I didn't plan on pitching softballs to my dying roommate. I'd be lying in a hospital bed, willing myself not to throw up. My left side had a worse track record than my right when it came to finding veins and putting in subclavian lines, but I didn't say anything. The radiologist explained that a PICC line was a small tube that is inserted in a peripheral vein in my upper arm and pushed through larger veins toward my heart. "Will it feel like getting a cutdown?" I asked thinking that it sounded similar, just higher up on my arm. The nurse's eyes flared a little.

159

"How do you know about them?" she asked.

"I had one," I said.

"This won't be as bad," she assured me. She gave me a shot to make the process easier on me and they started.

I could feel the cut, then the tube pushing into my arm. It hurt. Then, it hurt a lot more. The doctor and nurses both gasped simultaneously. There was more pressure. Medical words were urgently exchanged. The pain stayed the same as they tried to correct whatever hadn't gone as expected. "Whew, okay," said the radiologist. The nurse started putting a dressing on the line.

"What happened?" I asked.

"Don't worry about it. Everything's fine now," he said. "It's just that they don't usually do that. It's a good thing we did it here in radiology instead of bedside." Apparently doctors could administer PICC lines "blindly," hoping that tubes go where they should (toward the heart instead of up the neck). I was glad that Dr. Sure had not trusted that to work for me. It was over and my arm ached, but it was something I could deal with. The uncertainty and intense pain had passed. They wheeled me back to my room, but it was different—a single! My mother was there, smiling. She had made this happen. I could lie in a bed without listening to the young woman suffering in a bed next to mine.

I started getting hydration and I didn't throw up. When someone came to take blood from my arm, I said "Take it from the PICC line please." The PICC line was only for hydration, she explained. I said that I could do without hydration for the length of time it would take to draw blood. She was hesitant. Taking blood from the PICC line would require special permission from my doctor. She'd have to track him down and she was here to take the blood now. It would be easier if she just found a vein and drew it. I insisted that it wouldn't be easier for me, and that she needed to contact him. She did, if reluctantly, and the doctor gave permission for all of my blood drawing to come from the PICC line. This was a huge victory. There was nothing else to do but wait for my blockage to clear. The wait would last a week.

During that week, I walked the halls trying to stimulate my intestines. I got x-rays to see if there was progress clearing the blockage. I requested Ativan® to help me relax each night, so I could fall asleep. One of the nurses mocked me about this, but I ignored him. I got the Ativan® and it helped. I rejected medication that I knew was not mine. The nurse was initially annoyed, but then realized that I was correct: the medication would have undermined my recovery. I started to go through menopause. Sporadic, warm waves and brief, crying jags came in the evenings. I found them manageable. I was visited frequently by a nun. She told me about the cancer that she had survived. More flowers arrived.

Dr. Sure, Dr. Kind, and members of my gastrointestinal team visited me daily. Only two visits stand out in my mind. The first was early in the week with Dr. Sure. He said, "I know you are scared. I know why. I've seen inside of you." He meant this literally, but it felt like he was saying something profound. Wouldn't seeing the mess inside my abdomen suggest the deeper scarring on my soul? He continued, "I saw what he did to you." He was talking about Dr. Evil:

"He didn't know anything about the female body. He put things back in the wrong places. Your ovaries were stuck to your intestines. Your cords were twisted and your uterus was positioned incorrectly. After that surgery, you would never have been able to have children and the surgeon would have known that. On a more positive note," he added, "sex should be less painful now." I had never had sex before my appendix burst. I didn't know how uncomfortable it was or wasn't supposed to be. Dr. Sure continued, "Try to just remember that you would have died without surgery. That doctor prevented you from dying. That's all he did, but at least he did that." Then he asked if I had noticed how much better the scar looked. I said I had and I thanked him, knowing the pride that surgeons take in their incisions.

When Dr. Sure left, I remembered how I had felt when I finally left Dr. Evil's shabby, little office, convinced that he could no longer hurt me and that I had survived him. It had been an illusion. I had never been able to leave him behind. I carried his ugly mark on the outside of my body, and his misogyny was also within me. Was Dr. Sure right when he saw my abdominal chaos as evidence that "He didn't know anything about the female body," or was it actually evidence that he knew and hated the female body, *my* body . . . *me*? I wanted to feel purged of Dr. Evil with my new, more humane scar and without the organs that he had treated so cruelly. But I was still full of adhesions and endometriosis, and emptied of so much more.

The second memorable visit was from Dr. Kind. He told me that at some point soon, we'd need to stop waiting for the blockage to clear. He would need to clear the blockage surgically by cutting out a small section of my bowel and reattaching it. I was very calm during this conversation, but my mother's face turned red and crinkled up as she fought away the tears. He left, and I suggested that she go get something to eat. She hated crying in front of people, so she gladly left the room before breaking down. Across the street from the hospital, she cried her way through her fast-food dinner. I'm sure she wasn't the first mother to do this. I sat in my bed thinking, *He's not my doctor. I can refuse surgery. I'll stall them all until my body is able to clear this blockage. I don't need an operation.*

And I didn't. I refused the operation until my body cleared the blockage on its own. They released me after a week with a low-residue diet, a recommendation that I followed precisely. The diet consisted primarily of white food: mashed potatoes, Wonder Bread®, noodles, and things that could dissolve in my mouth. I started working on my next research article the day after I was released. I felt good enough to entertain visitors who came to celebrate my survival. I had received over one thousand dollars' worth of flowers during my hospital stay—a figure I calculated so that I could bask a little longer in the outpouring of support for me. In our final meeting before I was discharged, Dr. Kind reminded me that if I remained cancer-free for the following five years, then my chances of recurrence would be small. In response, I made a choice that was completely out-of-character for me; I chose not to worry that it might return. I was going to get on with my life.

It was time to plan my next year's sabbatical: a year for professional enrichment during which I would not have teaching or administrative responsibilities at school, but would receive half-pay. I wanted an adventure. I felt like I deserved one. I would have it— teaching and writing in Australia for five months.

Chapter 8: "An Undetected Cancer Tumor Could Be Sending Out a Flare": My Eye

Preparing to leave for Australia was a cherished preoccupation. Before leaving, I had to rent my house, move my possessions into a storage facility, and prepare to live in a country where I knew no one. I had projects that would follow me to another continent, including an article on the local 2002 congressional campaign and my own book, far beyond its due date. My editor wasn't worried. No one else was working on such a big project, so we didn't have to concern ourselves with competition. But I wasn't accustomed to missing deadlines and it bothered me.

Fresh off a brush with death and the end of my relationship with James, I still had found time to have a passionate affair with another unsuitable man. It wasn't right. It wasn't prudent. It wasn't careful or safe. In some ways it seemed like he could be my soul mate (a cringe-worthy, overused term that I can think of no substitute for). I thought he understood me, especially my pain. It was not just because he endured so much of his own, but because he seemed tragically wise, embracing the tragedies in his life with his eyes and mind open. He had made understanding suffering his life's work. He said that I made him feel again and those feelings included joy, excitement, and anticipation. He treated me with respect, and an attentiveness that made me think I could be deeply sad with him and not have to hide it, explain it, or apologize for it.

I left for Australia at the height of the relationship. Never one to pine, I seized the opportunity to reinvent myself. I was an independent loner: healthy, outdoorsy, and active. I didn't have a car, so my pace slowed down. I only bought what I could carry the hilly mile from the grocery store to my small but airy, apartment. I didn't want to carry lots of papers and books, so I worked in the university library like I had in graduate school, taking notes on the journal articles instead of copying and highlighting them. I made more progress on my book than I had in a year. I spent a lot of time in the gym working out and just as much time sitting on my balcony sipping tea. I kept a journal for the first time since I was a child. I had limited Internet access, and phone calls to the United States were expensive and inconvenient, so I made them rarely.

Although I went on weekend trips to Sydney, Cambria, and Melbourne I made sure to truly experience Brisbane, the city where I lived. I saw, smelled, heard, and felt that city like no other because I was alone; the city was my companion. I would spend hours walking, stopping to look, think, and sit whenever I wanted. I'd watch the mangrove roots emerge and recede in the mud. I awoke each morning to sunlight coming in the window and the sound of exotic birds calling. I delighted in the sound of a laughing kookaburra, the surprising sight of wild turkeys walking the campus, and huge low-flying bats in my neighborhood. I'd become more observant and more conscious. Rather than perpetually surveying the natural world for danger, I became more open to taking in the beauty that it offered.

It was hard to come back from Australia because the experience was an amazing one and I hadn't felt done with the adventure when the semester was over. I didn't want to give up feeling safe walking alone at night. I didn't want to leave a culture where people said "no worries" and meant it. It had been fifteen months since my hysterectomy. Returning to the United States also meant scheduling a CAT scan that would determine if the cancer had returned and spread. I hadn't spent my time dreading this scan, though. Brisbane was a balm for my anxiety . . . why not for my body as well?

I returned to Pennsylvania during cold and dreary December. Because my house was rented for the year, I was staying in one of the college's small apartments for the few days I would be in town before driving to Florida for the second half of my sabbatical. I returned for doctor's appointments. I scheduled the abdominal CAT scan, a dentist appointment, and a visit to Lens Crafters®. My teeth were in better shape than my vision was. My contact lenses didn't seem to be working very well. I assumed I needed a new prescription. I returned knowing, from the little communication between us, that my pre-Australia tryst was over. I wanted to understand why. I didn't want to hear general platitudes. I wanted a deep, heart-wrenching, truth-telling conversation that would be reflective (and respectful) of the relationship I thought we had. I was ready to sustain any emotional blow to understand why he had pulled away. I wanted to crawl into his brain and know every synapse that had fired (or misfired) regarding us. I scheduled a meeting with him but first, I had my appointment with the optometrist.

I was used to not seeing the great big "E" with my left eye when I wasn't wearing my glasses or contacts. I wasn't used to the smear of black and white that I saw through my left eye when the contact was in it. I was also surprised that I couldn't discern which little dot was the closest to me on the 3-D card. I always aced that part of the test. Yet, I still thought the problem was my lens until Dr. Sweet, my optometrist, told me that she thought I had suffered a retinal vein occlusion in my left eye. She showed me pictures of the left eye ball, the thick red of the blood at the center radiating out into lines of blood. She said that she needed to refer me to a retinal specialist. I asked what could have caused this. She was calm and sensitive, explaining that it *could* be related to blood pressure. Mine was high, but she said that could be due to the stress of this situation and that I should see my primary care physician.

Her calmness did not rub off on me. I was upset about my eyesight. I realized now that I was relying on my right eye for almost all of my sight. I was worried about what might have caused this, and what other problems it might cause. I was worried about getting access to someone in my primary care office and whether or not he/she would finally take my blood pressure seriously. I was worried about what the retinal specialist would say and do to me.

I still had the key to my office at Dickinson, so even though it was inhabited with the sports memorabilia of my temporary replacement, I could go in and use the computer.

Forgetting about my meeting with my most recent Mr. Wrong, I lost myself in the Internet's wisdom on retinal vein occlusions. It indicated that they were most likely to occur among the elderly, the diabetic, and the obese. This sounded like the uterine cancer crowd. *What does my body have in common with this group? I keep getting their diseases!* I wondered if diabetes was in my future as well.

Then, I read two things that concerned me more than root causes. First, it said that the problem was actually an indicator of a larger systemic problem like lupus. It also said that once you had one retinal vein occlusion, the likelihood of getting another occlusion in the other eye increased significantly. My whole life revolved around my eyesight. My career was all about reading and writing (with some television and film-viewing thrown in). My greatest pleasures were from my sense of sight—going to art museums, reading novels, and watching the ocean. How could I ever feel safe if I couldn't see? How could I ever be reassured? How could I live alone in my suburban house? I had accepted the fact that being in a wheelchair was my future. That would not have been a surprise, but I wasn't prepared for this. I pictured the vulnerable, unemployed, unhappy blind woman that I might become. I had to do something.

It was too late to start badgering my primary care physician's office for an appointment. I would see Dr. Sure the next day for an examination and find out about the CAT scan that I had taken the day before. I didn't feel right staying in my office, because it wasn't really my office anymore. I didn't want to call a friend and cry about my latest disaster. They were all still recharging their sympathetic batteries from my uterine cancer scare. Some had also endured the heartbreak tale. So, I did what any nerd would do to seek comfort: I went to the bookstore.

I wanted to find a book about going blind, preferably written by someone who had gone through the experience. I wanted to read, while I still could, about how frightened she was when she learned the news, how she adjusted to the knowledge, and finally how she prepared herself for blindness. Then I would have a blueprint of what to do. The health section (primarily diets) was not useful. I didn't have a name for this imaginary person who would help me, so the biography section was out as well. This was not the kind of research I was used to doing. So I went up to the information desk in the middle of the store. "Where would I find a book about how to accept and adjust to going blind?" I asked.

"I'm sure there isn't one" the woman at the desk replied. "Who could deal with *that*?" I ended up buying a magnifying glass to make reading easier. It couldn't make up for the sight I'd lost in my left eye, but it made me feel like I was doing something. As I left the store, disheartened and exhausted, a customer walking in chirped,

"Smile! It can't be that bad!"

The next day Dr. Sure examined me, asking how I was feeling. I said, "Desperate and afraid because I have a retinal vein occlusion." Then I started crying. He started writing. He wanted a blood test anyway, and now he was ordering the kind of test that doctors would want to see if I had a coagulation problem. This would save me time, he said, as he handed the prescriptions to me.

I thanked him. Then he told me that I would need to do another CAT scan in three months, and he wrote out a script for that. "Why?" I asked.

"Well, the scan revealed some lesions on your liver. They're small and they probably aren't anything, but we want to be sure."

"Sure that it's not the cancer?" I asked. He nodded. "Is this one of the places uterine cancer can spread to?" I asked.

"Yes, but try not to worry about it. It's probably nothing. You have enough to think about." I did. But my ability to worry had never been limited; it could expand to suit the size of the disasters.

I had an appointment for the next day at the retinal specialists. The retinal doctor was a wiry, little man who wanted to chat about my career. Political science had been his undergraduate major. What did I think about Bush? How did I like Dickinson? He wasn't the first doctor to treat me like a stranger he'd met at cocktail party. Dr. Bottom-Feeder had spent our entire last visit asking me for advice about where his son should apply to college. Yet, somehow I was still given a bill for his time and I couldn't bill him for mine. The eye doctor might have been trying to put me at ease with this chatter. If so, it wasn't working. I was here as a frightened patient, not a political scientist. I wanted him to get to the part about my eyes.

Eventually he said, "Let's see what we have here," and he pulled the big eyeglass machine in front of me. I gave him the piece of paper and said,

"I have a retinal vein occlusion in my left eye. I currently have these blood tests being run; I could have you copied on the results. These are the blood pressure readings from my last three years of doctors' appointments." He looked surprised. Perhaps when he said "Let's see what we have here," he had been talking to the ether.

"Let's not get ahead of ourselves," he said. "We don't even know what you have yet. You can't trust an optometrist at LensCrafters® for a diagnosis." I was glad Dr. Sweet couldn't hear that. The retinal doctor looked at my eye. "Well, look at that. She got it right. That *is* what you have. Either it will get better, get worse, or stay the same. There's nothing that can really be done about it." You'd think someone so disdainful of optometrists would have something more than that to offer.

"Do you think this is caused by high blood pressure?" I prompted. "Do you think there are some other blood tests that I should have?" He said,

"Why this happens isn't something I concern myself with. It happened and now we have to deal with it. But offhand, I'd say those blood pressure readings are high enough to be a potential cause. Most people who have retinal vein occlusions also have elevated blood pressure. You should probably get that under control, although, getting your blood pressure under control is not necessarily a guarantee that you won't develop another occlusion."

That wasn't very reassuring. He wanted to see me again in a few weeks. *Why bother*, I wondered, if nothing could be done about it? I told him that I'd be in Florida and that I'd see a specialist there. I'd see him again in six months.

The next day, the same morning I was scheduled to drive to Florida, I went to my appointment at my primary-care physician's office. I was determined not to leave without blood pressure medication. The wait was stifling. The waiting room was small, with a country farmhouse décor, and thick windows separating patients from the staff. The wood chairs were hard. A television blared drug advertisements. (I knew the practice was getting paid to subject us to this and I resented it.) A woman who seemed to be in her sixties was complaining loudly about having to wait. When she sat down, she turned to me and said, "Retirement isn't all that it's cracked up to be. You get old. You get sick. They make you wait. These are supposed to be the Golden Years." It seemed to escape her that she was talking to someone in her early forties who was also sick and waiting. It would have been a great relief to me if ill-health had only tarnished my Golden Years instead of so much of my life.

Eventually I was brought into the examining room. The nurse weighed me and took my temperature. She took my blood pressure and said, "That's high. You should watch that." Since she had raised the issue, I exploited the opportunity to continue the conversation:

"Yes, that's why I'm here. That's why I was here last time, too. I need blood pressure medicine." For emphasis, I added, "The doctors here need to give it to me." She didn't say anything. She had my file and asked to update it.

"You're due for a yearly checkup," she said accusingly.

"I've been busy with specialists this year," I replied, pointedly gesturing to my file, "but I'm here now." She looked over my file and asked the usual battery of questions including, "Are you pregnant?" Usually I don't sweat this question, but I was an emotional mess, and she'd already put me on the defensive. I thought, *What part of "radical hysterectomy" don't you understand?* It was all there in black and white. I was frustrated and a little ticked off, but I don't express anger very well. So instead, I cried. I hadn't even seen the doctor yet and I was crying. She scurried out of the room and another nurse walked in. She offered me tissues.

"Are you all right?" I think the answer was obvious. I wouldn't be crying if I were all right. I wouldn't have scheduled a doctor's appointment with three days' notice. I was not all right. I said,

"I have a retinal vein occlusion and it was probably caused by high blood pressure. I want blood-pressure medicine." Someone would be with me soon, she reassured. I should try to calm down.

It was hard to calm down, but hysteria wasn't going to increase my efficacy in dealing with doctors. I usually had organized my information for them and tried to present it efficiently and succinctly. If they didn't understand me when I used that approach, how were they going to understand me now? I had to get it together.

The doctor that day was a woman I'd never met before. She wasn't officially a doctor; she was a physician's assistant (PA), which means that she could practice medicine under supervision of a medical doctor. PAs go to medical school, but not for as long as doctors. I knew Almost-Doctor had the authority to write prescriptions. I had so many bad experiences with doctors, but a few good ones with nurse practitioners, optometrists, and physical therapists. I assumed Almost-Doctor would be a better listener than the doctors I'd dealt with. She asked me to fill her in on what was going on. I could tell by her expression that she had been briefed on my emotional state by the nurse. As quickly as I could, I detailed the uterine cancer, the liver lesions, the retinal vein occlusion, and the news that an occlusion could happen in the other eye. I explained that the occlusion was most likely related to high blood pressure. She said that my blood pressure wasn't actually that high. She considered it "borderline."

I reminded her of the number on the sheet of paper in front of her. The nurse had classified that number as high. Almost-Doctor dismissed it. The number was probably artificially inflated because I was in such an emotional state. I handed her my piece of paper with blood-pressure readings from the months that I was in the oncologist's care. They were all elevated, I noted, and the retinal specialist thought that they were high enough to cause the occlusion. She said that once you were on blood-pressure medicine you were usually on it for life, so it wasn't something that should be prescribed casually.

I countered that my brother-in-law had lower blood pressure than I did (I recited his numbers) and he was on medication. She said that men were not as good as women at following directions to change their lifestyles. As a result, men tended to get treated with blood-pressure medicine when women weren't. I couldn't believe what I was hearing. Women don't get medication *because* they are obedient? *I* was obedient. Was that why I hadn't been treated?

"If you look in my file," I suggested, "you'll see that two years ago, the doctor I saw in this practice noted that my blood pressure was too high, and recommended that I go off of the pill and lose ten pounds. I'm not on the pill now, and I lost the ten pounds. My blood pressure is no lower." Almost-Doctor didn't look at the file:

"We really don't like to prescribe medication if you are asymptomatic." I couldn't take it anymore. My voice got shrill and loud.

"I have a symptom! I am now blind in one eye! I don't want to be blind in the other! Please give me some blood pressure medicine!" Again I started to cry.

She looked upset. I apologized for crying and then begged for medicine. I think I said something about the appendix, the hip, and the cancer. I was a mess. She wrote a script for blood pressure medicine. Maybe my friend Sharon was right when she said, "Just demand drugs and cry a lot and they'll give you what you want to get rid of you." Then Almost-Doctor queried, "Have you prayed about all of this?" I couldn't believe she had asked. It was none of her business.

"I thought it would be more efficient to come to a doctor's office since I needed blood-pressure medicine," I retorted.

"It's just that you've been through an awful lot." *Yes*, I thought, *that's right.* Maybe she was just being understanding and compassionate? Perhaps I should overlook her inappropriate use of religion to express that? But she continued,

"I just think that with all that you've been through God is trying to tell you something and you're not listening. You should pray to understand Him."

I practically ran out the door to the pharmacy. I was glad to drive out of town. When I stopped for lunch, I read the drug warning materials. Anyone allergic to sulfur-based antibiotics wasn't supposed to take this. That would be me. I had seen the "Allergy Warning" sticker on the outside of my file. Almost-Doctor hadn't read it.

I didn't have a cell phone then, but I still managed to call the office three times each day as I drove to Florida. I never got connected. No one returned the messages I left with the answering service. Even the one message I left that said "I'm feeling tightness in my chest," was ignored. I wasn't bluffing. I had worked myself into frenzy. I saw a cardiologist in Florida. I had to pay out-of-pocket because I couldn't get a referral from the primary-care office that wouldn't answer the phone, but I thought it would be worth it. The doctor in Florida prescribed Lisinopril and my blood pressure went down.

* * *

It was easy to choose and get seen by a retinal specialist in Florida, because my sister-in-law was his nurse. This doctor was chatty like the other retinal doctor, but he lectured me about politics instead of asking me questions. He had a lot to say about the Abu Ghraib prison torture scandal in Iraq: "They're in prison and they're enemies. We can do anything we want to them. I have a prison-guard patient and I said to him, 'When no one is looking, you beat them up don't you?' He said, 'Of course we do.'" Then, the doctor chuckled knowingly. I tried to tune him out as he spoke with pleasure about prisoners deserving to be humiliated. I had decided long ago not to use a morality yardstick to measure medical professionals. I feared that if I did, I might end up without a doctor.

Dr. Torture was not *as* bad as the pseudonym I have given him would lead you to believe. He was another one of those doctors who did things to me because he could learn something from what he did, and not because these procedures were likely to help my condition. Whereas my first retinal specialist was comfortable assessing the eye by looking at it when it was dilated, Dr. Torture wanted to shoot a dye into my vein that would allow him to take pictures. I had read on the Internet that many doctors didn't do this because it didn't prove particularly useful after an occlusion. When I voiced my concerns, Dr. Torture emphasized that we needed a benchmark. He *had* to do the test. So I let him.

I felt railroaded regarding the test, but at least the nurse had admitted that my arm veins weren't promising and had agreed to use a butterfly needle for my hand. Then Dr. Torture stormed in, "What's taking so long?" He scoffed when he heard my veins were causing the delay. "What do you mean you can't use the arm vein?" he asked, interposing himself between the nurse and me. "I can find the vein." He missed the vein . . . twice. I ended up with the butterfly needle in my hand. We got some vivid pictures of my eye, but no additional information on the occlusion, and the test was never repeated, so it was hard to see why I needed it as a benchmark.

The other procedure that Dr. Torture did was even more distressing. He said that sometimes the occlusion was resolved faster if there were steroids administered to the eye. I hoped the steroids were administered as a cream. It didn't. It meant an injection. He reassured me that the injection was done after a cream was put on the eye to desensitize it. Just in case I tried to blink at the wrong time, he needed to put me in an eye clamp. That's probably not the right word for it, but anyone who has seen *A Clockwork Orange* knows what I'm referring to. It's an apparatus that keeps the eye open.

He was right that the shot did not feel like I was stuck in the eye with a needle. It felt like a sharp stick. He did it twice. It took days for the soreness to go away. In addition, my eyesight got worse before it got better. Since the occlusion began, it had been difficult or impossible to see anything that I looked at directly. Now I could see lots of little bat-like shapes in the bottom of my vision and floaters everywhere else. There were lots of drops; I wore an eye patch to deter infections. Dr. Torture admitted that the steroids hadn't helped and in the same breath pronounced them, "worth a try." I wondered how often the steroids had to fail for Dr. Torture to determine that they *weren't* worth trying. I suspect that we would have disagreed over what would constitute an acceptable rate of success.

I wanted to know why I had a blood clot in my eye, so I went to the hematologist practice where my father had gone. I gave him the extensive blood tests that Dr. Sure had ordered, and told him my medical history. The hematologist was concerned that the blood clot might have been an undetected cancer tumor sending out a flare. To test his hypothesis, he ordered more blood tests, another CAT scan, and a brain MRI. To me, his fears about an undetected cancer tumor sounded like something my body would do and something most doctors would miss; to my health insurance company, this sounded like a series of unreasonable tests. The battle began. There was eventually a compromise. They could do one type of brain MRI, but not another. The technicalities eluded me, but the price did not. I was out-of-system in Florida, and responsible for 20 percent of the bill after the deductible.

I had the CAT scan and the MRI scheduled for the same day. It took a few tries to get an IV in so I could receive the contrast for the abdominal CAT scan. They ended up using my hand. After a lot of waiting and getting sick to my stomach, it was time for my brain MRI. They needed to find another vein. They couldn't. They sat me in the hallway as they searched for a phlebotomist. While I sat, I noticed my hand and arm getting black and blue. It seemed like a lot of bruising and it was getting worse. I stopped the next doctor who walked by.

"What is going on with my arm?" I asked. He looked at it.

"It's black and blue and getting worse by the second," he reported.

Exasperated, I clarified, "What's *wrong* with it, I mean?" He didn't know. I said, "You're a doctor. How would you suggest we find out?" He sat down and asked me to wiggle my fingers.

"Was there tingling?"

"No."

"Was there numbness?" Again, the answer was no. I suggested that it might have been from the IV that I had gotten that morning for my abdominal CAT scan. He said, "Oh, you're the liver-lesion lady. I looked at your scan. I think your arm is fine. Don't take any aspirins for the next day or so." Then he walked off. *The liver-lesion lady?* That didn't sound good. Dr. Sure had hoped the lesions would not be on the second scan. But apparently they were visible *and* memorable. *Is the cancer back?* I worried. *Is this the site of the flare?* I felt the weight of the potential bad news.

Around this time I told my mother that I felt like the "pace of my destruction has accelerated." I called my investment broker and switched some long-term stock investments to bonds that would pay dividends each year. I vowed to spend the dividends. I had spent my life being very cautious with money. Always carefully saving for the future, I was starting to think that I wouldn't have one. I needed to have more fun with my money. I would buy some new furniture when I got home. When I left the hospital that day, I bought a one-hundred-dollar dress. It might have been my first.

As if to mock my spending spree, there were no lesions on my liver. My MRI and my blood tests were normal. The swelling was going down in my left eye and nothing bad had happened to my right one. I would never regain the loss of sight in the center of my vision, where the vein had clotted, but it was workable. Resolved to enjoy the reminder of my sabbatical, I decided to stop thinking about what would happen next.

Over the summer my renters moved out, and I moved my things back home to Carlisle, PA. Some of my furniture was damaged, so it was a good thing I was ready to spend some money. I prepared for classes and hoped to get my life back on track.

One night, I was having dinner alone at a sushi bar. The man next to me was outspoken and gregarious. He offered me wine. I took it. When we got around to discussing our professions, he said something like, "Does it matter?"

"No. Not really . . . as long as you're not a doctor. I can't deal with doctors." Even though I had not been joking, he laughed.

"I am a doctor." I scolded myself internally: *How embarrassing. How am I going to get out of this one?*

"Okay, some doctors are fine. As long as you don't work for my primary care physician's office. They are horrible."

It turned out that he was the newest member of their staff.

I said, "It might just be me," and we got to talking about how confusing my problems had always been to doctors. I told him about my last ordeal—all the tests that were done to reveal little more than what I had known leaving LensCrafters®. I said, "I've adjusted to the diminished eyesight. I'm hoping for the best.

They couldn't find an answer and I can't find one myself. So, I decided that I was done."

"I don't think you should stop looking," he said.

"Do you want to take a crack at it?" I asked, with equal parts flirtatiousness and trepidation.

"Hell no. You are way too complicated for me." My unsuccessful searches for a significant other and decent healthcare had collided at the sushi bar. I wondered if the explanation for why both eluded me was that simple. Was I just too complicated?

The evening wasn't a complete bust. The doctor-in-disguise referred me to a physician he knew at Johns Hopkins.

"She's brilliant," he promised. "If anyone can figure you out, she can." So I went to Johns Hopkins.

The brilliant doctor looked at my records. She listened to my story and asked me a few questions. She ordered a few more blood tests. Ultimately she said, "Sometimes things just happen and we never know why. If you ever have another blood clot, you'll need to be on Coumadin®." It was a drug that my father, uncle, and aunt had taken. It seemed likely that it would be in my future.

When I walked out of my appointment, I marveled again at David, the man who had offered to accompany me to Baltimore. I didn't have to ask—he offered to go with me after just a few dates. It didn't seem hard for him. He was upbeat, but not too cheerful. He was confident that they would find my vein on the first try without belittling my doubts that they might not. Even when I didn't make a lot of sense to him (he had never been a worrier), he took cues from me, adjusting quickly to what I needed and wanted. What I didn't know then was that David would want to spend his life with me regardless of how complicated I could be. David would become my second husband.

I had been looking for someone with luck like mine, suspecting that only a man who had experienced pain and betrayal could cope with my anxieties, as well as my past, permanent, and future complexities. David possessed the resilience I longed for, but it came from an unexpected source: good luck and a rare, genuine lightness, and joy. That's what had stood out when I met him at a speed dating event. We only had six minutes to talk, and I don't think either of us said anything particularly interesting. But we had smiled a lot. He made me smile, not because he was funny or charming or flirtatious (although he could be all those things), but because he glowed with happiness, warmth, and openness. Nothing about me scared him. He would take care of me regardless of what my physical problems were.

"Even if I can't walk anymore?" I asked, testing him.

"Yes," he said, so I upped the ante.

"Even if I go blind?"

"Yes."

"Even if the cancer returns?" The answer was always an unhesitating, unremitting "yes." If I had been testing him with my truths, he passed the tests without having to study or fret about them. David had a well of certainty that "we," yes, *we*, in spite of our individual deficits, would make a great team. His smile, the cute little glasses, the soft blonde hair, and the kind blue eyes were the first thing I thought of when I woke up the next morning. All I had to do was think of him and I grinned. I still do.

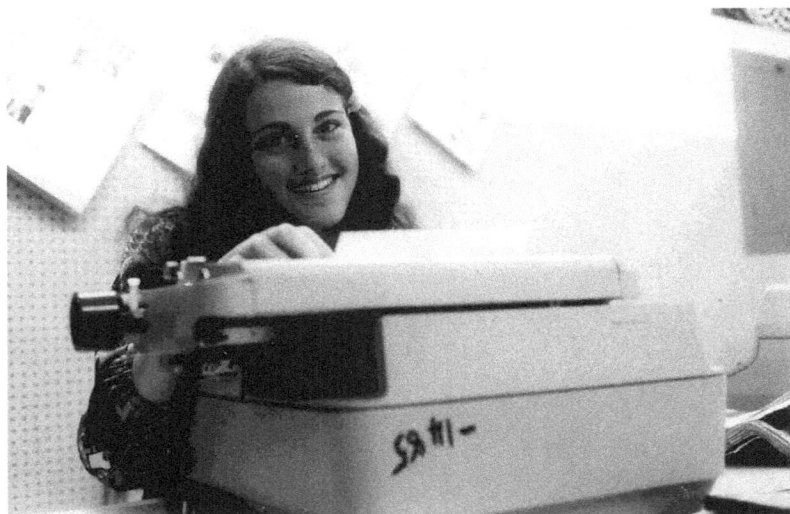

Stephanie in her early teens, working on the school newspaper.

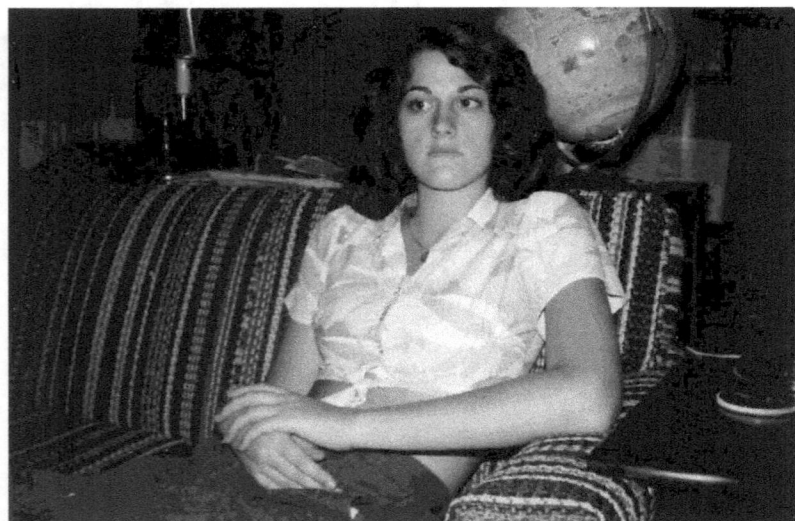

In high school, after a haircut.

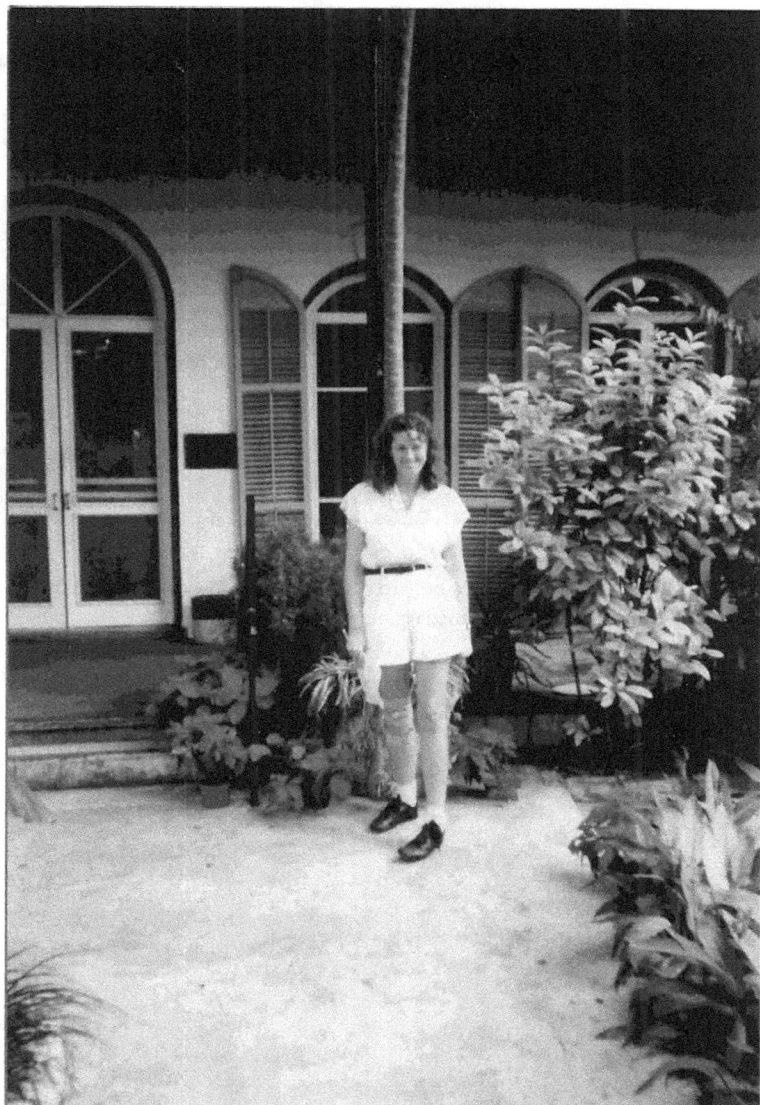

Stephanie with the knee brace that she wore for ten years.

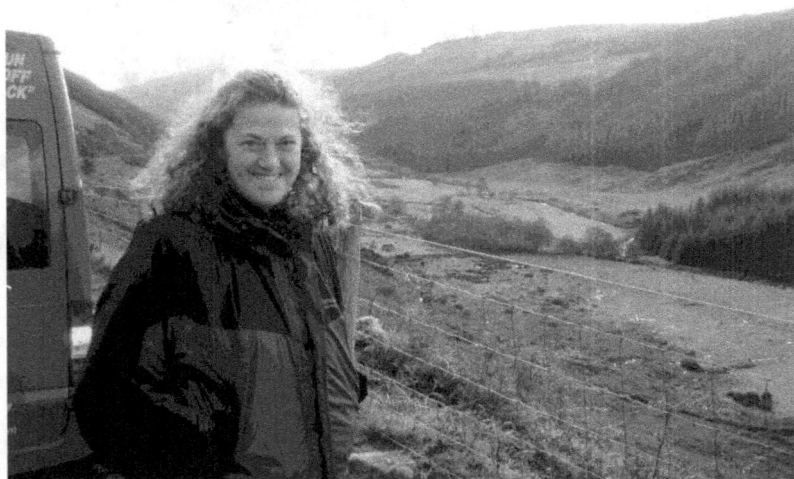

Stephanie in Ireland four days before getting the food poisoning that led to the discovery of her peritoneal cancer.

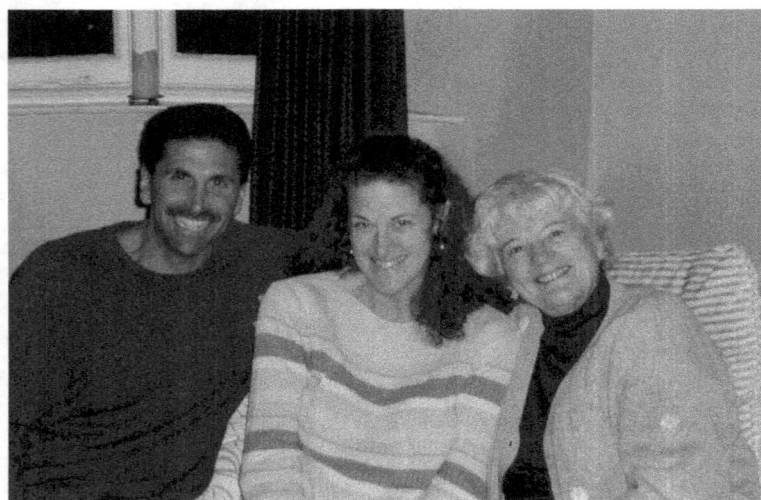

With Diana, her mother, and Marcus, her brother, after being released from the hospital in early 2007.

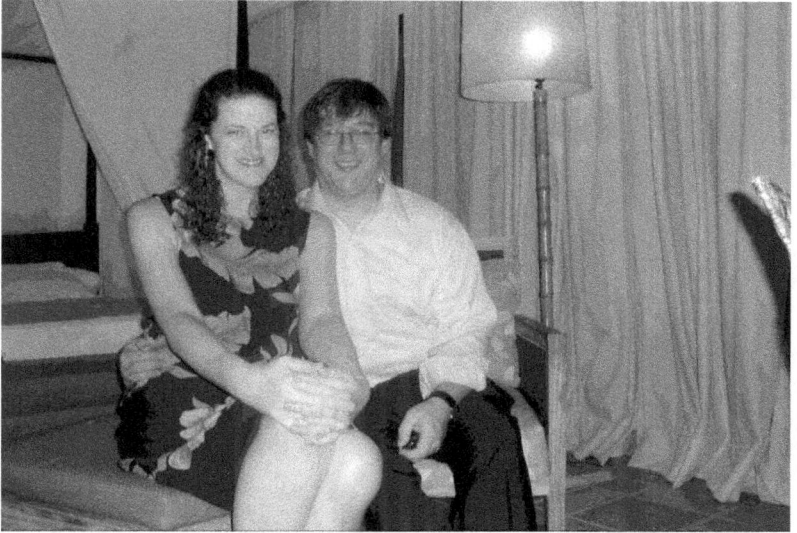

Stephanie with David, her husband, in Tenerife on the first of many mini-vacations taken while undergoing chemotherapy in England in 2007.

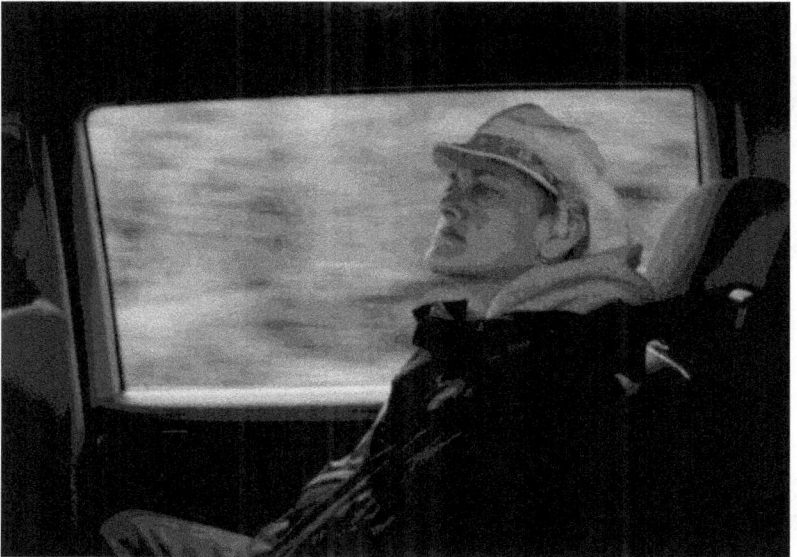

On a tour in Madeira in 2007. Even during chemotherapy, Stephanie actively explored new places.

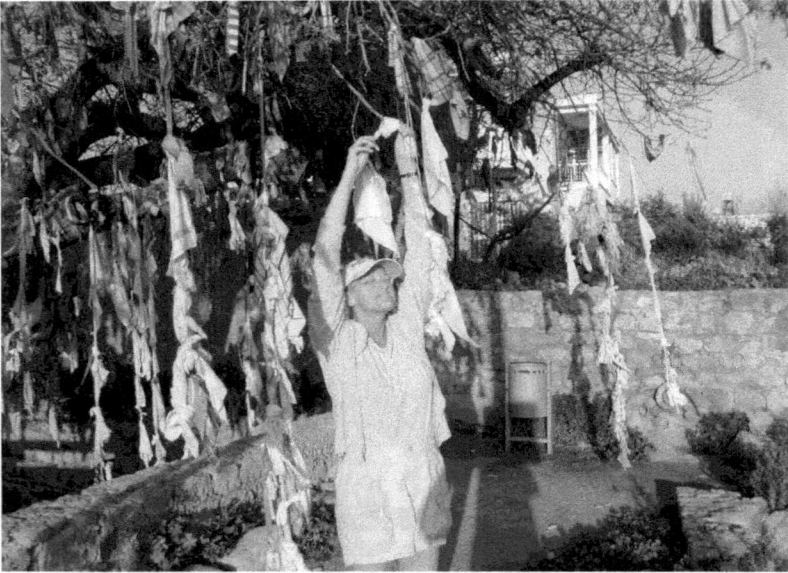

At a prayer tree at the Agia Solomoni Catacomb in Paphos, Cyprus in 2007.

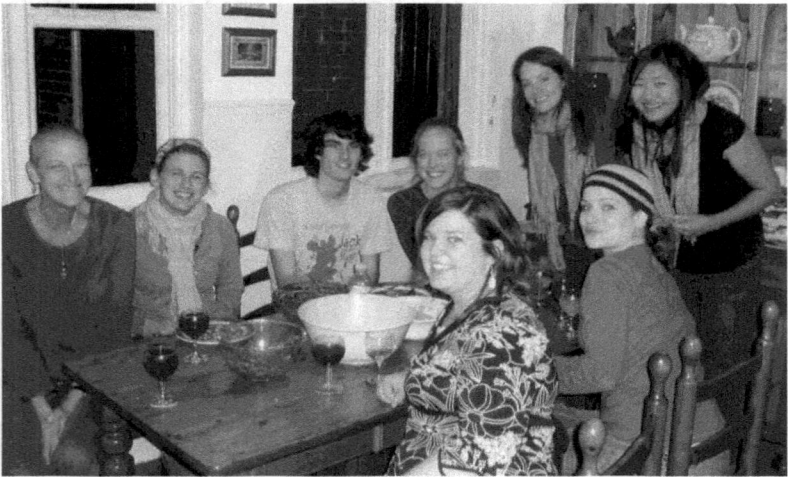

Stephanie with students around Easter in 2007. Sitting next to Stephanie is Meghan Allen, the editor of the book.

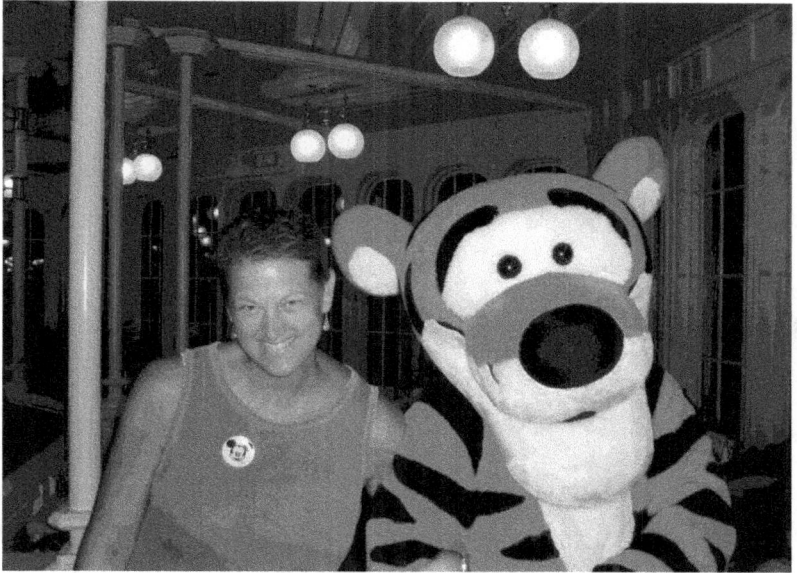

Stephanie with Tigger in Walt Disney World in 2008 while on a break from chemotherapy.

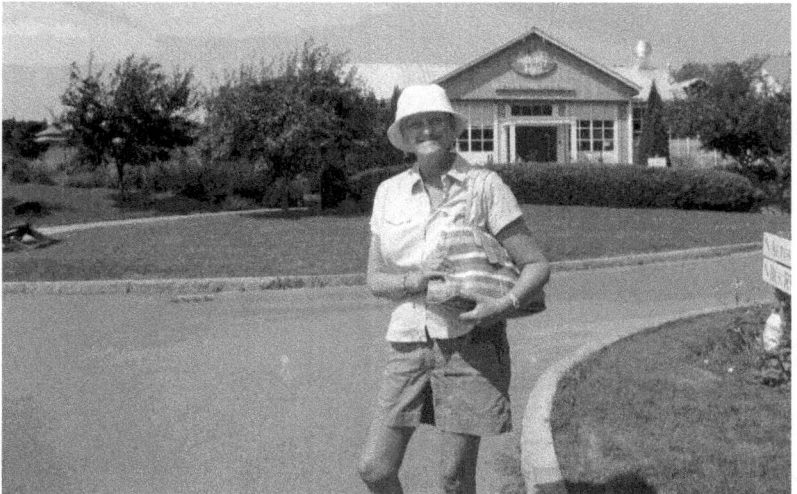

During a vacation in the Finger Lakes in 2009.

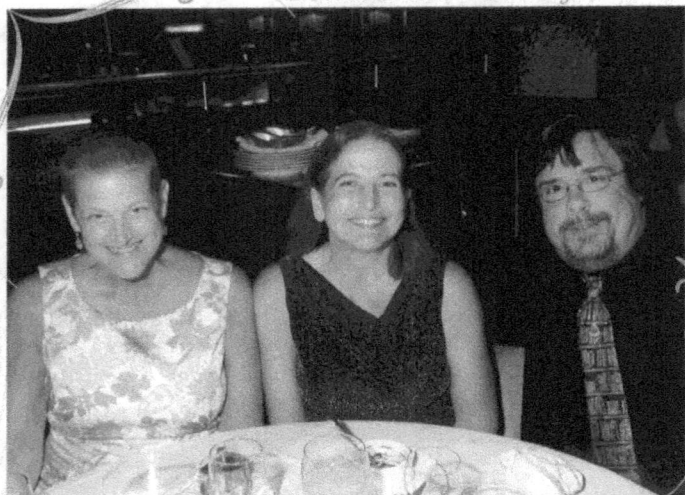

Celebration Dining Room

Stephanie with Connie, her sister, and Meade, her brother-in-law, on a cruise in November 2009, a month before Stephanie visited the Burzynski Clinic for the first time in Texas.

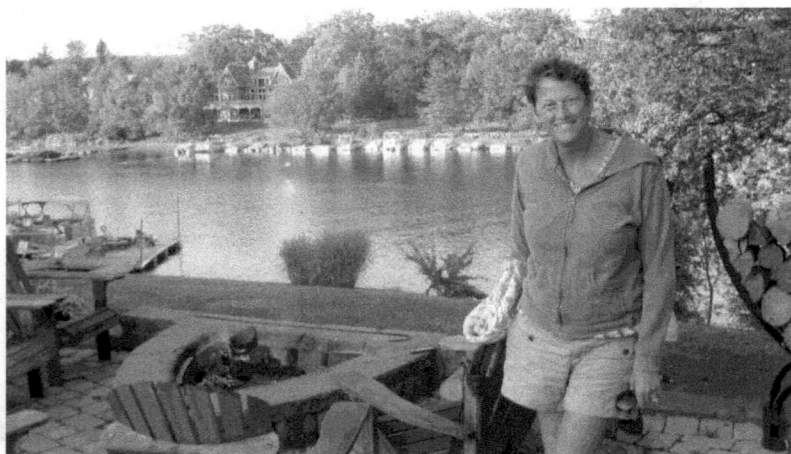

In 2010, during one of her last vacations. Stephanie stopped chemotherapy two months later.

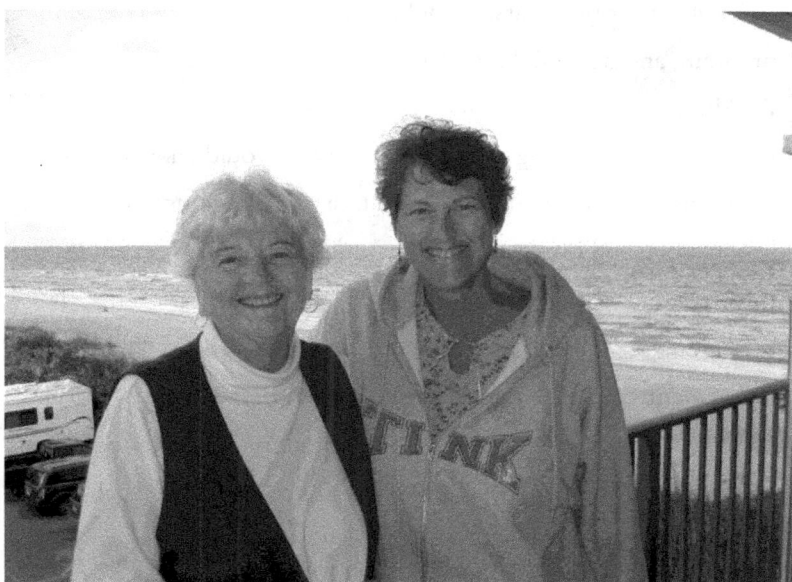

Stephanie in Florida with her mother in January 2011. This is the last photograph of Stephanie.

Chapter 9: "You have Months, Not Years, to Live:" Ovarian Cancer in England

In the summer of 2006, I was preparing for another adventure. This time I wouldn't be alone. David and I were going to England for two years. I would direct the Dickinson Humanities program, and he would look for a job. The program was for Dickinson juniors who would take classes for two semesters at the University of East Anglia in Norwich. They would take two classes from me—one in London in August, during which time we'd all live in a bed and breakfast together, and another in Norwich during the academic year. David and I would live in Dickinson's big, old house in Norwich and host the students for social and cultural enrichment events. Our plan was to get married when we returned.

I was exhausted before the summer preparations began, because it had been a particularly stressful school year. As chair of my department, I had led a ten-year, self-study and an evaluation of a colleague for tenure. Persuaded by a generous fee that would be our European travel fund, I had written a workbook for Advanced Placement (AP) United States Government and Politics in just a few months. I was in the midst of packing up my household goods, getting my home ready for renters, finalizing travel documents, and preparing for the class I would teach in August. The class was to use London as the setting to understand the literature, art, culture, and history of a country I had never studied before. I was reading and learning about England and London at a pace that I hadn't since graduate school. It was exhilarating.

David was putting everything he had on the line for us. He sold his house, his boat, and his car. He found new homes for his cats and quit his job. He did it all unconditionally and eagerly. It was a dramatic contrast to dating men who couldn't commit, or would only do so if it meant they didn't have to change anything except their availability to other women.

We were having problems getting David the right visa. He would have to enter the country on a tourist visa for six months, and then try to convert to a work visa after finding a job. I realized that as a tourist David would not be covered by England's National Health Service (NHS), and he no longer had his American insurance. He trusted that it would be fine: he'd never even had an IV. I, on the other hand, lay awake at night wondering what would happen if he got sick or had an accident. I suggested we get married at the county courthouse before we left. That would solve everything. We were already engaged. I didn't have any doubts that I wanted to marry him. We would simply forgo a wedding and reception. He suggested that we keep the marriage a secret and have a wedding when we returned in two years. We could have it all— security and fun.

Amid the boxes, debris, and stench of cardboard, we dressed up for our ceremony. We used my mother's eternity wedding ring that I had always loved. After the ceremony, I would put it on my right hand, and put the engagement ring David had gotten me back on the left hand. A tall, old judge presided. His secretary was our witness. When the judge was reading the "Do you take this woman" part, David regarded him intently. The judge and I both knew he was supposed to be looking at me. I watched him stare earnestly at the judge and say the words that he was supposed to be repeating to me. I thought what a lucky woman I was to have found such a genuine, sweet, and loving soul.

The judge congratulated us and gave us a small bottle of chilled champagne. We took it to the lot that we had purchased. We planned to build our dream home there when we returned from England. We popped the cork over the lot and toasted our future. Then we went to my favorite spot on Dickinson's campus. It is known as the Morgan Rocks—named after the terrain and a nearby dorm. There's a tree there that was planted in honor of Matthew, one of my advisees, who died during his junior year abroad. It had been a perfect spring day when we planted and dedicated that tree. The breeze had made the older trees' leaves rustle in that soft, ethereal way. For me, this had become a place of quiet contemplation and peace. David and I finished off the little bottle of champagne and I gave him one of those singing cards. We danced to the first two lines of "Unchained Melody" over and over again, repeatedly reopening the card to create a makeshift melody. Then we got back to work preparing for the move.

* * *

During the months of preparation, my digestion had been off. I tried not to worry. There were plenty of reasonable explanations. In the chaotic preamble to leaving for England, I was under a lot of stress. I had a compromised abdomen and I was aging. When I considered going to the doctor, I recalled my late thirties, when I had experienced diarrhea so frequently and cramping so severe that I worried I might have colon cancer.

I had gone to the doctor, equipped with a food diary that he barely glanced at. I said that the only pattern that I had observed was tomato products, but eliminating them from my diet hadn't seemed to help. He said that women in their late thirties tended to have a lot of stress in their lives with the pressures of career and family. That could explain the problem. But I was on sabbatical when this started, I explained. I was living in a beach house, sleeping nine hours a night, going to the gym four times a week, and writing a book on public opinion at a leisurely pace. I was free of teaching and administrative stress. I didn't have children. "It could be because you are a Type-A personality," he said, seeming uncomfortable that I had questioned his judgment.

"I've always been this way. So why would my personality suddenly cause me such digestive problems?" I asked. "More importantly, how do I get this to stop?"

"There really isn't anything you can do," he said. "Just try to relax." I did relax when I realized that garlic usually accompanied my consumption of tomatoes. A little experimentation revealed that it was the culprit. When I stopped eating garlic, my digestive problems stopped as well.

"I love garlic! How can you live without garlic?" friends would ask when I meticulously ordered food without it at restaurants. *You should see how I live with garlic*, I'd think.

* * *

Now, I was in my mid-forties, and it seemed normal to add to the list of things I couldn't eat. I started the list after rejoining the "land of the eating" post-appendix rupture. Pancakes, cabbage, broccoli, cauliflower, Brussels sprouts, and cucumbers all went on the list. After a particularly difficult night, I added orange juice. I wasn't sure why I would occasionally feel full after eating a reasonable amount. Every few weeks I would go on a bland and minimal diet for a day or two to get back to normal. Although troubling, it wasn't anything I couldn't adjust to.

The digestive problems continued in England. Every few weeks, I would have a hard night of digestion. It didn't surprise me. Most of the time it seemed to follow an Indian dinner. Maybe they used a spice that needed to be added to the list?

I had already chosen a primary-care office (what the British call a "surgery"). It was easy to get an appointment. If you called in the morning, you got an appointment to see a doctor that day. If you called in the afternoon, you might have to wait until the next day. The office was a twenty-minute walk from the Dickinson house. The doctor whom I saw explained that I didn't need a mammogram because England recommended them every other year (rather than the yearly ones I had been getting). She examined me and gave me a new prescription for blood-pressure medicine. She said that adjusting to a new country's food could take time. But before I knew it, the Christmas holiday was approaching and I still hadn't adapted the way the doctor predicted I would.

In December, after the fall semester, David would fly to America a week before I would to secure the paperwork for a visa and to visit his family in New York. We would meet up in Florida to celebrate Christmas with my family and then fly back to England together in January. Before the students scattered for the break, we invited them to meet us at the cutest pub in town. We ended up taking those who stayed the longest to dinner at the closest restaurant. Because it served Indian food, I knew this was risky for me, but I tried anyway. That night, I awoke feeling terrible. I vomited a few times. Then, David got sick. We were miserable throughout the day. We suspected that we had gotten food poisoning from my chicken dish. That would explain why we were both sick. My tumultuous digestive history explained why I was so much sicker than he was. Still, he managed to drag himself to the train station to get to London so that he could catch his flight to America. I stayed in bed sipping water.

Two days later, I was weak from hunger and glad that I felt hungry. But not long after I ate, I was vomiting again. After a night of severe abdominal pain that reminded me of my post-hysterectomy pain, I knew I needed help. I booked an appointment with my doctor and called a colleague's wife to see if she could drive me to the office. The walk that had seemed so manageable before was impossible in my current condition. Getting dressed and downstairs was a chore. On the short drive, I told her how concerned I was that there was something seriously wrong with me and the doctor would think there wasn't. She seemed a little confused. She trusted doctors and hadn't had any major problems. She thought the doctor would take care of everything and I would be fine.

The doctor saw was an Indian man, which made telling him how this had started a little awkward. I agonized about whether he would think I was blaming his national cuisine. I told him that I had had an intestinal blockage before and in some ways, this felt very similar. He listened to my symptoms, had me pee in a cup, felt and listened to my abdomen, and concluded that I was dehydrated from food poisoning or a virus. He wanted me to drink more and avoid solid foods. He thought I would be fine. "Good news," said my friend. I wasn't so sure.

I decided to err on the side of caution by not eating solid foods for two and a half days. On the first day, I did a little paperwork and went to the office to meet with a few remaining students. On the second, I took a bus into town and ran errands, buying Christmas gifts for the gardener and maid. I was exhausted and weak, but I would sit down to rest often and sip water. I was afraid to eat, but I knew I had to try. I boiled a handful of egg noodles and put a quarter of a teaspoon of butter on them. Eating reminded me of how hungry I was. My body wanted food. My mouth wanted taste. I finished the noodles and indulged myself, eating three mini-chocolate chips.

Soon I was projectile vomiting with fire hose-like force. I had never vomited like this before. How could my body be so weak and so powerful at the same time? How could such an innocuous little meal result in such fury? I slumped over the toilet bowl, resting between assaults. I was alone in a body that needed help and seemed destined to be misunderstood.

Eventually the vomiting stopped and I was left with excruciating abdominal pain. The worst of it came in waves, but it was never entirely gone. I called David, but what could he do from across the ocean? I planned to ride this out for the night unless new symptoms appeared. Then, I would call my local doctor's office again and see what he advised. I was sure that I needed to be admitted to a hospital. I would try to convince them in the morning.

I didn't sleep at all that night. There was too much pain. I read during the calmest periods to distract myself. I wasn't able to comprehend much of what I read, but there was something oddly hypnotic about the process of consuming each word carefully until the spasms would cause my eyes to accelerate, as if to outpace the pain. I would stop reading and scream until the wave abated. It was a long night.

I called the doctor's office as soon as the night answering service said they'd be available. I was instructed to go to a local clinic, which served as a triage center over the weekend. A doctor there would decide whether I needed to go to the hospital. I called a cab, managing to put on shoes and a sweatshirt. I would have to stay in my sweatpants; bending to take them off hurt too much. In any case, I doubted that I would be able to get jeans over my swollen abdomen. The clinic wasn't far away and the cabbie wished me luck.

The waiting room was full. There were lots of children crying and coughing. I sat doubled over on a hard chair, trying to regulate my breathing to endure the wait. I assumed it would take hours to be seen. But somehow I was the next one admitted. I must have looked awful for the British to allow me to jump the queue (cut in line). The doctor who examined me was another Indian. Again, I hated to include that the Indian food was the origin of my problems, but I had always been thorough when talking to doctors. It had been almost a week since that meal. This had to be something else.

My hysterectomy scar was clearly visible, but I made sure he knew that it masked the earlier appendix surgeries. I offered my intestinal blockage theory to him, trying carefully to be deferential in my tone and speculative in my suggestion. He listened carefully, examined me and explained that he felt my symptoms were consistent with food poisoning. I would be better soon, he predicted, but there was a hint of hesitation in his voice. There was an uncomfortable silence between us. He looked at me and I looked at him. He saw my desperation and I saw his compassion. He felt my abdomen again and said, "It is not really my decision whether you are admitted to a hospital. But I can report to them that I do feel some resistance in your . . . ." The words washed over me. I didn't care what he told them. I just knew that he would try to get me into a hospital. He made the call and got me admitted.

Doubled over, one hand pressing on my abdomen, I asked the front desk to call me a cab so I could go to the hospital. A man standing there said there was no need for that, he would drive me. He didn't seem to work at the facility, but he didn't seem like a patient either. When he said that a cabbie would probably drop me off at the wrong place and he could get me there sooner, I accepted the ride. Upon arrival, I was admitted to a ward with seven other beds, a few with patients in them. I was given an IV for hydration and examined by a doctor who took notes as I told my story. I didn't want to scare the other patients with screams and moans when the waves of pain intensified again, so I just sobbed as quietly as I could, rocking back and forth while holding my abdomen. A woman in another bed told a nurse to get me something for the pain, and without any explanation or persuasion from me that is what she did. Later I was given an x-ray. Eventually everything calmed down and I slept through the night.

In the morning, I was feeling better. Since it was the diagnostic ward, I thought I would spend my time diagnosing my companions. The woman next to me was just old. She kept forgetting to push the button to alert the nurses when she needed a bedpan. She might need a nursing home. The man diagonally across from me, who had been fitful all night, clearly had had too much to drink. I had an intestinal blockage. I had no idea what the woman across from me had. She didn't know why this was taking so long, or what was wrong with her, but she did know she was tired of being in the diagnostic ward. Maybe it was an ulcer or a gallbladder problem.

I was at the Norwich University Hospital, which is a teaching hospital, so a host of doctors-in-training trailed after the senior doctor responsible for the ward I was in. Bobbling about at his heels, they reminded me of chicks chasing after their mother hen. Consequently, I thought of them as his "baby doctors." The senior doctor had assigned each of them to one of the patients in the ward. As he completed his rounds, he listened as the baby doctors reported what they had gathered, observed, concluded, and would recommend. After each report, the senior doctor would ask a few questions and make his own diagnosis. The first baby doctor suspected that the drunken man had appendicitis. (*No way*, I thought). The senior doctor corrected him, providing technical reasons for why that assessment was wrong and concluding that the man was dehydrated from too much alcohol. (*Baby doctors: zero. Me: one.*) The woman across from me was a mystery to all of us, and the senior doctor couldn't tell what was wrong with her either. He ordered more tests. The woman next to me didn't belong in the hospital. (We all got that one right.) Then, the gaggle came to my bedside. My baby doctor summarized my condition and concluded that I had food poisoning from "spicy food foreign to her." He noted that my surgical history and food allergies made my reaction more acute in duration and severity. The teacher asked,

"Really?" in the way teachers do when we mean: wrong. "What do the rest of you think?" That was another technique I used in the classroom—having them correct each other. But none of them had anything to add. *No overachievers in this crowd*, I thought. *Or maybe it's a British thing?* If these were American students, they each would have wanted to throw in their two-cents' worth even if they had no idea what was wrong with me.

The doctor asked about the x-ray. A technical answer followed. It must not have been the answer he was hoping for, because he suggested that they all go look at the x-ray. When they came back he explained, "You have a partial blockage of the small intestine. This is probably caused by one of your adhesions. We will give this twenty-four hours to resolve itself with hydration and if it doesn't we'll need to operate." I asked if I had bowel sounds that had complicated the diagnosis. Was that why the other doctors had missed this? He turned to the baby doctors and said, "That's an excellent question. What's the answer?" They didn't know. I was glad that I had graduated to the senior doctor's attention. He explained that when the small intestine blocked, the large intestine could still be working on what had gotten through before the blockage. This type of circumstance could result in bowel sounds.

I was moved to another ward with patients who had digestive problems. The woman who had not been diagnosed was moved with me. We did not have to talk to understand how our respective health stories were unfolding. We could all hear the doctors. I knew that she was concerned about what was wrong with her (although she didn't seem fearful), and frustrated by how long it was taking to diagnose her. She looked away when she thought I needed privacy, and looked at me sympathetically when she thought I didn't. She wished me good luck when I was wheeled to the operating room, and again when she was released. The first was said with hopeful enthusiasm, the second with resignation. Both were appropriate. Both were appreciated.

Soon after my transfer, Kim, the wife of my colleague, came to drop off a few of my things. Her number and those of my students were practically the only ones in my cell phone. Kim told me that she had spoken with David. He and my mother were having trouble getting to England because of bad weather. She brought me some clean underwear, body lotion, a pad of paper, and the small stuffed toy that I had requested. It had always been comforting to have something soft to hold on to in hospitals. I didn't realize how soon I would need it, until a nurse came over to explain that the doctor had ordered a nose tube for me. She could see from the look on my face that I knew exactly what she was referring to and what it would feel like to have it inserted. She said that nurses realized how hard on the patient this was, so she had already asked the doctor if it was necessary. It was. I asked the nurse how much practice she had doing these and how many times the tube had come out of the patients' mouths. She reassured me that she had a lot of experience and that she'd *never* had a nose tube come out of a patient's mouth. She found that the calmer the patient, the easier the tube went down. I asked if I could have water to swallow. I could: it would just come back up the tube if it couldn't get through the blockage. She'd give me a little time to get used to the idea. As she left, she drew my curtain.

I held the little, stuffed bear rubbing his stomach in a steady rhythm, forcing myself to breath in and out in the same beat. In my head I repeated the words, *Don't panic.* I couldn't say or think it would be all right. I knew it would be awful. But I also knew that there were degrees of awful, and the compassion of the person subjecting you to the awful thing made a difference. This kind, woman who tried to prevent this from happening to me and was giving me this time to compose myself, wasn't a torturer. She would make it as easy on me as she could. *Don't think of the other time,* I instructed myself mentally. But my mind did not obey my wishes. The roughness, the rush, the cracking sound, the gagging, the lack of air, the scraping of my throat, the harsh directives to "swallow," the feeling that I was being killed—all came back. I told myself to breathe in and breathe out. I told myself: *You are not that young girl dying in that hospital bed anymore. You are a middle-aged woman. You can help yourself by being calm. Be calm. Be calm.*

When the nurse returned, she asked me if I was ready first. What could I say? Never? She spoke softly and encouragingly. I was as calm as I could possibly be while she inserted the tube up my nose and down my throat. She told me when it was almost over. When she was finished, she told me that I had done a good job. I told her that she had too.

I walked the halls a lot that night because I knew that if the blockage could pass this might help. It was something that I could do to try and help myself, but I was almost positive that it wouldn't matter. I was sure that I would have surgery the next day. I wasn't exactly looking forward to it because I knew the risks and the recovery challenges, but I wanted to be out of limbo. After successfully getting the attention I needed and surviving the diagnosis stage, I wanted to move on to the fixing and healing.

After a long night, I awoke to a hasty preparation for surgery. A new doctor explained that I was having emergency surgery because they didn't want to allow the blockage to continue. Food rotting inside of an intestine could cause all sorts of problems. I knew that, but wondered why they hadn't been worried about it the day before. I had been ready since I arrived. If they'd thought it was such an emergency they could have knocked me out, put the nose tube in while I was unconscious, and cut me the day before. I would have preferred that.

This new doctor was not doing the surgery, but he was on the team that would. He had come to tell me about the surgery, review the possible complications, and have me sign release forms. I was not surprised to hear that I might wake up without an intestine. I asked him what the chances of this were and he said that he thought they were low. I could stipulate that they were not permitted to go forward with that procedure regardless of what they found, but they could still perforate the colon accidentally and be unable to repair it. I told him that I dreaded getting a colostomy bag, but I wasn't going to prevent them from giving me one if that's what had to happen. There were other questions about what I would permit them to do and what I wanted done. I had always been rushed through this process in the United States, and there seemed to be only two choices: operate or let me die. Here, there seemed to be a middle ground. I asked him if I would have to have drainage tubes inserted in my sides. He didn't think so, but if there were complications, it was a possibility. I signed the papers stipulating that I didn't want to be kept alive in a vegetative state. I certainly hoped it wouldn't come to that!

Everything else preceding the surgery was familiar: I received a sedative through my IV and went into surgery. Wholly *unfamiliar* was my experience waking up in recovery. As soon as I started to come to, a nurse was at my side. She said, "Stephanie, you're in recovery. You do not have 'the bag' or any drainage tubes. Go back to sleep." I felt immediate relief and gratitude that she had told me this. I marveled that the doctor had told her what worried me. This communication touched and startled me. I was not used to kindness in hospitals. I slept.

* * *

The next morning the surgeon who had operated on me came to my bedside with three other doctors. They introduced themselves and I immediately forgot their names. He explained that the surgery had been successful at relieving the blockage. They had cut out a few inches of my small intestine and reattached it. "It was not blocked by an adhesion as we had expected," he began. In the movies, this moment is typically depicted in slow motion. The doctor's voice fades. Instead, the audience hears the high-pitched mechanical whine that Hollywood has assigned to accompany the delivery of bad news and (aptly) the aftermath of explosions. In real life, there is no slow-motion respite, no prophetic whine.

The next words I heard were, ". . . blocked by a tumor growing on your abdominal wall that had wrapped itself around your small intestine. We called in a doctor from the gynecological oncology team while we were operating. He will come to see you later today. Until you recover from the surgery, both teams of doctors will be working on your case. Then you will be in their care exclusively. Do you have any questions about the surgery itself?" I had the presence of mind to write some of the technical words that he had used on my note pad. When David arrived, I wanted him to have those. He could explain what they meant after researching them on the web. I did ask if the cancer was inside of the colon. He said it wasn't. I asked if he had taken the cancer out. It wasn't operative because it was part of the abdominal wall. Any other questions about the cancer should be saved for the oncologist.

Even though I was talking to the doctor, part of my mind was busy handling my surprise. I calculated that it had been a little more than four years since the hysterectomy. I was mere months away from the five-year mark, the time when oncologists generally agree that the active threat for a reoccurrence has passed. I remembered how attentive my father had been to his five-year clock after he went into remission. It was this memory of his vigilant anxiety that had motivated me *not* to obsessively watch the clock, but as always, the clock watched me. I was disappointed and exhausted. Hours before, I had been at the end of another medical nightmare. Now, I knew that it was just beginning. Since the cancer wasn't operative, I suspected I would have to have chemotherapy. I knew my veins would not cooperate.

I didn't cry when I got the bad news, or after the doctors left my bedside. *Only a masochist would cries with a nose tube*, I told myself. I wished David were there, but also knew that keeping my composure would be harder once I saw him. I called Kim, told her the news and requested that she email David. I spelled out the technical words, including the name of the operation and the name of the cancer cell. He and my mother would be arriving from London that evening and would be coming to the hospital. I hung up and turned my attention to actively (and anxiously) awaiting the expected visit from the oncologist.

The oncologist arrived with his executive nurse. He explained that I had metastasized ovarian cancer, somewhere

210

between stages IIIB and IIIC. This meant that the cancer had spread beyond the ovaries into the abdomen, but not to the other parts of my body. If it had spread to my lungs, brain, or into organs (like the kidney), I would have been stage IV (the final stage). I said that I had never had ovarian cancer, so I didn't understand how it could have spread from my ovaries. I must have had it, insisted the doctor gently. They looked at cells from my tumors under a microscope to type them. They were ovarian cancer tumors. The largest one had caused the blockage, but there were many, many more. They were scattered throughout my abdomen, appearing where the upper rim of my uterus had been.

He told me that the gynecological oncology team would meet the following day to discuss my case and develop a recommendation. The nurse would tell me what they decided. I was surprised. I didn't understand why a team discussion was required to determine my course of treatment. Wasn't chemotherapy the obvious course of treatment? I asked him what options they would be considering. "Whether chemotherapy makes sense in your situation," he replied. I wondered why it wouldn't make sense. *Isn't that how they fight inoperative cancer?*

"You mean instead of radiation?" I asked, thinking that might be another possible treatment.

"No, radiation is out of the question because of where your tumors are." *So why would they not do chemotherapy?* I was only forty-six years old, and there was nothing else wrong with me. I could take it. I didn't know how to phrase the question. So I just asked,

"How bad is this?"

He hesitated—"Do you really want to talk about this now?" The last time I had heard an answer like that, I had learned that there was no such thing as Santa Claus.

"Yes, of course."

"It is terminal; it might not be helpful to have chemotherapy. That's what we'll discuss tomorrow." He left, and I told his executive nurse that I wanted to know as much as possible from the meeting: what they recommended; why they recommended it; and what assumptions they were using. I wanted to know how long they thought I had. She said she would try.

It was worse than I had imagined. At first, I didn't think about how it would kill me, just that it would. I had only gotten to enjoy David for a small amount of time, and I feared that the rest of our lives together would be overshadowed by this death sentence. I wanted to sob, but I wouldn't let myself. Gagging on my nose tube would only make things worse.

That afternoon I received a phone call from the executive assistant of the Political Science Department at Dickinson. I had worked with Vickie for the last fourteen years. She was on a phone that was brought to me from some far away nurses' station (as there weren't phones by our beds). If anyone could manage the labyrinth to make contact with me in a hospital across an ocean, it was Vickie. Her competence was only exceeded by her persistence and compassion. She said she needed to know how I was. I think I said, "This is the one that's going to get me." I do remember telling her that at least I wasn't going to have to teach "Introduction to

American Government" anymore. It was good to hear her voice, but the nose tube scratched my throat as I talked.

David and my mother arrived that night. There was barely enough room for them to stand by my bed. My mother's eyes were red. How could I tell her this was terminal? She'd already watched my father die from cancer. Children aren't supposed to die before their parents. It was easier to look in David's eyes. They were as loving and peaceful as usual. I needed to tell him how bad this was without alarming my mother. I wanted her to have time and privacy to process my diagnosis. I didn't think David needed my protection. He somehow knew I needed to be alone with him, so he said that he was going to drive my mother back to the bed and breakfast and return to spend a little more time with me.

When David returned, I told him it was terminal. He already knew. He had read about my cancer cell when Kim emailed him the diagnosis. He sat by the bed and held my hand, and I allowed big tears to roll down my face. I changed my own rules: tears were allowed. As long as I didn't sob, involving my throat, nose, and chest, crying with a nose tube didn't hurt.

The next day the executive nurse told me that based on my age and overall good health, the team had recommended chemotherapy. They would do six treatments, one every three weeks if I could tolerate them, (which they assumed that I could). If the chemotherapy didn't diminish the activity of the cancer, then treatment would be terminated. Chemotherapy was unlikely to cure me, but it might extend my life or make the time remaining more comfortable. I asked her how long they thought I had. The doctors had been reluctant to answer this question, but she had pushed them based on our conversation from the day before. "Months," she replied grimly, "not years."

* * *

I ended up spending ten days in the hospital, during which I experienced a few debacles. They weren't as horrendous as what I had gone through when I was twenty, but they were upsetting. There was a miscommunication between my two teams that allowed a CAT scan to proceed too early. I tried to protest the timing, but the train kept on rolling. After I drank the nasty, chalky, white stuff, I got sick and the scan wasn't clear. They tried to do another one days later, once I was officially allowed fluids by mouth, but by that time all of my veins had collapsed and they couldn't insert the contrast dye.

There was also a nasty baby-doctor who overruled a phlebotomist. The phlebotomist was waiting for a butterfly needle to use on a vein in my foot. The baby doctor went for the vein with a full-sized needle because she liked them better. She had no regard for how much easier the experience would be for me if we waited for the smaller needle. I sobbed; David yelled. I later complained about her to the lead doctor.

"She is very new," he said, "and she makes mistakes. But," he continued, "That is not an excuse, just an explanation." I was satisfied with his response, and appreciated the fact that I never had to see her again. I was not sure if that was by decree or coincidence.

There were also problems hydrating me. Since I couldn't drink anything until my bowels had recovered, and they couldn't get fluids to me through IVs once my veins shut down, they tried to put a patch on my leg to hydrate me. The patch had lots of little pins that inserted into my skin so that fluid could slowly irrigate below it. I was warned by the nurse who put it on that this could do some damage, and for that reason, I should immediately report any swelling or pain in the area of the patch.

Unsurprisingly, the slowest nurse was on duty when it started to swell and ache. She said she could not help me until she finished her medication rounds (not a brief task, even when done by a more efficient nurse). The problem kept getting worse as I waited and worried. I started to hyperventilate and gag on the nose tube. I had vowed not to fit the demanding-American stereotype, and I think I succeeded until that night when I hysterically tracked the nurse down in the hallway. It wasn't my finest hour, but I got the patch removed.

Despite these missteps, the hospital stay reflected well on the United Kingdom and its medical system. On the whole, the medical staff was patient with the recovery process and respectful of patients' autonomy. They also assigned value to modesty and privacy. The system's virtues were exemplified in an interaction I had near the end of my hospital stay.

Early one morning, my favorite night nurse came into my room and asked if I would prefer that she take out my staples, rather than the day nurse. It was nice to be given a choice. One of the hardest things about hospitalization is losing all of your

215

freedom. Things are done to you without explicit permission and according to a schedule that is not your own. The nurse allowed me to choose the order she would pull the staples out. Skin had grown over some and there were sore indentations with blood in the corners of others. I would alternate between choosing worrisome-looking ones and those that looked easier. I was particularly concerned about the one inside of my belly button. The nurse remarked, "I don't know what the doctor was thinking with that one." She didn't tell me it wouldn't hurt because she knew it might. She didn't rush because that would have made it hurt more. She didn't treat me like an object, like a dress that she was taking a hem out of. She didn't try to distract me by chatting about something else. Instead we talked about each staple. "That was a hard one," she'd say.

"That one was easier than it looked," I remarked.

"Sorry about that one," she'd say after it started to bleed.

I could articulate my discomfort without having to apologize. It felt like we were working on something together. To be worked with, instead of worked on, was refreshing. It allowed me to feel like a human instead of a broken machine.

* * *

I had two weeks after I was released from the hospital to recover from the surgery before I started chemotherapy. As usual, my incision was improving much more quickly than my intestine. Eating seemed like a good idea in theory. I had lost a lot of weight since that dinner at the Indian restaurant. I missed food, but my body didn't seem to remember what to do with it. While I struggled through this, I decided to write letters. I composed an email to people with whom I was in regular contact in order to update them on my situation, tell them how I felt, and what I needed (and didn't need) from them. I tried to console them towards the close of the email by saying, "Part of me believes that I was supposed to die when my appendix burst in 1980, and I've had the gift of twenty-seven additional years. I feel like I've used them well, and am at peace with that."

I also used fancy stationary to write to friends who were important, but not necessarily present in my daily life. I would probably never see them again and I wanted them to know how important they had been to me. The letters took a lot of energy to write, and I didn't get through the long list of people I had planned on writing to. My mother would tell me, "You don't have to do that. No one expects you to do that." She didn't understand that the letters were not just for my friends, they were also for me. I didn't have much I could do, so these letters allowed me to visit and respect the past without hiding in it or being self-indulgent. I also got some lovely letters in return.

The chemotherapy that I received in England was Carboplatin® and Taxol®. It was administered at the hospital every three weeks. Privacy and efficiency dictated the arrangement of the room; chairs were scattered throughout a large space, far enough from each other that I never heard another patient's voice. Each patient's recliner had a visitor's chair next to it, so patients could bring a friend or relative. There was a doctor there, but I only saw him once when my IV gave out. Otherwise, we dealt exclusively with the nurses. They were quiet, serious, kind, and they always sent one of the senior nurses to insert my IV. The nurses knew that finding a vein would be difficult, and their efforts did not always go well, but we had an understanding. We both knew it would be tough, and we both knew it was necessary. They were patient with this procedure, allowing me to soak my arms in warm water to bring my pathetic little veins out. When I'd cry after they missed the first two times and would have to move on to my hands, they would quickly draw a curtain around me. Even with the enforced solitude that tears would bring, I felt like it was all right to cry in the English chemotherapy ward. No one took it personally. No one became angry, defensive, or distant. Most significantly, no one made me feel like there was something wrong with me or my body.

There was a beautiful women's cancer support center at the hospital. It had a counselor whom I chose to see a few times, a relaxing lounge with cookies and tea, and a consultation on tying scarves. In England, you receive a free wig with your first chemotherapy treatment. The day after each chemotherapy infusion, a nurse would call me to ask how I was doing. I was relieved that they didn't expect me to assess the seriousness of my own side effects and decide whether or not I should try to get medical attention. I was assigned a home nurse who could visit me weekly if I wanted. It all felt humane and non-judgmental. I was sick; they wanted to help. Even though I couldn't be cured, I felt cared for in England.

Chemotherapy kills off fast-growing cells in the gastrointestinal system, blood, and hair, so there is a lot of collateral damage. People know that chemo patients are often bald, but that's only true of some chemotherapy. It was true of the frontline drugs for ovarian cancer—Carboplatin® and Taxol®. They lowered my resistance to germs and caused tingling in my fingers, joint pain, exhaustion, and digestive problems. My mouth had a metallic taste that combined oddly with foods. I would yearn for a certain food and then not want it after one or two bites. I was thirsty a lot. Steroids and anti-nausea medicine prevented me from throwing up, but they also caused me to be anxious and weepy.

I spent the first week after treatment in bed. It's probably obvious why that would be the case. I was tired. Everyone's been tired before, so they think that they can relate to this. Yet it was substantially different from any other exhaustion I had ever known. It was not like staying up all night working on a term paper and then needing to function the next day. It was not like drinking until three in the morning and then having to get up for work in a few hours. It was not like having someone kick your seat when you flew from New York to Ireland on the red eye, after which you had to drive on the "wrong side" of the road for four hours to reach your destination. I had done these things. Exhaustion had always been something that I could will myself through. I tried to do this after chemotherapy, but it didn't work. The fatigue that I felt on chemotherapy was not caused by a lack of sleep. I would usually sleep ten to twelve hours a night and often took a three- to four-hour nap in the afternoon. But I was still tired. The exhaustion that I felt on chemotherapy felt like every cell in my body was screaming for rest. I suppose that they were, since chemotherapy depletes platelets and platelets carry oxygen to every cell in the body.

More than a week after my first chemo treatment, I thought the worst was behind me, and I longed to get out of the house. I wanted to go to a boutique chocolate store and buy the students some Valentine's Day candy. It sounded like a manageable excursion. We had a car. They had a parking lot. I rested up for the adventure; David and I stopped and sat on a bench between the car and the store. The store was smaller than a classroom and it wasn't crowded. But soon, I was just completely depleted. It wasn't that my legs were tired or that I was dizzy or faint. It was simply impossible to stand another moment. *I can't sit down right now,* I thought. *I will be okay . . . I just have to wait.* But there was no negotiating with my body. I sat down on the floor of the store. It was embarrassing, but I didn't have a choice. I didn't need to explain—the English look away when you do something embarrassing in public. If I had had to explain, I'm not sure I would have had the energy to try.

For a few days during the third week after chemotherapy, David and I went on a trip. Unlike the frugal vacations of my past, we spent a lot of money to make these trips as easy and wonderful as possible for someone as weak as me. Our first trips were to places I would never have planned to visit. But our goals were different than they would have been had I been well. I wasn't looking for education or adventure; I wanted to escape the wet, grey winter of Norwich, where the sun would go down around three in the afternoon. I needed sun, water, and calm. Our first trip was to Tenerife in the Canary Islands.

We had a driver take us to an airport outside of London. David stood in most of the lines while I rested on benches. I didn't eat until we arrived, and then napped after some scrambled eggs. I tried to walk down to the beach, but it wore me out. Our room was lovely with a canopied bed, a big tub, a rain shower, and a hot tub on a private patio with a view of the ocean. It was ideal, since I would spend most of the vacation there. The dinners were buffets that dazzled David and allowed me to taste and sample. On the first night my hair started to fall out in big clumps. Each day I lost more of it.

Since we spent the whole vacation at the resort, we decided to sign up for spa treatments. I was to get a scrub, a shower, and then time in a warm, saltwater, infinity pool. My attendant didn't speak any English and I didn't speak Spanish. But it wasn't hard to communicate that he needed to stay away from my abdomen. My scar was still red and puffy, and my midsection was bloated. I don't recall finding the scrub very relaxing. The shower wasn't pleasant either. I stood about ten feet away as the attendant literally hosed me down. I didn't know how to ask him to adjust the water pressure so I gritted my teeth until it was over. Later I heard David's surprised shrieks and giggles when he had his hose-down. When I heard him, I couldn't help but laugh along with him (as did his attendant). It was another illustration of our contrasting natures, and it reminded me of just how perfect he was for me.

It wasn't until I got in the pool that I relaxed. It was warm and bubbly with a perfect view of the ocean. Cool raindrops fell softly around me. I couldn't remember the last time I had felt that good, but I knew it was before the killer Indian dinner. I saw David walking from our room toward his appointment at the spa. He was in a big robe and slippers that were too small for his feet. He bounced happily on the balls of his feet as he tried to avoid puddles. As I thought, *He is so beautiful,* he looked up and saw me smiling at him. He smiled, too, happy to finally see *me* happy. I was struck by the realization that I was glad that I hadn't died on the operating table—that this moment was worth all that I had gone through. I had been working so hard to live, but I hadn't really been living. In that pool I realized that in this new existence there would be moments of pure joy, peace, beauty, and love. When I could find those moments, they would make enduring the rest of the nightmare worthwhile.

* * *

The months of chemotherapy in England took on a predictable pattern: a week of complete exhaustion and discomfort; a week at home with some distractions; and in the third week after chemo, a trip somewhere wonderful. Those trips weren't easy. I spent more time in airport, hotel, and restaurant bathrooms than I want to admit. Eating was often difficult, especially in Madeira where I kept finding garlic or cabbage where I didn't expect it. In Cyprus, I couldn't seem to avoid little, deep-fried, whole fish regardless of what I thought I had ordered. I didn't have the energy to see most of the sights, although I did better in Prague and Amsterdam than I would have in larger cities.

In all but a few of our pictures, I am bald. In the most breathtakingly beautiful location we visited (Positano, Italy), I looked the worst. We have the pictures to prove it. There I am: pale, thin, without a hair on my head—one eyebrow drawn on crooked and the other rubbed off. But there's a huge smile on my face. This was the destination I had longed to visit since seeing it in the insipid and irresistible romantic comedy *Only You* (1994). All the trips were worth the trouble. They gave me something to look forward to and something to remember. They made memories that David will have long after I am gone. After chemotherapy, we were able to enjoy more active vacations in Rome, Paris, and Switzerland. I felt my best on a cruise of the Mediterranean that I took with a girlfriend while David went fishing in Scotland. Each trip had moments that reminded me of why I was trying so hard to stay alive.

In between resting and travelling (week two), I spent time at home, with quiet distractions that also brought me joy. I could spend more time out of bed, and I could eat more than I had during the first week after chemotherapy. I would go downstairs and read novels or watch television. Sometimes David would take me for a short drive in the countryside. We watched DVDs of *Buffy the Vampire Slayer*, a show I had never seen before. I also watched episodes of *Charmed* in the afternoons. Not only did I enjoy watching the sarcastic, attractive sisters fight evil, but the message of an afterlife and the healing power of goodness appealed to me.

One of the main characters was a guardian angel who married one of the sisters. He would put his hand over the girls' injuries and heal them with his white light. Some nights I would ask David to give me white light, and he would put his hand on my abdomen, and we would think positive, peaceful thoughts of healing.

I also watched some British television namely, the affable Jamie Oliver, who I loved to hear enthuse, "The herbs are brilliant!"(He pronounced the silent "h"!) I also watched *Deal or No Deal*, which allowed me to make comparisons between the Australian, British, and American versions of the simplistic show. The British version was hosted by a low-key, short man, and the suitcases were held by average Brits who urged each other on. There were no beautiful models in high heels and glittery dresses, flashing lights, or sight gags. The British contestants were a bit awkward and humble. They hoped for the best and accepted the worst without whining about it. It was an approach that resonated with me and my cancer experience in England.

David and I played *Dr. Mario* on an old Nintendo game system. It was oddly diverting to match the three colors and eliminate viruses with pills that Dr. Mario dropped into a pillbox. I had first discovered this game in the late 1980s when it was new. I would play with my friend Carolyn during her son's afternoon nap. We'd eat popcorn, Peppermint Patties®, and play. She was pregnant with her daughter at the time and needed to have an amniocentesis because something didn't seem right to the doctor. The call telling her that the baby was normal came when we were playing *Dr. Mario*. It was a moment of absolute joy and relief that somehow became embedded in the game for me. News from doctors didn't always have to be bad and sometimes the good news was correct (as it had been about my friend's baby). The carnival-like music of the game would get stuck in my head at night and I'd watch imaginary pills squash viruses until I fell asleep. I pictured the chemotherapy working like that on my cancer cells, making them magically disappear upon contact.

Part of my responsibility as Director of the Humanities program in Norwich was to host the Dickinson students for social events. It was during this second week after chemotherapy and the early part of the third week before we traveled, that we did this. We had students over for dinners, parties, or to watch NFL football or movies. We brought back cheeses from Amsterdam and had a wine-and-cheese party. We cooked together—pizzas, sausage balls, and Chinese dumplings. The students would cluster in the kitchen like conspirators, bent seriously over their respective food preparation tasks. They played badminton in the backyard when the weather got nice. They would tell me about their classes, roommates, travels, and on occasion, ask for my advice about their love lives or lament their recently-broken hearts. On my birthday, they brought over a cake. We had a hotdog-eating contest, which ended with David and I exchanging wedding vows, so we could finally put on our wedding rings. In our candlelit backyard, the students were reverent, many of them crying quietly while David and I promised (again) to love, honor, and care for each other always.

Only one of my treatments needed to be delayed because of my blood work. That was only for a few days. Every three weeks they took a blood test to see if the chemotherapy was doing any good. This CA125 tumor marker measures the activity (not the size) of the cancer. The goal is for the number to get smaller and eventually sink below thirty-two. For the first four times mine was measured, the number went down. Then, after the last two treatments, it leveled out around forty-one. Six weeks after I finished treatment and right before I left to return to the United States, they took the CA125 again. The results weren't ready when we met with the doctor. They'd email the number to us. The hope was that it would be stable, allowing me to feel good for a few more months.

I also had another CAT scan. Once again I was required to drink a glass of chalky, white fluid for the scan to work. The waiting room was full of patients who had glasses and pitchers of the same vile beverage. I remember saying, "This looks like happy hour in Hell," but nobody laughed. I was ready to get back to the United States, where almost everyone talks to strangers. I was also ready to see my friends and claim my things. My plan was to spend a few weeks in Pennsylvania and then go to Florida when the weather turned cold. I didn't expect to outlive my medical leave for the fall semester.

No tumors showed up on the CAT scan. This was a good sign, but it didn't mean that the cancer was gone. More likely it was still there, but too small to detect. The doctor said that the next few months would be critical. If the CA125 stayed low, then I had a good chance of living longer than they had originally thought. If it went up again, I was platinum resistant. "Platinum resistant" meant that the best drugs wouldn't work for me and there was no reason to keep trying. The toll they would take on my body would not have enough of a payoff. The doctor wished me luck and thanked me for being such an agreeable patient. In his experience, Americans were a demanding people, quick to assume that the doctors weren't doing everything they should be doing. He warned me that "In America, they'll tell you we did everything wrong and then they'll try to chemo you to death." I would soon find out that he was right.

Chapter 10: "Someone Told Her She Was Dying": Chemotherapy in America

My first week back in America was joyful. I felt healthy, saw friends, and without many digestive problems, ate foods that I had missed. I appreciated Carlisle, the beautiful little town where I had been happy and active for fifteen years. David and I moved into my house and repacked some of our things for Florida. The plan was to move there during my medical leave and stay in a condo on the beach that my mother had renovated for me—she had been sending me paint swatches and pictures of furniture to choose from while I was in England. If I lived longer than the five-month leave, then I assumed I could go on permanent disability and live off of our savings. I assumed that healthcare was part of disability, either through my college's insurance or Medicare. Since I was operating with a months-not-years mentality, my vague sense of how it would all work didn't worry me. I had done the chemotherapy and now I could only hope it would delay the inevitable end. I would try to enjoy what I could of my last months (or more, if I got lucky). I felt well enough to picture a time when I would see some friends, enjoy the beach, and maybe go on a final cruise to the Caribbean with my family. That was my plan and I thought I was at peace with it.

Then I got the email the British doctor had promised. According to the research I had read, ovarian cancer patients whose CA125 stabilized after initial chemotherapy treatments were more likely to live an average of twenty-one months after diagnosis. But my CA125 score had not stabilized. In fact, the email indicated that it had almost doubled in six weeks. My cancer was platinum-resistant because the most useful drugs for managing this cancer's growth hadn't had a lasting effect.

Maybe I just need a little more chemotherapy, I thought. I knew that was not what the British doctors would have advised, based on their research of the disease. There, they prioritized quality of life over quantity of days lived. Since my quality of life would certainly decrease with more chemotherapy, and my lifespan might only extend a little, I would not have had the option to choose more chemotherapy. But I was back in America now, where doctors were more aggressive. I should at least hear what they had to say, and I needed to have forms filled out by a doctor to establish disability. I called Dr. Sure's office and set up an appointment. That decision, born of fear and necessity, would put me on the American path of trying to beat a cancer that scientific data indicated wasn't beatable.

The first thing Dr. Sure did was correct my diagnosis. He said that I didn't have metastasized ovarian cancer. He had removed my ovaries and they had been cancer-free. I had primary peritoneal cancer. The good news was that it had not yet spread. The bad news was that this rare type of cancer was immediately staged as IIIB. He confirmed that the protocol used in England for metastasized ovarian cancer was the same one that would have been used in the United States for primary peritoneal: under a microscope the cancers were the same. He did say that he would have used different doses and would have varied my treatment plan when my dropping CA125 had reached a plateau after the fourth treatment. He claimed that he would have known I was platinum-resistant from that leveling off.

Dr. Sure was confident that I had many previously unexplored options for treatment. Some women responded to different drugs than Carboplatin® and Taxol®. He wanted me to think of this as a chronic disease rather than a terminal one. Together, we could drive the cancer back so that it wouldn't kill me . . . yet. We could manage the cancer, but not long enough for me to have a normal life span for a woman born in 1960. I decided to inhabit the middle ground and think of the disease as both chronic *and* terminal. The chronic treatment didn't *prevent* the dying, like it might for other diseases; it just *might* delay it.

Of course, there was also a possibility that the treatment would be too aggressive and would kill me. Dr. Sure didn't say that, but I knew from everything I had read about treatment that it was true. When I asked him how he could safeguard against the chemotherapy killing me, he replied, "We give smaller, less toxic doses, more frequently than you had in England. That helps. We take blood tests, CAT scans, and PET scans. We adjust as we go along. Of course, there is no guarantee."

Of course. He said that even though I would probably need chemotherapy *for the rest of my life*, he administered it in such a way that this life could be "full." (*That was an odd expression.* I resisted unpacking the assumptions behind it—*what did he consider a "full" life? What did I?*) He told me that some patients had remissions between chemotherapy regimens that lasted for years, and that some women never got remissions, but they lived for years because their bodies tolerated weekly chemotherapy. He closed his pitch by encouraging me to think of cancer like diabetes. I was skeptical.

This wasn't diabetes. This wasn't consistent with what I had read or what the doctors had said in England. They had warned me that when I returned to America, "they'll try to chemo you to death."

I also remembered that the British doctor cautioned me to expect American doctors to criticize him. That's what Dr. Sure did next: it was a good thing I was home so I wouldn't be another casualty of the socialized healthcare system in England, which in Dr. Sure's opinion, "rationed healthcare." He blamed the English for scaring me and intensifying my distrust of doctors. "The British," he pontificated, "have a stiff-upper-lip approach to cancer. That's why you have such a gloomy outlook." He wanted me to have hope. When I asked him about the statistics (that supported a more grim interpretation of my prognosis), he told me about a woman who had been coming to him for thirteen years. I knew about this persuasive technique from being a communications major—when the statistics don't support your assertion, rely on anecdotes. Anecdotes are true, compelling, and if the audience wants to believe your point, they can project themselves onto the story you tell them.

I didn't think that one woman's experience was enough to discount the thousands of others who had bleaker stories. He probably saw the skepticism on my face because he said, "I know one thing for sure—I can't help you if you don't believe I can. A good attitude is essential." He had hit my Achilles' heel. I hated being told that something was my fault, and I certainly didn't want my own death on my hands. Even though I did not believe that chemotherapy's effectiveness was based on the hopefulness of the patient, I wasn't going to argue with him about it. Then he'd have more evidence that my attitude was the problem. What good would it do to challenge the widely-held myth? I had one decision to make: more chemo his way, or a relatively immediate and untimely demise.

I decided that I would give him a chance to get the CA125 down, while silently disagreeing with his opinions of socialized medicine and the power of positive thinking; I would try chemo American-style. During the months of treatment that followed, he would make derogatory comments to me about Obama, England, liberalism, and healthcare reform. I got in the habit of mentally recalibrating what Dr. Sure said, adding words like "hopefully," "maybe" and "sometimes" to his declarations. *Maybe* I would be able to live with cancer and continue working. *Hopefully*, I could live for years. *Perhaps* they should not have given me such a bleak prognosis in England? I doggedly reminded myself that he was an excellent surgeon who knew my medical history.

Dr. Sure ordered smaller, weekly doses of chemotherapy instead of larger doses every three weeks. It would include Avastin® (not approved for treatment in the U.K.), which would cut off the blood supply to my cancer tumors. First, I would need a brain MRI, an abdominal CAT scan, a blood test, and surgery to insert a PowerPort® in my chest. This device would allow drugs to be administered without accessing a vein. I was familiar with how all of these procedures would feel except for the PowerPort® surgery. Dr. Sure said that there was nothing to it. Everything was scheduled for the following week.

A friend of a friend had been treated by Dr. Sure for ovarian cancer for a few years. I was told that she was doing wonderfully and would be happy to talk to me. I was told a lot of things. She hardly ever missed work. She didn't seem depressed and talking to her wouldn't be depressing. She had lots of confidence in these doctors and their approach to treatment. People couldn't imagine that she had a terminal illness. If I had what she had, then I would be fine, too. I was doubtful, but I did want to know what the PowerPort® operation and recovery was going to be like, so I took her up on the offer to talk.

When David and I went to the woman's office, she was cheerful, energetic, and confident about the treatments. She said everything was working out well. But as she told her story, I couldn't help but think that the evidence didn't support her interpretation. She had surgery to remove a tumor (something I couldn't have), and then chemotherapy that got her a remission (something I didn't get). About a year later, the cancer returned. She had more surgery, and more chemotherapy followed by a second remission. She had been in remission long enough to need a haircut. She felt hopeful that this remission would transform into a cure, but she knew it might not. I doubted that she was done with cancer since I had read that each time it returned it was more likely to return again (and faster). The cancer would build up a resistance to the chemotherapies. I assumed she knew this, but had chosen optimism.

She said that she loved the nurses at our practice, in part because they were lots of fun. She adored our doctors, and I shouldn't be worried (as she had been initially) whether Central Pennsylvania doctors would be as qualified as those in big-city medical centers. In fact, she had gotten a second opinion from a doctor at a major teaching hospital but had been turned off by him. She said he had "tried to scare me with bad statistics. I didn't want to hear those." She loved the patients she met in the chemotherapy room. They were upbeat and laughed a lot. They were great to be around. They brought in homemade baked goods. Sometimes they dressed in ridiculous costumes to amuse each other. From doctors to patients, this sounded like a group I would not fit in with. I wasn't upbeat. I didn't want to pretend to be, or to be disregarded because I wasn't. I didn't want to make new friends in a sorority that I hadn't chosen to pledge. I would wear no funny hats.

Finally, she spoke about the PowerPort®. Getting the PowerPort® "was nothing," she advertised. She was back at work the next day. (I was already on medical leave and hadn't resumed treatment yet.) The shots were a little inconvenient but they were just shots and helped boost her energy. (*What shots?* I wondered. There weren't any shots in England. I hated shots.) She ate what she wanted, drank a glass of wine in the evenings, had to sleep a bit more than usual, but other than that, her lifestyle hadn't changed. I was skeptical. Were the weekly doses that much different from the three-week doses I had gotten in England? Or was her body much stronger than mine? Was she trying to soften the blow for me, or was this just a fairy tale that she wanted to tell herself?

When we left her office, David and I agreed that it was nice of her to share so much of her time and her story with us, but we were both exhausted by it. I felt that she had charged me with the task of becoming more optimistic about American-style chemotherapy, but I suspected that my body (and my mind) wouldn't live up to her positive spin. She was the type of patient that doctors and nurses loved. I was not. I had proven that often enough. It seemed hypocritical and futile to try to exude cheerful enthusiasm when that wasn't how I felt. I didn't know how my cancer would react to the new chemotherapy, but I suspected that getting it would make me sick, sad, frightened, and annoyed. I felt demoralized already.

* * *

The afternoon of my PowerPort® surgery, it took the nurses three tries to find a vein for the IV. I could feel the pressure as the doctor inserted my PowerPort®, but the pain didn't come until later when the drugs wore off. There were days of aching and pulling in my shoulder, but having a PowerPort® was well worth what I went through to get it. It eliminated the stressful and frustrating searches for veins. Since my body had been surgically altered to facilitate treatment, it reinforced what I already knew—I was the property of the medical world.

I got my American chemotherapy in what was once the living room of an old mansion that faced the Susquehanna River. It had a gas fireplace, wood floors, and big, glass windows with tasteful drapes. Sometimes a harpist played for us. The big, comfortable reclining chairs were positioned side-by-side along three of the walls. There were snacks in the corner, sometimes homemade by the patients receiving treatment that day. There were no additional chairs for visitors, individual television sets or curtains for privacy. The nurses were jovial—often boisterous—as they escorted us to and from the examining rooms, accessed our Mediports® or PowerPorts® (two different versions of the central lines) and brought our bags of treatment. Just like the setting itself, they encouraged us to talk to each other—to be a community. These were the unwritten house rules: get comfortable; be cheerful; and make friends.

It was so different from England. I missed the quiet, the privacy, and the permission to acknowledge the sadness and seriousness of the experience. Although I had primary peritoneal cancer and most of the women there had advanced stages of ovarian cancer, there was not much difference between our prognoses. Yet I never feel like I fit in. I was not sure when or how I would die from this (would it travel to my kidneys or my lungs?), but I knew that it was in the cards and beyond my control. I didn't want to pretend it wasn't. And yet, I felt that my unwillingness to pretend disturbed everyone else's good mood. It distracted them from the illusion that there was nothing wrong here. But I couldn't forget.

Even though they had been in treatment for years and their diseases had metastasized, the other women would talk about what they would do when they were cancer-free. I grew weary of hearing patients attribute their dropping CA125 and their robust blood cells to what they were eating, their good attitudes, or how God-fearing they were. If someone (usually new and not-yet-socialized to the ways of the Mansion) said something about how hard chemotherapy was or how sad she was, the other women would say things like, "We should thank God for these doctors," "You've got to be patient; you'll get through this," or "Life is hard; this is no better or worse than what other people face." I didn't share these opinions, but I kept my mouth shut. I did once disagree with a woman who said that she hated it when people complained about their illnesses. I thought that when you were this sick, I said, you were entitled to complain all you wanted.

I did enjoy talking to one other patient who I had known years earlier, when she worked at Dickinson. We didn't have the same approach toward the disease—she believed that doctors knew best, but seemed to enjoy hearing my frank observations. She was an intelligent woman, but had decided against researching ovarian cancer. "I don't want to know what I don't want to know," she told me one day. The last time I saw her at the Mansion, she was eager to try another type of chemotherapy and to get her abdomen drained of fluid emitted from her tumor; but she had to wait until the blood clot that had formed in her foot went away. She was less upbeat than usual, but still probably more optimistic than I was normally. It was the lack of chemotherapy that frustrated her. She died a few months later.

I wanted to talk about death: how long it would take and what it would feel like. The published studies said the median survival for what I have is two years. I didn't hear that from my doctors at the Mansion; I had to sneak out of their house first, and go to the Internet, like a teenage boy looking for pornography. The doctor in England said that half the women with my cancer fade away instead of dying in pain. What would "fading" feel like? I wanted to know more about that, but it seemed as though there was no need to talk about death when they could talk about the "thirteen-year woman."

The thirteen-year woman was legendary. She had been in treatment since before the practice moved to the Mansion. Referring to her seemed to energize the patients. Some were reverent in the way they talked about her, making her seem mythical. Others talked about her like she was a role model that they were trying hard to emulate. Once again I felt like an outsider, because I thought of her as a Powerball lottery winner. I was happy for her, but had no illusions that I was likely to follow in her footsteps. Certainly you can't win if you don't enter, but most people will lose the lottery, even if they exhaust their bank accounts trying. Eventually, I met the thirteen-year woman. She was small, old, and wearing a baseball cap over her bald head. Standing in line to be weighed, she announced with pride that she was having her 170th chemo treatment that day. Instead of feeling inspired, I wished that I were in England again, with a curtain of privacy that would give me permission to cry.

I hoped that when I was officially handed over to hospice care, that I would be allowed to talk about death and ways to find peace with it. But while I was in the Mansion, talking about death would constitute evidence that I didn't want a remission badly enough. Because our culture separates living and dying, it seems to deny that they are connected. One day I overheard one of the nurses hang up the phone and impatiently demand, "Why is she still calling us? She's in hospice care now." Apparently this nameless patient didn't understand her place. She was not supposed to reach out to the place where she spent so much time fighting for life in exactly the way she had been instructed. She was supposed to stay within the system that does not characterize dying as a failure (for the patient and the healthcare providers).

Like the woman on the phone, I, too, was a problem. The nurses did not like my winces when they gave me the shots intended to boost my white and red blood cells. Apparently, it was not polite to remind them that some parts of treatment were painful. Other patients continued to talk and joke through their shots, or closed their eyes and gritted their teeth silently. But my greatest transgression was that I never forgot what I had learned in England—that the cancer was terminal. That set me apart from everyone. When I said, "That's a pretty good break," to a patient who had returned from a six-month remission, one of the nurses gave me a dirty look and told the woman,

"Don't mind her. Someone told her she was going to die."

* * *

After receiving chemotherapy at the Mansion, I would go home to a small life that would get smaller the longer I was in treatment. I couldn't leave the house, and I felt too sick to entertain guests, even though my friends said that they just wanted to see me. There was nothing "just" about that. Being able to sit upright somewhere besides the toilet was a prerequisite for socializing. It was stressful to predict when I might be well enough to enjoy seeing them and not depress them. Imposing a social quarantine was much easier. Besides, I always had David to distract me when I felt up to it.

David quickly grew to know what he could do to help me. He got better at accepting that sometimes he could do nothing, and I needed to be left alone. His patience for hearing me remark upon, complain about, and worry over the same side effects seemed endless. Fortunately, like many men, he found digestive body functions interesting and amusing. So we had something to talk about even during my worst side effects. But often, I would be too weary to talk or even to be observed as I relived the same agonizing nightmare. A life of constant chemotherapy was simultaneously horrible and boring.

Most of my chemo world consisted of me, my bed, my bathtub, and my toilet. On a good day, confinement in my bed would be made more bearable with mindless television, computer games, and my laptop computer. Time in the bathtub could be accompanied by light reading, and time on the toilet could include a game of Yahtzee® (on the battery-operated, hand-held game—

the best ten dollars I ever spent), or looking at a crappy magazine (no pun intended).

I missed being able to eat out. It was something I had done often in my life. Even when my first husband and I were just starting out—he, unemployed, and me, on a graduate school assistantship—we would go out for pizza or nachos a few times a week. When we moved to Gaithersburg, Maryland, the increased cost of living, our fiscal conservatism, and our modest salaries left us in no position to go to the extravagant restaurants that the D.C. area had to offer. But each year the *Washingtonian* magazine published an edition in which they listed the "Best Cheap Eats" in the metro area. This became my eating-out bible. Each month, I tried at least one new restaurant on the list. I kept records of where I went and rated the experiences. My first husband was game for the American and Italian places, but for anything more exotic, I needed to find a friend to accompany me. (I eventually became comfortable trying the noodle-bar-type restaurants alone.) It would be wrong to say that our palates broke up our marriage, but my desire to experience new things and Scott's aversion to anything different helped us drift apart. After our divorce, I became comfortable eating alone in any type of restaurant.

During my pre-cancer years, to counter-balance my penchant for eating out and keep my weight down, I'd have a no-dessert month. It was usually in March, after my birthday and Valentine's Day had extended holiday-season excess and made sweets seem like the mandatory end of a meal. The month was always hardest in the beginning, but I was disciplined. Friends had lots of cheating suggestions: "Eat cookies first and they won't technically be dessert"; or "Go crazy today and just add a day in April to make up for it." But I knew that I needed to follow the letter and spirit of my own rule to recalibrate my eating habits. I'd usually lose about five pounds, and was more thoughtful about what I ate until Christmas celebrations began.

Even as my dietary restrictions grew over the years, going to restaurants remained a priority. I was simply more careful. This was also true during periods of chemotherapy. As soon as the chemo side effects eased enough for me to leave my house, the first stop was a local diner where I would have French toast and bacon. It was not food that I would have eaten often before chemotherapy, but it was high in calories (which I desperately needed) and easier to digest than most things. This was often my only restaurant experience. It would be midday Sunday, which was late enough in the week that I could stomach it, but too early for the distress of digestion to interfere with teaching.

During my sickest chemo days, I would watch a lot of mindless television. I had to take too many inconvenient bathroom breaks to follow much of a story line. The *Food Network* was ideal, with its continuous loop of how-to cooking shows, competitions, and restaurant advice. So what if I missed seeing Rachael Ray chopping the green beans, or telling us again to use extra-virgin olive oil? My favorite show was *Diners, Drive-ins and Dives,* on which a cheerful, chubby guy with funky hair and a big grin goes around the country in a red convertible eating comfort food. His infectious enthusiasm for food and life, and his ease with strangers reminded me of my husband. During my chemo weeks, I watched this stranger eat more food than I was able to eat. It made me happy to see the juicy hamburger grease run down his arm and hear him exclaim, "Wow! That's good!" over and over again. It didn't make me feel sorry for myself because I couldn't eat. In fact, I was like everyone else in the television audience—none of us could smell or taste the food. Some of the appeal of the show was probably nostalgia for a life in which I went out to eat, and could finish off that huge, combination Mexican platter. But some of it was probably hope; in spite of my realism, I would write down names of restaurants that I longed to visit. When I turned off the television, I had to tune into chemotherapy's twenty-four-hour show, featuring: side effects.

Exhaustion is always a consequence of chemotherapy, but in the United States, it became problematic in new ways. In England, they accepted the fact that drugs killing off all the fast-growing cells in your body would fatigue you. They did not expect people to keep working during treatment. If you were sick, you could stay home—away from germs that would make you sicker. In the United States, you were expected to work. Chemotherapy was not an excuse to press pause on a productive life. Moreover, unless you were sixty-five or older, you *needed* to work to pay for the health insurance that paid for the chemotherapy. So I knew that if I lived long enough I would have to go back to work.

But it was hard to imagine feeling or remaining well enough to work. Chemotherapy depletes white blood cells, which are responsible for fighting infection. To counteract this dip, weekly chemotherapy was followed by two to three shots to rebuild my white-blood-cell count. If it was chemo every three weeks, I would get one Neulasta® shot. When my counts were lowest, I would catch any and all germs that I can into contact with. In the winter, just getting my shots led to catching viruses, because there was usually someone sick at the Mansion. Although these were mostly colds (coughing, sneezing, body-ache-types), some of my worst vomiting wasn't a direct side effect of the chemo. It was from catching a bug I was too weak to fight. I didn't catch flu in England, but I got sick a lot during the chemo in the United States.

As much as Dr. Sure believed in the weekly schedule, it did not work well for me. There were no shots, foods, or vitamins that replenished platelets. Although some people claimed that cat's claw (an herbal remedy used to treat arthritis, chronic fatigue syndrome, digestive disorders, and cancer) helped, it didn't help me. When my platelets stayed low, I would not be eligible for the next week's chemotherapy. This happened often. Only once was I able to get three weekly chemotherapies in a row. By my second week of treatment, I was already off of the schedule. My platelets took longer than most patients' to come back. As one nurse put it, I had a "longer nadir." While I waited, my blood wouldn't clot very well, and I'd get nose bleeds, bleeding gums, and bruises. Thankfully, my platelets always bounced back in time to keep me from having to get blood transfusions.

Pains in my legs, head, back, and chest bone were common. Some of these were caused by the shots. They stimulated white blood cell production in bone marrow, which caused deep bone aches in large bones such as the sternum, pelvis, and skull. The nurse's warning gave me an accurate sense of the severity of these bone aches. "Some patients go to the emergency room because they think they're having a heart attack," she explained. "But it's only the shot, so don't be alarmed." (Apparently, there's no need to be alarmed if you feel like you're dying . . . so long as you're not.)

I was not alarmed, just immobilized. Headaches sometimes robbed me of entire days. The longest, searing headache I had on chemotherapy was two and a half days long. At its worst, the leg pain could make me sob and shake, but usually it just kept me from walking and led to warm baths. Tylenol® with Codeine No. 3 was prescribed to help with this problem, but it came with its own side effects (constipation and bloating).

Mouth sores, nausea, vomiting, acid reflux, diarrhea, constipation, bloating, and abdominal pain were all on the lists of side effects for chemotherapy. They resulted from the gastrointestinal tract's fast-growing cells being killed off. Most patients I knew experienced some of these, but not all. It seemed that whatever part of your digestive tract was already the weakest would give you the most problems. That's why some patients complained most of vomiting, and others of reflux. My weakest organ was my intestines. I had no problems thinking about or smelling food, unlike many patients who couldn't stand the thought of food in their mouths, or became nauseous just smelling it. I just had a hard time digesting it. Even without the chemotherapy, the intestinal resection and the peritonitis in my abdomen limited my ability to digest many foods. Add poison and eating became a crapshoot (pun intended this time). I'd be fine for the first thirty or forty-five minutes after eating, and then things would get ugly.

I became an expert on my own bowel movements. I documented what I ate, when I ate it, what drugs I took, when I took them, when I went to the bathroom, and what the experience was like. I could describe color, consistency, smell, duration, urgency, extensiveness, density . . . simply because I hoped someone could use this information to advise me. I talked to two oncologists, one surgeon, a gastrointestinal specialist, countless nurses, and a nutritionist. No one was interested in hearing details. They would occasionally test me for a *C. diff* infection that results from the good gut flora being killed off, but I never had it. The chemo doctors dismissed my plight as a side effect, if an uncommon one, of chemo. Instead of focusing on my side effects, I should be glad that I wasn't constipated. But I had the bloating and cramping that comes with constipation, so I wasn't particularly thankful.

"Eat intuitively," advised the nutritionist. "Ask your body what it wants and then eat that, no matter what other people might say about it. If it tells you to have cake every meal, then do that." The gastrointestinal doctor's advice conflicted with the nutritionist's. Instead of "asking your body what it wants," he encouraged me *not* to over think what I ate.

"You will drive yourself crazy," he cautioned. His parting words were, "Sometimes a food will digest, and sometimes it won't. Shit happens." (Yes, those were his exact words.) Sometimes he would prescribe a drug that would cut down on my bad gut flora, and the bloating would improve. But like most doctors, he seemed to expect me to play the stoic and handle the discomfort on my own.

The digestive problems were relentless. I had more in common with the radiation patients than most of the chemo women. For me, going to the bathroom (meant here as a euphemism . . . you know I wasn't brushing my teeth) became a full-time job. To say that I had diarrhea is to call a hurricane a rain shower. I would expel frequently, urgently, and violently. I once found an entire cube of watermelon in the toilet bowl an hour after I had swallowed it. I could go twenty times in one day, and I routinely went three or four weeks without having a single formed stool. My record was two months. Often I had only a minute or two of warning. Of course my inability to digest food further exhausted me, because I wasn't getting nutrients from what I ate. When I could get away from the toilet, I was too tired to do anything. I felt like a prisoner, sentenced—in a body that was deteriorating—to a tiny room with a lot of running water.

The bathtub became my favorite running water in this prison. I would soak my raw bottom, my aching legs and back, and my bloated abdomen. Bloating is another one of those things that sounds routine and tolerable—not worth putting on chemo's hit parade. But again, the frequency and the degree of the problem is what challenged this interpretation. Like most women, I have a closet full of clothes of many sizes—fat jeans and skinny jeans, for example. Since I lost weight during chemo, I was thinner than the smallest sizes in my closet. This allowed me to document the degree of bloating. About an hour after eating, the bloating would start; within fifteen minutes I would bloat more than two sizes. I would go from having lots of spare room in my size twelves to being uncomfortable buttoning sixteens. My large abdomen was as hard as a basketball. The only thing that would relieve some of the pressure would be to immerse myself in the bathtub and wait. It would typically take about eight to twelve hours for this to end—in violent, but welcome, diarrhea. The whole time I would be listening for bowel sounds and feeling for grumbles that would reassure me that I wasn't having another intestinal blockage.

I spent so much time in the bathtub during chemotherapy weeks that I bought artwork for my tub area, so I could look at something peaceful when I was in too much agony to read. While I was in the bathtub my husband felt free to play his Xbox Live®. It kept him busy and gave him a virtual social life when my condition prohibited a real one. I think it also allowed him to feel effective. There was nothing he could do about my cancer, but he could reach new levels of game achievements. Sometimes he would get loud enough so that I could hear him shouting orders to the other players. Just as frequently, I would hear him lecturing them, "No need for that language," or "I can't play with just you; we need to include Billy." Other times his directions were about the game— "Cover me," he'd yell (when he played the war games like *Call of*

Duty®), and, "Smoker's got me," (when he was trying to survive zombie attacks on *Left for Dead*®). For most of these games, a character could be killed and then reanimate moments later. If they got shot or attacked, but not killed, they could use health packs to regain their full strength. A player could only carry so many health packs, so a good, cooperative team would share theirs with each other. One night, when I was soaking in my tub—bald, bloated, and exhausted—I heard David yell to his team, "Does anyone need to be healed?"

"I do," I whispered to the pink tile that encased my bathtub.

* * *

I had developed a routine to manage my digestive nightmare, but I was never able to persuade my doctors to manage my blood pressure fluctuations. Every week my blood pressure was higher. The nurse repeatedly suggested that I manage my blood pressure through my primary-care physician. I was reluctant. By this time in my medical adventure, my primary care physicians' office was a filing cabinet for copies of all my blood tests and scans. None of the doctors there knew me. I had graduated to specialists.

I did have a cardiologist, Dr. Young, from when I returned to town after the retinal-vein occlusion. He had given me extensive blood tests, an echocardiogram, and maintained my Lisinopril prescription. He admitted to not knowing anything about chemotherapies, but resisted changing my blood pressure prescriptions because the high blood pressure was due to the chemo and not my heart. He was afraid that the chemo and blood pressure drugs would pool, causing damage. It didn't make a lot of sense to me, but he was steadfast.

Again I was told at chemotherapy, this time by both the nurse and Dr. Kind, that I should see a doctor about my increasing blood pressure. To the best of my ability, I explained Dr. Young's concerns about pooling. Dr. Kind disagreed with Dr. Young's assessment. He hadn't been impressed with cardiologists. Even if the high blood pressure was artificially high because of the drugs, it was dangerous. I should go back and explain this. I told Dr. Kind that he would need to do the explaining, because I had no credibility with Dr. Young. I had already tried and failed to get him to do something. Dr. Kind promised to call the cardiologist. But he never did.

My first chemotherapy regimen in America started on August 29th, 2007. I was on medical leave then, so I didn't teach. I was taking Cisplatin, Gemzar®, and Avastin®, trying to do a three-weeks-on, one-week-off schedule. The second week, my platelets were too low to stay on the schedule, and the nurse announced loudly that my platelets "aren't good enough" for treatment. I had failed another test. I felt like a loser. True, I couldn't study for these blood tests, but that didn't make me feel better. I needed chemo, and I couldn't get it because my body lacked the ability to do what most of the women at the Mansion seemed able to do. This drug combination allowed me to keep my hair, but it completely exhausted me, hurt my digestion, and made me weepy from the steroids. It also increased my blood pressure. After ten treatments of Cisplatin, seven of Gemzar®, and seven of Avastin®, my blood wasn't able to rebound enough for additional treatment. On December 4th, 2007, the doctors discontinued this regime.

On January 2nd, 2008, Dr. Kind brought out the big guns—Carboplatin and Taxol®. These were the drugs that had brought down my CA125 in England. Dr. Kind hoped that the weekly schedule and the addition of Avastin® would make these drugs work even better than they had on the three-week dose used in England. I lost my hair, had worse digestion, continued to have high blood pressure, and anemia. I was so weak that I developed anticipatory anxiety about all the germs I knew I would catch from my students that semester.

As the end of my medical leave approached, I realized that going back to work would literally mean that I was working to live. I needed health insurance to pay for treatment. David was still looking for a job after giving up his previous position to follow me to England. Medicare wouldn't take me until I'd been on disability for two years. COBRA was expensive and would only last eighteen months. No private insurance would accept me with all of my pre-existing conditions. It wouldn't have been affordable if they had. I prepared for the spring semester by organizing my eating and getting sick time around windows of opportunity to work. I didn't do this to prove anything to anyone. I didn't do it because my work brought me great joy. (It had when I was healthy, but I wasn't healthy anymore.) I didn't do it so I could feel normal (because nothing about chemotherapy felt normal), or to persuade myself that I *could* get better. I needed to work to receive chemo. After my medical leave was up, I needed to get back into the classroom.

It wasn't easy working again, but fortunately I could do all the preparation and grading at home. I still needed to be in the classroom for six hours a week. I'd get a blood test Monday, and teach Monday afternoon. Thankfully, the Monday class was seminar-style, so it wasn't unusual for me to teach the class from a seated position at the head of the table. Monday night, I'd have a moderate-sized, mild-tasting dinner, followed by chemo on Tuesday. Chemo took most of the day and I'd sleep the rest of the time. On Wednesday, I'd sleep late and then teach in the afternoon, seated and a bit hyper from the steroids. The steroids delayed the worst side effects until Wednesday night. Thursday and Friday were bed and bathroom days with minimal food. I also dragged myself to the doctor's office for shots. Saturday I could make it to the living room and eat a bit more. Sunday I would enjoy French toast and bacon at the local diner. I'd do it all again the following week.

By February 19th, five treatments of Carboplatin/Taxol®/Avastin® and too many coughing students had left me so weak that I couldn't sit on the examining table to wait for Dr. Kind. I remember laying there and hearing him say that, although all of my blood counts were low, none of them were so bad that I couldn't have more chemotherapy that day. He was concerned about my blood pressure, advising, "You don't want to maintain a blood pressure that high or you'll pop."

"Do you mean I will suffer a massive stroke?" I asked. There was no need for euphemisms when I felt this badly.

"Umm . . . yes," he replied a bit sheepishly. I asked him what the cardiologist had said about changing my medication. He looked confused. Careful not to let my frustration creep into my voice, I gently prompted,

"Remember, you were going to call him?" I was asking a question I already knew the answer to.

"Was I? When was that?" he asked.

"Before you went on vacation to San Diego," I recalled. He corrected me,

"That wasn't a vacation. That was a conference. I don't actually remember calling him. I don't think I did."

By this time, the CA125 was still going down, but only by a small amount and not every time we measured it. I still wasn't close to a normal CA125, but it felt like taking the drugs was causing me to lose myself. I could picture myself treading water in the middle of the ocean, and there wasn't a rescue ship on the horizon. If the ship wasn't coming, how long should I continue trying to stay afloat? It didn't make sense to tread water if the only thing left in life was trying not to drown.

Dr. Kind looked at me and said, "I can see from the look in your eyes that you need a break. So let's not give you any more chemo. We'll take a break for three months."

"What will happen to the cancer?" I queried, hopefully.

"The cancer will do what the cancer will do," he said. *If this kills me,* I thought, *it will be my fault because he was going to chemo me, but my eyes said "no."* David saw it differently.

"He just needed to come up with a reason for why he was changing his recommendation," he assessed. "He should have been looking at you the whole time. You are in no shape for more chemo." I was both worried and relieved. I decided that if this break was my last hurrah, then hoorah! I was going to try to enjoy it.

* * *

During the first few weeks of this break, I was still too weak from the damage chemotherapy had done to notice much of a difference. I continued to use all my energy to be effective in the classroom. But before long, I felt like myself again. I had energy. I could eat and digest food. I started accepting invitations to social and professional engagements. Everyone seemed happy to see that I was back, interpreting my return as a sign that I was beating cancer. I was determined to correct this misperception, even though I felt like a disappointment to everyone.

I constantly reminded myself that this was a hiatus from feeling ill, not a recovery. I hoped that if I kept this in mind, my return to chemotherapy (or the progression of the cancer) wouldn't be as disappointing or tragic. At the same time, I vowed not to squander my good health. It wasn't enough to just return to a pre-illness work day and social life in Carlisle. I wanted to go places and do things.

First, I went to Las Vegas with my friend Lydia. We stayed at the Venetian, spent hours sunning by the pool and sitting in hot tubs. We ate at wonderful restaurants and saw an expensive show with Beatles music and acrobats. We drank mojitos. Cancer didn't ruin our vacation, but it didn't disappear there either. If it had, we probably wouldn't have talked about what we thought happens after you die while we watched the water show in front of the Bellagio one night. She didn't believe in heaven. I thought that was sad, but I wasn't sure if I disagreed with her. Many of my smartest friends believe that when your heart stops beating you no longer exist—anywhere, in any form. I don't want to hear the rational explanations for why they believe this, because I do not want to be convinced. I prefer to believe in an afterlife. I love hearing my husband talk about it.

David is completely convinced that death is not the end. He believes that we are part of spiritual families, who stay together throughout lifetimes. This lifetime he was my husband. In our next, he might be my daughter. Between lifetimes, souls can choose to stay in heaven to rest, reflect on their lessons, or help other souls. He believes that learning and perfecting ourselves is what living is for, and that we choose before we're born what challenge we'll face. Some are harder than others. There's no guarantee that we'll learn in one lifetime what we need to. Sometimes we have to repeat ourselves. He says that my soul has chosen a hard lesson for this lifetime and that's why my health problems and experiences with healers have been so relentless and challenging. "Of course it doesn't seem fair," he says. "During one life span, it's not. But

255

when you consider the entire spiritual journey, it is. We all have hard lessons that our souls will get to eventually." It is comforting to think I can have (or have had) lives where my body worked well.

My brother is sure that we get only one life and when it ends, we go to heaven or hell. Heaven is so wonderful that issues of fairness on earth are irrelevant once we get there. He believes that it is a place where our souls are content because we are close to God. A friend who is a priest says that heaven is not just a place for souls. In heaven we will have our own perfected bodies. He will have hair; I will have strong knees. Between the time that I was a child who thought of heaven as a place where angels sat on clouds, and when I was an adolescent targeted for conversion by born-again Christian friends, I developed my own theory of heaven and hell. If you were (mostly) good, you got to relive all the good times in your life. If you were (mostly) bad, then you relived the bad times. Now, I'm not sure what to believe, so I just hope.

David and I went to Disney World during this chemotherapy break. Since I had grown up in Orlando, I had been going to Disney World since it opened in 1971. I remember my parents taking me out of sixth grade on the afternoon that it opened. We had reservations at the Contemporary Hotel for that evening. The school principal refused to count the trip as an excused absence, so we were delayed while I took a geography test. I remember my mother saying that that would be the last time that she ever told the truth to get one of her children out of school. From then on she'd claim we had a dentist appointment. The next

256

day we went to the Magic Kingdom and I was swept away by its magic. We would return often.

Disney World was where I celebrated my adolescent birthdays. It is where my family took long weekend vacations. It was one of the first places where I felt free and independent, walking around by myself because my parents were convinced that the Magic Kingdom® was safe. I remember seeing George McGovern campaign on Main Street, USA. I went to Disney World on the first Valentine's Day I had a boyfriend. We listened to Blood, Sweat, and Tears sing "You've Made Me So Very Happy," and made it our song. Disney World was where Scott and I spent a romantic weekend before I moved to Tallahassee. We ate prime rib in Cinderella's castle, and stayed at the Polynesian Hotel as "Mr. and Mrs." even though we weren't. The fake authenticity of Epcot's® World Showcase introduced me to an idealized England, France, and Italy long before I visited those countries. Since this chemotherapy break could have been my last healthy time, I thought it was important to spend some of it at Disney World.

We spent the whole week there. We stayed at the Wilderness Lodge, went to all of the parks, and ate at some of the best restaurants. I drank Long Island Iced Teas by the pool one day while David went fishing. It was glorious. He had only been to the Magic Kingdom® and I had done everything but the Animal Kingdom®. I liked the combination of familiarity and newness, and being able to guide him through the experience and see it through his (new) eyes.

Although I am embarrassed to admit it, the trip made me as happy as any of the European vacations had. I am reminded of that every time one of the many photographs of our trip flashes on my computer screen saver: David head-butting Winnie the Pooh; me, in a white sundress, sitting at a fountain in the Floridian Hotel's gardens; us, with sunburned noses and oversized t-shirts, in front of Epcot's golf-ball structure. You could not tell that the smiling woman with very short hair in the pictures had the health equivalent of a time bomb ticking in her abdomen, with no idea of how long it would be before it detonated.

Chapter 11: The Power of Positive Thinking . . . to Piss Me Off: Reflections on Attitude Control[4]

People ask me what it is like to have terminal cancer. I tell them it's awful in ways that I expected *and* in ways that I hadn't anticipated. I expected it to be deeply sad and sometimes overwhelming to know that I will die soon, that I will not have a future, and that I will miss out on enjoying the decades that an actuarial table tells me that I should have ahead. I expected it to be scary: to have sleepless nights wondering what death will feel like, what happens next, and exactly when it will happen. I expected to be frustrated and pained by the physical decline that I would undergo. I expected to be disgusted and sometimes embarrassed by what my body would be transformed into by the disease and the treatments. These are responses that people can understand. People are less likely to comprehend my bitter criticism of the American medical system.

---

[4] Editor's Note: I used a hybrid of American Political Science Association (APSA) Style (the style Larson preferred) and the Chicago Manual of Style (CMS) to cite sources in the References list. I relied predominantly upon 7th edition of *The Political Science Student Writer's Manual* for this task. When I felt that APSA did not offer the reader all of the information that Larson provided about a source, I consulted the CMS to develop citations as necessary. In-text citations, however, follow the author-date method—a method accepted by both APSA and CMS.

People who have had limited, indirect, or positive experiences in the healthcare system feel that my anger, fear, and frustration are overblown. They believe a series of myths about the American medical system, beginning with the conviction that the United States has the greatest medical system in the world. You are in good hands as long as you have access to medical technology, American-trained doctors, and drugs. Scans, robots, and lasers help doctors know all kinds of things they didn't know ten years ago. American doctors are sympathetic and attentive. Even if they cannot cure you, they are doing the best they can. Drugs prevent, cure, and soothe. People trust the system that they don't have to spend much time in (or that they are in, but not scrutinizing). My experiences have eradicated that trust, and I cannot help but dwell upon the ways the medical system, which is supposed to help me, has relentlessly hurt me.

Not only are my attitudes about healthcare at odds with most people's, but my attitude about my attitudes seem to be as well. The language surrounding how we talk to and about cancer patients, specifically our calls for them to "stay positive", seeks to comfort and uplift people. Healthy people believe that encouraging a sick person to stay positive is the same as giving the sick person a measure of control over an ultimately uncontrollable situation. If I stay positive, everything will improve—I'll be happier while having cancer, and if I *believe* that I will get better, my body may miraculously heal. These recommendations make me feel blamed. If I refuse, falter, or ultimately fail to stay positive, am I complicit in my own demise?

Because I have incurable cancer, I see the role models for cancer patients with positive attitudes everywhere, and because I am a political scientist, I can't help but analyze what these prototypes imply and wonder where they come from. Role models for a positive attitude towards illness are on television, on the Internet, in books, at the Mansion, and at my college. People point these cancer patients out to me as if I don't see them on my own; see how *she's* handling it? Even this seemingly innocuous question implies that my approach to cancer is inadequate.

For example, when a teacher says, "I like how Marie's hands are folded," she is inviting the rest of the class to see the error of their own unfolded hands and follow Marie's obedient lead. Anyone who fails to fold his or her hands is surely a vehicle of his or her own destruction. "She's cheerful," they say about positive cancer patients, and "productive," they add, "working every day!" This suggests that all cancer patients are capable of keeping normal routines. "She's not letting cancer define her" is my least favorite compliment. The verb "to let" suggests that cancer patients can *choose* whether or not they are utterly overwhelmed by their cancer ordeal. It implies that the gradual, hurtful, and occasionally humiliating degeneration that cancer incites is dependent upon the permission of the patient—thus implicating the patient in his or her own decline. The word "define" strikes at the very core of individual identity, signifying that dying from cancer is a resignation of one's very self.

"I'm not sick. I just happen to have cancer," I hear women at the Mansion say.

"Don't pity me; I just have cancer," says another. They are brave. They are strong. They are going to make it. These are the upbeat, model patients I'm supposed to emulate. I don't even try. And so, I feel blamed for having cancer. I feel blamed for how I think about cancer, how I talk about cancer, how I haven't beaten it, how bad my side effects are, and how I've allowed my side effects to limit my activities.

My frankness about the nightmare of cancer and my unwillingness to believe in the possibility that I could recover makes healthy people uncomfortable. Healthy people want sick people to be well. They don't want to believe that this could be happening and that there are no cures. They don't want to think that going to a doctor will not be a solution. They can't bear to think of themselves in our shoes, so they encourage us to dress up our realities with optimism about our outcomes. This masking is recursively referred to as "the power of positive thinking." My unwillingness to think positively makes me feel like a loser in a society that only believes in winners. I feel like a victim, but people don't want me to use that word. When people compliment my bravery, I feel like a fraud. I'm scared and I would love to run away from this nightmare. I feel frustrated because I am a can-do person who can't do anything about the biggest problem I have ever had.

The positive-thinking crowd cites, but never produces, the research that shows that people with positive attitudes are more likely to get well. I've looked at some of the research, including the studies that refute it. Positive thinking looks, to me, remarkably like wishful thinking. The research isn't strong, and there's just as much work that fails to find a relationship between attitude and cancer survival. One of the more helpful things a friend has said during my illness was, "I read that research when my sister was dying of breast cancer. There's no clear evidence that positive thinking makes a difference." Then she said, "Don't let them make you feel responsible for having cancer."

Positive-thinking rhetoric insinuates that the victim has a degree of control over an incurable disease. But I don't have control. I am the victim and neither optimism nor pessimism can change my outcomes. My approach to having cancer may not be sanctioned by the mainstream cancer community, but it works for me. I feel like a realist who is in a bad situation. I want to be both hopeful and truthful. I don't want to ruin the moments when I feel well by being sad about my illness or anticipating the resurgence of the pain. But I can't say that I'm fine when I feel like shit. I want to try to extend my life with whatever drugs or operations are most likely to help, but I also want to acknowledge when they are ineffective and stop using or having them. I don't want to pretend that my life hasn't changed and try gallantly to do what I did, like I did it before—determined, but inevitably failing. I want to accept that this is how things are now, and be myself, my authentic self—not defined by what I do or don't do, but who I am—in whatever constraints my illness presents.

If I can only watch television, I will try not to do it like a mindless couch potato. I will try to do it *actively*, and with all the critical-analysis techniques that I brought to my profession. If I'm going to have a conversation, I'll make it an honest one. I want the

essence of Ill Stephanie to be as close as I can get her to Well
Stephanie. Not by making her try to do the things she used to do
(with all the stress and incompetence that a diminished body brings
to an active lifestyle—Look at me! I'm at work . . . throwing up!),
but by allowing her to be *authentic*. What she feels, she's allowed to
feel. What she wants to say, she can say. Let her do what she needs
to do. Don't judge her by old standards.

   A friend of mine calls me "resilient," and I like the sound
of that. Not only does it ring true to me, it avoids the labels of
optimism and pessimism. I consider it a compliment since
resilience isn't easy. It was hard to come back from each romantic
break-up, the restrictions my injured knee imposed, my limited
eyesight, and the loss of reproductive capacity. I had to rebuild my
world, accept it, and grow to love it in spite of what it lacked. I
tried to think about what was still possible as being greater than
what was impossible. That approach no longer works very well
because the limitations are so great. I can no longer live the
energetic, active, and full life I had before this cancer (and its
treatments) demolished my intestines. Trying to hold on to that
life, or fantasizing that I'll return to it, makes the life I have now
even harder. This life is as real as the one I had before, even
though it is admittedly less happy, less free, and more troubling to
society. I need to embrace it. The call for positive thinking as a
solution minimizes the validity of my approach and the severity of
what I'm going through. It denies my reality and characterizes the
important and difficult adjustment that I am trying to do as giving
up or letting the cancer define me. I am not giving up. I am not

letting the cancer define me. But the American cancer culture doesn't seem to have language to describe people like me.

* * *

I know that the cancer culture isn't explicitly telling me that I am a failure, but its language is, and the assumptions embedded within that language are. Culturally-approved models for what to say to sick people can be found in greeting cards. They are supposed to help people who desire to communicate concern, but don't know how. The Hallmark® store has lots of get-well cards that make me cringe because they are full of denial.

Many of them try for a laugh, and often it is at the patient's expense, demeaning the severity of the illness and medical treatments. The jokes that I find the most disturbing are the ones that include healthcare professionals. These are sober reminders of the power of medical professionals and the vulnerability of patients. For example, one card's front says, "Thanks to modern medicine, you're getting better," and inside, "And thanks to that weirdo in radiology, pictures of your colon are now circulating on the Internet. Hope you recover quickly!" (Hallmark, n.d., C-739-6).[5] There's one that shows a clipboard that reads, "Your

---

[5] Editor's Note:

In some cases, Larson's notes on cited sources did not provide enough information to locate and verify those sources. In other cases, sources she analyzed are no longer available or accessible. As the editor, I was charged with retaining as much of Larson's voice as possible; thus, I refrained from removing or reworking analysis of sources that I could not trace. Sources located are cited in full. Untraced sources are marked as such in footnotes that contain the information Larson provided.

Operation Check List: Room: Covered; Operation: Covered; Meals: Covered; Bedpan: Covered." The inside of the card reads "Your butt, not covered. Hope you recover soon." The drawing is of a frowning dog with an IV stand and his bottom showing (Hallmark, n.d., C-738-9). Another says on the front, "Four out of five doctors want you to get well immediately!" Inside it continues, "That fifth one thinks you might still have a couple bucks somewhere" (Hallmark, n.d., ZZF-328-1). That one actually makes me smile because it mocks doctors. A number of cards make jokes about getting shots. The cards poke fun at humiliation, a lack of privacy, financial ruin, and pain. Why aren't I laughing?

Many get-well cards insist that the recipient of the card get well quickly. These cards assume that illnesses are a temporary and undesirable condition that people have the power to escape. "There's no speed limit on the road to recovery!" one card urges, continuing, "Travel as fast as you can!" (Hallmark, n.d., C-253-0). A monkey in a chair has this message: "Just sittin' around waitin' for you to get better! Hurry up, cause my butt's gettin' sore!" (Hallmark, n.d., C-352-4). Maxine (the cranky, old lady on many

---

I was only able to locate one (of fourteen) of the Hallmark cards Larson analyzes in this section. If she had them in her personal possession, her husband, David, was unable to locate them. It is possible that Larson never owned the greeting cards and that she simply visited the local drug store and took notes without purchasing the cards. Neither APSA nor CMS provide a method for citing greeting cards. But because they constitute published material, I have cited them under References with "Hallmark" in place of an author. Per the CMS, I have denoted my inability to locate publication dates for each card with "n.d." (no date). I have placed the first line of the card in quotation marks to signify as a title, and immediately following each title, I cite the card number as provided in Larson's notes. In text, I have followed the author-date method as closely as possible by crediting Hallmark, specifying "no date," and noting the card number.

cards) points at the reader and says, "You better get well. There aren't that many people I like" (Hallmark, n.d., ZF-181-14). Chronic and terminal illness doesn't allow me to go anywhere; I'm not getting well. The cards remind me that I'm failing because they indicate that staying ill is inconvenient and disappointing for others.

Get-well cards depict medical treatment as easy and assume that drugs and operations fix everything. "Finish all your medicine and get well soon" is accompanied by the song "A Spoonful of Sugar" (Hallmark, n.d., 499-GNG-317-8). "People who think laughter is the best medicine apparently never had morphine. Take your drugs and get well" (Hallmark, n.d., ZF-290-4), jokes another. "Get well soon! Meanwhile enjoy the things you see on medication," reads a card with a sunbathing frog wearing sunglasses and hair braids (Hallmark, n.d., ZF-290-6). But, chemotherapy drugs are nothing like the medicines that cards glorify. Chemo drugs made me feel sicker, and they don't cure me. Some cards try to charm their recipient to recovery in iambic pentameter: "Glad your operation is in the past, but don't be impatient to get well too fast. Just relax, take it easy, get plenty of rest and before long you soon will be feeling your best" (Hallmark, n.d., C-592-6). My last four operations were followed by chemotherapy. No one gets to relax when they have cancer: there's too much to do—chemo treatments, shots, trying to eat, recovering from eating, monitoring your condition, challenging the insurance company, scheduling appointments, and just trying to function. Chronic and terminal illnesses don't have the happy endings these cards assume. The cards deny my experience. Receiving them makes me feel misunderstood.

Hallmark® has recently gotten into the niche market of cancer cards as well. There aren't many to choose from, but I suppose I shouldn't complain because many stores don't even carry cancer cards. I hoped that one labeled "Fighting Cancer" would get it right. It read: "Why? Somewhere in your heart, you're probably asking this question. Though I don't have an answer, I do know you're a strong and determined person who will get through this. No matter what lies ahead, I'll be caring about you . . . surrounding you with positive thoughts and prayers" (Hallmark, n.d., ECG 8-4). I like the part about "caring about you." I understand and appreciate the desire to surround me "with positive thoughts and prayers," even if I'm sometimes skeptical about their utility. What I don't understand is how anyone could say that they "know" I'll "get through this." Even the cancer card pretends that illness is temporary.

What about serious-illness cards? Are they better at finding appropriate words for the terminally and chronically ill? One reads: "We're thinking of you. Sometimes it's easier to keep a positive attitude when you know that people care about you. This is to let you know that we do" (Hallmark, n.d., TOY 225-7). I'm glad they're thinking of me and they care about me, but I don't want that to be an investment in or contingent upon my positive attitude. What does the card labeled "Serious Illness—Religious" offer? "Sometimes God can use a difficult time to challenge us . . ." the card opens, painting cancer as an experience with a limited time frame, which can be overcome. It lists the benefits of having cancer for me and my relationship with God: "to stir up new strength we didn't know we had . . . to make the power of His love for us a very real blessing in our lives." Finally, it concedes, "It can be hard to cope with an illness like this—no matter how strong your faith," and finishes by recommending, "Praying the Lord will be with you every day, adding His strength to yours" (Hallmark, n.d., TOY 867-4). I am no theologian, but I find this card unsettling and contradictory. Is it saying that God wanted me to be sick? Is it asserting that if I'm strong enough, I'll get well? Is the logic that people feel God's love the most when they are sick? Or that God's strength wouldn't be with me unless a friend was praying for me? Is it implying that my strength is greater than God's by saying that His strength will augment mine (instead of the other way around)? While thinking about this card might distract me for a little while, it wouldn't bring me the comfort it was trying to deliver.

Although the care implicit in the act of sending cards can negate their imperfect messages, it seems safer to just send ones with simple messages. Cards that try to reassure me that I'll be all right aren't the right cards. Cards that try to make me laugh usually won't. Cards that tell me to do something that I can't do aren't uplifting. I would rather people send me a card with a pretty picture on it that says they're thinking of me and hoping for the best. Those cards are not easy to find, but there are some. If I were sending myself a card, it would be the one that reads, "When life hands you lemons, make lemonade;" and inside it says, "But when life hands you a load of crap, don't make anything. Trust me on this one" (Hallmark, n.d., ZF 177-2). Not only does this make me smile because its message comes as a surprise, it also acknowledges that I'm up against something ugly, and mocks the cheerful can-do culture that wants to pretend everything will be okay. I don't know how it could be okay—not this time, at least.

* * *

Another way that words seem to fail the terminally and chronically ill is through labeling. People want to call me a "cancer survivor," but that does not feel right. Cancer hasn't killed me yet, but it will. To be a survivor, I would need more assurance that I could come out the other side with cancer behind me. I'd need to feel like I wasn't walking around with something growing inside of me and substantially altering how I want to live my life. "Living with cancer" doesn't feel right either. It's so casual and cavalier— so dismissive. The phrase makes it sound like ugly shag carpet in the family room ("I'll live with it"). Besides, it doesn't always feel like I'm doing much living during chemotherapy, when the tumors are getting big enough to stop me from digesting food effectively, or when the heart failure from the chemo is making it hard to breathe and impossible to sleep. "In treatment" sounds like I'm getting psychotherapy or in drug rehabilitation. It also erroneously implies that at some point I will be out of treatment, and that I chose to be in treatment in the first place. It is equally inaccurate when I'm taking breaks from chemotherapy. "Fighting" or "battling cancer" assumes constant action. What about the times I am too weak for chemotherapy? Is that a cease-fire? And how could I be at war with my own body? I would like the cancer cells to calm down, multiply less often, and stop sending out demanding messages to my vascular system. I would like to peacefully co-exist with all parts of my body.

I'm more comfortable with the term "cancer victim," but that term is passé. It has been stripped from the discourse by those seeking agency, and ironically, by those who want to empower us. If I call myself a cancer victim, people get unhappy. They don't want to think of me as a victim. I don't fit the cowering, helpless stereotype they have in their heads. So they correct me: "You're no victim"; "You're still here, aren't you"; or the generic "Don't say that. You have to stay positive." So if I'm not a victim or a survivor, and I'm not really living with cancer or necessarily in treatment, what am I? I'd say that I am a "cancer sufferer." I am a cancer sufferer. I have cancer. I suffer from it. I am not always fighting. I am not always in treatment. I am not yet dead from cancer, but I will be in months or years, and until then, my life is fundamentally altered by the presence of cancer and the medical protocols for treating it. I am a cancer sufferer. Like fools, I don't suffer it gladly.

* * *

The positive-thinking advice has a lot in common with the power-of-prayer rhetoric. The former assumes that the curative power lies within me, and the latter believes it lies with God. They are both well-meaning, but they both require that I do something, and do it correctly, in order to be saved. I've been told not to lose my faith by people who know nothing about my faith, nor whether it has been put in jeopardy by cancer. I have been advised that the prayers should *claim* a miracle, as in, "I claim a remission in the name of Jesus," because these sorts of prayers demonstrate my faith in God. Others say that I should *ask* God for the miracle, since it is His to give, but I need to be very specific. I need to have a *purposeful* prayer that asks God for exactly what I need. I should say something to the effect of, "Lord, make my CA125 go down to twenty-four." I need to pray often and with certainty for it to be effective. Once again, I feel like people are saying that if I die of cancer, it is my fault. It's because I didn't pray correctly or often enough; failure to recover is a failure of genuine faith.

Email chain letters indicate that asking for God's help will not be effective because whatever hardships we experience were intended to teach us lessons. One mailing included a list of prayer requests ("I asked God to . . .") followed by explanations for why God rejected each. The passage that irritated me the most read: "I asked God to spare me pain. God said, 'No!' Suffering draws you apart from worldly cares and brings you closer to me." I don't think the person who wrote this ever experienced excruciating pain. If so, he or she would know that "worldly cares" remain. It is the pain itself that consumes every thought. Every breath is focused on enduring. Pain does cause you to leave behind worldly cares like what to eat for dinner, but it also causes you to leave the world beyond your body. All that exists is your body. You're not feeling spiritual, enlightened, or open to learning anything about God. All you want is for the pain to stop. I don't think God would do this to someone He loves in order for them to feel closer to

Him. That's not the kind of dysfunctional relationship that I expect God to want.

People ascribe all kinds of divine and spiritual intentionality to cancer. It could be that: God is mad at me (cancer as punishment); God is teaching me something (cancer as lesson); God is testing me (cancer as challenge); or God is calling me home (cancer as love). Since the last one is at odds with the other ideologies that prioritize life over the afterlife, I suspect that people won't interpret my cancer as God calling me home until I'm weeks or days away from death. But, I do not find any comfort, wisdom, or use in the idea that cancer has anything to do with God punishing, testing, or rewarding me. That doesn't mean that I have rejected God or am disillusioned about Him. My faith is not contingent on outcomes. (If my faith required a fair world, I would not have needed cancer to dishearten me; instead, my faith would have been shaken early and easily by the injustices in the world. Why is it that so many people's faith is shaken by their own tragedies, but not by those of strangers?)

I believe that God knows I want the cancer to go away, regardless of whether I talk to Him about it. I believe that time with Him is better spent in quiet, peaceful togetherness, than attempting to berate, beg, or bribe him into giving me what I want. After I am dead, He might explain how or why this happened to me. That explanation might have a logic or lesson to it that I wouldn't understand now. But I think it's more likely that He will say, "Life's not fair. You had more physical pain than most people. I know that was upsetting." I'll be satisfied with that. I'd appreciate the understanding and acknowledgement. I'd be relieved not to hear him say "Look on the bright side . . . ."

* * *

In many ways, being a cancer sufferer is not consistent with the can-do version of me that my friends and family miss. But my problems now don't have solutions. I try hard to remind myself of this, because after years of practice, it feels instinctual to figure things out and fix any problem that arises.

Although so much of our upbringing seemed to be background noise to my sister, the can-do attitude of my father got through to her. She's a powerful woman. She's successful in her career (computer science), her volunteering (Head Start®), and her home life (managing the lives of her husband, her mother-in-law, and her son). When she develops an interest or a hobby, it is with intense identification and unbounded enthusiasm. She has embraced my cancer with the same intensity, telling my mother that she was determined to "Get Stephanie a miracle." She has me on prayer lists, and she sends out updates to keep the people praying motivated. She emails me web page links to treatments that might work, and she sends me flowers during chemo weeks. She calls to see how I'm doing, gives me pep talks, and tolerates my moods.

As I approached three years since my diagnosis, she concluded (justifiably) that chemotherapy seemed to be hurting me more than it was helping. She admitted that this was a disappointment, but she said that *she* still believed that I could "get that miracle." If would help, she thought, if *I* also believed that I was going to get it. However, I could still be helped even if I wasn't a believer, but she was still sure that believing would help. She explained it to me this way: "It is like what they told us [she and her husband] when we sold Amway®. We learned then that what you expect is what you get; what you put out there is what is returned to you. If you think that you won't make a sale, you won't. If you think you will, then you will." I politely didn't correct her by saying, "You mean when you *tried* to sell Amway®." That would have been rude, but truthfully, it had not been a successful venture for them. They had enjoyed it, though. Going to the conventions, touring houses they'd be able to afford if they were successful, meeting so many go-getters. It was pretty good stain remover, but it had not become the family business she had hoped and expected.

My father would certainly have endorsed her logic for how to succeed at sales. He once tracked down a door-to-door magazine salesman whom my mother had sent away. She had actually wanted to buy a magazine subscription, but the salesman had apparently been rejected too often to believe that. After she answered the door, he had simply asked, "You don't want magazines, do you?" My mother had found herself parroting him—shaking her head—no, she didn't want magazines. When my father heard about this, he went out into the neighborhood, found the defeated young man, and gave him a here's-how-you-do-it demonstration. I don't know if the guy became a better salesman after all of my father's advice, but he at least sold a subscription to the Greco household.

My sister didn't just internalize my father's messages. She embraced America's, because these are core values of our culture. We are a can-do, bright-side nation. We have a Protestant work ethic, which indicts the individual in his or her own success or failure. If you fail, it is because you didn't try hard enough or were in some way undeserving. If you succeed, it is because you worked hard and earned it. In other words, Americans tend to think you get what you deserve. Competition permeates our culture. You can ask for help, and people might give you some, but only to a point, because inevitably the outcome is up to you. These ideologies motivate us. They justify our public policies. They've also made it difficult for us to talk about chronic or terminal illnesses and death.

The competitive, can-do, individualistic ideology worked pretty well for me as a middle-class, educated white person with agency and opportunities. But it isn't working for me now that I'm powerless and limited by my illness. People cringe at the term "powerless." There must always be something that can be done, they think. But I am powerless to stop my cancer from growing. I am powerless to stop the side effects of chemo from disabling me. I cannot change how sick I am, or that my sickness will prevent me from working the job that pays for my health insurance and my monthly fifteen-thousand dollar chemotherapy bill. I am powerless over my platelet and red blood cell counts, and over whether or not the chemotherapy will be effective. I am powerless over which healthcare reform Congress passes. My cancer cannot be persuaded to go away, either by me, the drugs, or by all the good will and optimism that people direct at it.

I try to translate the blindly optimistic and naïve things that people say to me so they don't make me feel badly. When people ask me how I am doing, I try to remember that what they mean is that they hope I am doing well. When they ask what my doctor says or if I've gotten a second opinion, I remind myself that they want someone to cure me. When they tell me that I have to believe in miracles, I know they are saying that they don't want me to die. If they are also thinking that they don't want to get what I have, that's okay, because I don't want them to either.

* * *

Not only does a culture of can-do-ism and individual responsibility require that your cancer can be cured (by your doctors, by your attitude, by God, by the universe), it also believes that there was a reason that you got sick. *Why* you have the disease becomes important. People don't feel comfortable asking me this directly, but they do feel comfortable asking if the doctors have any idea why I have this. They may just be curious, but I think at some level they just hope that I have an answer that will disqualify them as possible victims.

The idea of personal responsibility for health is common in our culture. It assumes that people are sick because they smoked, didn't exercise, had unprotected sex, drank too much liquor, did drugs, didn't eat right, didn't get checkups, or ignored their doctors' recommendations. It's reassuring to assume that as long as you play by the rules, you'll be okay. Unfortunately, I'm dying proof that it doesn't always work that way. My friends know me well enough to know that I had a reasonably-healthy lifestyle.

So they can't be reassured by the assumption that my ill health is due to obviously-bad choices. If it was something I ate, then it is probably something in their food, too. If it's something I breathed, it's in their air.

People aren't necessarily disappointed when they find out about my unimpeachable lifestyle, but they are uneasy, so they rarely allow the inquiry to rest. Casting about for a safe place to put the blame, they turn triumphantly to my genetics. I know what people are hoping to hear when they ask if cancer runs in my family. If it does, then they can feel safer. It doesn't affect them since they don't have my genes. Looking for genetic explanations can also feel like blame. Even though I may not be expected to have any control over my genes, it says that the cause of my problem is who I am.

People want to make sense of my illness. They want it to make sense within their pre-existing worldviews. That often leads them to a dead end. They ask if it drives me crazy, not knowing why. But I'm not preoccupied with the question. To me it's no more valid than why *not*? Bodies are complex and delicate. The fact that so many last for so long is more of a mystery to me than the fact that mine is sick again. While the mysteries of my body don't torment me, the reasons for my dysfunctional relationship with doctors do. Sometimes I think that maybe Dr. Evil is to blame for why I have cancer (again). My abdomen was brutalized, and that's where the cancer is. This theory could reassure people (My appendix didn't burst, so I'll be fine), or disturb them (If I can't trust doctors, who can I trust?). So I don't often share this idea with people. When I do, they always ask—where I was in 1980? Who was this doctor? They're glad it's not 1980 in Orlando; things must be different now, and he must be an exception. My experience tells me otherwise, but I usually don't debate the point. Why give them nightmares? Besides, I don't want to talk about the appendix anymore. I'm tired of thinking about the appendix.

Some people make sense of my cancer by saying that I'm unlucky. I find that answer credible because it doesn't deny what is happening to me, and it doesn't come with a prescription for how I need to think or act to fix the problem. The idea that there are lucky people and unlucky people has a certain appeal. It can feel a little blaming, because it is still about me, but at least I'm being blamed for something that is beyond my control. The luck explanation admits that the situation isn't fair; it's just random. Thinking that unlucky people get cancer can also be reassuring to healthy people because, as long as they resist thinking of themselves as unlucky, they can feel safe. Thinking of cancer as an unlucky thing that comes along and happens to people is less reassuring. Yet I find that a reasonable explanation, too. It satisfies the why-me question that I've been told I'm supposed to be asking, although asking seems arrogant and rude—as if this happening to someone else would make it okay. I don't spend much time wondering why this is happening to me, because I believe it is unanswerable; the answer wouldn't change that it *is* me.

* * *

The epitome of rugged individualism and can-do thinking is the cancer-as-fight metaphor. People encourage me to keep fighting. They tell me they *know* I can beat this. The analogy feels wrong to me in so many ways. It assumes that I have agency when I don't. This isn't a fight that I can train for, work at, or win with my brilliant strategizing. I have a terminal cancer. I'm still alive, but that doesn't mean I'm winning. Fighting the cancer or not fighting the cancer, I will lose and so the language of this metaphor sets me up as a failure. The cancer is taking whatever time that it will take to kill me. I have to explain this to people when they say that I must being doing great because I'm still here. I'm not actually doing so well if you assess my quality of life, the size of my tumors, or my prognosis.

The fighting language also transforms me into someone I don't want to be—a warrior. Not only does the language force me to be combative just because I have cancer, it positions me as at war with my own body. If I'm at war with cancer, and the cancer is me, then my body is my enemy. But I've always tried to love and accept my body regardless of its limitations. So, the fighting metaphor is an uncomfortable one. My cancer cells might be destructive (and ultimately self-destructive), but they're not intentionally out to get me. They're just confused (What are we supposed to be doing?), hyperactive (multiplying too fast), and needy (We must have more of the blood! We must have more of the nutrients!). They're like me on a first date in the 1990s, the decade after my divorce. They don't know what they want. They're trying too hard. They're too eager, too demanding. Like me, they're going to ruin the chance of a potentially good long-term relationship. I am not happy about that, but I can't vilify them for it.

If I am at war with cancer, then I was drafted. I did not enlist. If I had a choice, I would run to Canada. I would wait for an amnesty, or somehow adjust to the cold winters and stay there. If this is a war, then I wasn't trained to fight it. The only weapons I've been given to fight this war are poison and a pep talk. It's not poison that I can release into the enemies' air and slip away. I cannot hide in a bunker while the poison chokes my enemy. We have to stand together and breathe in the fumes. Yet it seems as though the enemy has a gas mask, and I do not. That's how many of the chemotherapies end up working—they are killing me, but not the cancer. If I am at war with cancer, then it is at war with me. But it also has a peculiar battle plan. It embeds itself in its enemy, and dies when it wins. It cannot survive without me. What a strange war we are both waging.

No, the fighting analogy doesn't work for me. I think of war enthusiasts as those who want to show off their ideological certainty and military superiority. Those are the American wars of my lifetime. I think of the war policies as going into little countries to dominate and control with fancy equipment. I can't relate to that; I'm a woman who wants peace. I try to take a more historical perspective and see if that improves the utility of the war analogy. What if I equate my cancer with Nazis in World War II? But for Americans, even that war was over *there*, and certainly I am suffering *here* within myself. Perhaps, I can think of myself as London during the Blitz. But that analogy still breaks down. I am not protecting the homeland from an assault because the cancer is not coming *in*; it is *from* within. The chemotherapy is from outside, and I know my body is resisting that, but isn't it the good guy? Maybe I am on a battleground, but I am not a warrior there. I feel like the naked, crying Vietnamese child, covered in napalm, running down the street toward nowhere safe.

American culture calls me and other cancer patients "brave." I don't feel brave. I am afraid, tired, and desperate. I think bravery is a choice. It is going into the burning building to save someone when you might die trying, and you didn't have to do it. Bravery is risking your life for someone else or for an ideal. I didn't have a choice. If I did, I would choose another option. I would choose wellness and forgo the compliments. All I'm trying to do is endure.

Supposedly chemotherapy is a choice, so perhaps the bravery comes in subjecting myself to its wrath? But the way the doctors talk about it, it doesn't feel like a choice. They say it is the only option to possibly extend my life. Maybe I'm not being courageous, and I'm simply too weak to resist their authority? Or maybe I'm frightened to face death? Or maybe I'm too stupid to understand the terrible statistics on what chemotherapy buys a person with this cancer? If friends mean that I am courageous because I've decided to have a treatment that will extend my life while it makes that same life so miserable, they're saying that my choosing to try living regardless of the costs is inherently the brave thing. But I thought that bravery was facing death? Isn't that a contradiction?

Wouldn't refusing to chemotherapy be more courageous? It's got characteristics that sound brave—honestly facing death, doing something on your own terms despite criticism, challenging conventions, and not allowing fear to distort decision-making. But resisting doctors' recommendations is not typically met with congratulations. It tends to be seen as foolish, shortsighted, or even suicidal. It can also be seen as selfish—letting your family down by not fighting. If I ever make the choice to stop chemotherapy, then you can call me brave, even though it will provide little consolation.

Overall, I don't prefer self-deception and delusion to truthfulness, but it feels like I'm expected to. I feel misunderstood (I *am* dying); undervalued (*this* version of me is still worthy); and judged (what I *should* be is what I *am*). If I buy into the argument that my thinking can heal me, that the Stephanie before cancer is the *real* Stephanie, and that I have to hold on to every aspect of her, then what am I supposed to think when I don't get healed and I'm diminished by cancer and the side effects of chemotherapy? I will have no choice but to feel like I failed.

Chapter 12: "Are you Depressed?": More Chemotherapy and Collateral Damage

In May of 2008, after the three-month respite from chemotherapy was over, I had another blood test to see how the cancer had reacted to the break. Surprisingly, the number had remained stable, and I was given another month off. By the end of the month, my digestion had gotten worse, and the CA125 went up a little. A dose of Avastin® didn't help. Dr. Sure ordered a CAT scan. It didn't show any cancer, but it did show gallstones and damage to my bone marrow. It seemed to me that I should wait until the CA125 went higher before taking more chemotherapy. I had read somewhere that some doctors waited until the number was over one-hundred before resuming the treatment. I thought that the more time I could spend feeling reasonably healthy and allowing my body to get stronger, the better.

Dr. Sure disagreed strongly. He said something like, "Sure, we could use that approach, if we didn't care if you live." I was used to his certainty, but not this sarcasm or bluntness. He seemed a little angry—as if I had asked him to euthanize me. He quickly calmed himself, and he explained that treating the cancer as soon as the CA125 went up and long after it was in the normal range resulted in longer survival rates than other approaches. Then he ordered a PET scan. It didn't show any cancer. The CA125 crept up a little more.

In my experience, doctors don't like to watch and wait—it's contrary to their training. They want to *do* something. So I wasn't surprised when my oncologists tag-teamed me in order to persuade me to have surgery. Dr. Kind said that I should get my gallbladder taken out because sometimes diseased gallbladders could inflate CA125s. He had an anecdote to prove it. And as long as I was having surgery for my damaged gallbladder, Dr. Sure chimed in that he wanted a second look to see if he could locate the cancer. This would also allow him to collect some samples, and send them to a lab that would determine what kind of chemotherapy would work best on me. I wasn't certain what good it would do for Dr. Sure to confirm the location of the cancer. But if there was a type of chemotherapy that would work "best" with my body, I wanted to know about it.

Dr. Sure thought that the results from a cholescintigraphy scan would help convince the gallbladder surgeon that I needed surgery. He wrote the script ordering the scan, seeming pleased that he could expedite the process. I should have reminded myself that surgeons like to operate and doctors get paid for ordering tests. It was unlikely that I needed this test—we already knew that I had gallstones and digestive problems. But instead of questioning the order, I dutifully went to the hospital to get the test. After lots of waiting, I was told that it would be necessary to find a vein because a radioactive tracer needed to be inserted, and they didn't want to put that in my PowerPort®.

The technician went through a checklist. He got to the question: do you have gallstones? I said that I did. He looked up from the list, surprised. "We don't give this test to people with gallstones. It would be extremely painful," he said. He began to tick off the steps we would have to take to perform the test: "We'll need to call your doctor and get approval to go through with it. You'll have to sign a release form." The good girl voice in my head said, *You have to do this because it's what the doctor wants. You can endure it.* But the scared, little girl, or maybe it was the skeptical adult, did not want to proceed. I went back to the waiting room to tell David about my anxiety. David said,

"This is absurd. Dr. Sure doesn't know what he's talking about. You're not going to do this test unless the gallbladder surgeon insists on it." Without truly understanding why I was doing it, I began to argue with David. Dr. Sure had written the order, and he wanted expediency. The technician was already making phone calls. We had been at the hospital for hours. What if we left now and it turned out that I needed the test? I wasn't sure how to stop the process, even if I wanted to! David said, "It's easy. We say, you are not going through with this, and we walk away." And that's what we did. It turned out that the gallbladder surgeon didn't need the cholescintigraphy test; the CAT scan was enough for him. Surprisingly, Dr. Sure never asked why there were no results in my file for a test that he had ordered. The surgery was set for mid-August, precariously close to the start of the fall semester.

The surgery preparation was the same nasty purging of the intestine that I had before the hysterectomy, but the purge didn't seem that bad this time. Chemotherapy had recalibrated my perception of what was unpleasant, what was painful, and what was intolerable. Intestinal pain and diarrhea were my new normal. Surgery revealed that my gallbladder had been completely shot. I had apparently suffered more than one painful attack, but I wasn't aware of it. Who knows which pain had been related to the gallbladder?

Dr. Sure had seen my cancer, but the surgery didn't fulfill any of his additional hopes. He reported that none of it was big enough to send to the lab for the test—the test that had convinced me to have the operation, and since the CA125 was going up, it was time for more chemo. From what I could gather, he had learned nothing new from the surgery. But now we had colored pictures of my cancer. It looked like pimples on my abdominal wall and my liver. If it had shown up on a CAT scan, it would have looked like a lesion on my liver. Where had I heard that before? Could this have been from the uterine cancer? Dr. Sure was positive it wasn't. This must be a second, primary cancer because he had removed all of the first cancer during the hysterectomy.

Unfortunately, my body did not adjust well to losing the gallbladder. Everyone says that you don't need your gallbladder, yet it does serve a purpose. The bile that is released from your liver is stored in the gallbladder and then released into your intestine when it is needed, like after eating a fatty meal. Without a gallbladder, the liver dumps the bile directly into the intestine, which is supposed to adjust. Mine had not adjusted. I had to figure this out on my own from reading web pages, because the post-op visits to the surgeon weren't helpful.

Every week I would go to the surgeon, and we both hoped that it would be my last visit. He was always distracted and in a hurry, leaving the examining room quickly and without a goodbye. This drove my husband crazy. As a salesman, he believed in pleasantries. "I'm sure he's coming back," David said, bewildered after the surgeon abruptly left the examining room during my first post-op visit. I didn't think so, and I was right. Once, we had to follow the doctor out into the hallway to make sure he would answer a question. It surprised and disturbed the doctor. He looked at us like a hunted animal might have.

During each visit the doctor would ask me how I was doing, and I would tell him about my horrible diarrhea. I would try to describe its frequency, urgency, consistency, and how different it was from types I'd had in the past. (I later realized that my post-op diarrhea was pure bile.) I thought this detailed information would be useful to him. He didn't agree and would always cut me off. For the first three weeks, he told me that I should feel better soon. I didn't. I was completely immobilized by the diarrhea, which had urgency like no other had in the past.

At the next meeting, the surgeon said that some people needed to take a drug to help their bodies adjust to the bile, and that this was usually a temporary problem. He prescribed packets of Cholestyramine powder that I was to mix in water and drink. They mercifully allowed me to teach my classes without running out the door. Yet they didn't solve the problem for more than a few hours. So the next week, he told me to take a larger dose. The following week, he told me to increase the dose again, but the level he suggested was the same level he had prescribed to me at my previous visit. I knew he wasn't listening very closely to me, but I was surprised that he hadn't listened to himself either. I didn't want to spend another week on the toilet, so I corrected him—I was already taking that dose and it didn't seem to be working. Did he still want me to increase the dose? "No, don't take any more than that," he reneged, clarifying that an increased dosage "would be dangerous." I was glad we'd cleared that up.

The next week, I reported that I was still having diarrhea and he asked, "Are you sure?" I had to laugh. Yes, I was sure. It ruled my life. How could my authority on this be questioned? So the next week, I brought in my detailed eating, digestion, and drug diary. I tried to give it to him, but he put his hands up and asked, "Why don't you just summarize it for me?" I did. Maybe there was something else wrong with my digestion, he suggested. He couldn't believe that these problems were due to the gallbladder surgery. We couldn't keep having all these appointments, which were not billable because they were part of the surgery and post-op fee. I should go to a gastrointestinal doctor. I told him I'd done that— the gastro-intestinal doctor said that my adhesions were probably interfering with my routine digestion, and more surgery would likely make it worse. His eyes lit up. "Oh, I don't know about that," he cajoled. "I could do the surgery." He had never been so solicitous.

"No, thank you," I said, and as usual, he beat a quick retreat. That was the last time I went to his office. I did see him in the hospital a few weeks later, but he didn't recognize me when I greeted him.

I went to see my gastrointestinal doctor instead. He confirmed what I had learned on the web. A fraction of people who have their gallbladders removed need to take something to bind their bile. He could give me a bile-binding drug that wouldn't interfere with the other drugs I was on. I didn't understand what he was talking about and I said so. Cholestyramine didn't interfere with the efficacy of my other drugs. Yes they did, he said. I argued that my gallbladder surgeon had *not* warned me that I shouldn't take the powder *within several hours* of any other drug. That was an oversight on his part, noted the gastrointestinal doctor. I had been weakening the effectiveness of my other drugs for weeks. I wondered if it had been undermining the new chemotherapy that I had started taking a few weeks after surgery. The new drug was called Doxil®. It would become my least favorite chemotherapy. But I didn't know that yet.

Doxil® was a second-tier drug, which had a lower success rate than the platinum-based drugs that I had already tried. It would be administered every three weeks in addition to Avastin®. Neither caused hair loss, and they were supposed to be easier on platelets than the drugs that I had taken intermittently over the twenty months since my diagnosis. It sounded like it would allow me to teach on Monday and Wednesday afternoons. A few of the downsides of Doxil® were that it might cause swelling, rashes, mouth sores, and heart problems. In fact, before starting the drug, I had to get a test to see if my heart was healthy enough to start treatment.

When I went to the hospital for the test, I learned that they couldn't use my PowerPort®. They needed to find a vein. After all the unsuccessful sticks that I had received from radiologists, I practically begged the technician to get a phlebotomist. But he was sure that he could hit the vein in my right arm. I warned him that it was my only good arm vein, so it would be better to get Chris from down the hall. She knew me from the weekly blood tests that I needed for my previous chemotherapies. She would walk me to Day Surgery with the paperwork and vials for my blood so that the chemo nurses could access my port. She knew about my health and my fears. But the radiologist had a schedule to keep, and didn't want to wait. He was sure that this would be quicker and easier.

As soon as he missed the vein, I started sobbing. I couldn't stop. I could barely breathe. He was shocked. He wanted to give me a minute to get myself together, but too much anxiety, exhaustion, and grief were built up behind the dam that had just burst. No matter how many times I saw him peek into the room through the small window on the door, I kept on crying. I remember thinking that I didn't really need the test because I'd be willing to try this chemo without reassurances that my heart could tolerate the treatment. I'd rather die of a heart attack than cancer anyway. I cried some more.

I cried because of what was going to happen next and for all that had happened before. I cried because I couldn't do anything about my veins or my cancer, my past or my future. I cried because I still hadn't recovered from surgery and I was going back into chemotherapy. I was still crying when Chris walked in. She was able to calm me down by reminding me that we had done this once before, and we could do it again. She told me that she was confident that the vein in my hand just below my middle finger would do. She showed me the butterfly needle she would use, reminded me to breathe, and mercifully, got the vein on the first try. I immediately stopped crying. As she quietly talked me through the remainder of the procedure, I took deep cleansing breaths. Cancer hadn't diminished my horror over something as routine as finding a vein.

Doxil® was administered through my PowerPort® once a month. It meant I was a bit hyper and on edge for one Wednesday class. Doxil® kindly did not make my hair fall out, so I wasn't marked as a cancer patient. I think the students only noticed that something was off once, when I told a student to shut up. In my defense, it was a student who always asked a lot of questions, and then talked while I answered. I immediately apologized; "Sorry about that. You do need to listen, but I would have said that much more nicely if I wasn't full of steroids." The Monday class after chemo was lower energy than usual, but I was able to manage. I was also battling the bile problem at the beginning of the semester, so I was forced to get most of my calories Wednesday night through Sunday morning when I would be home for the fallout.

That kept me from running to the bathroom in the middle of class, but it also meant that I couldn't stay and talk to students for very long after class without feeling faint.

I probably should have guessed that Doxil® would be problematic when it immediately caused me to develop a rash under my wedding ring. I had to stop wearing my ring and the red mark around my finger lasted for a year. The first week that I took Doxil®, I threw up so much that I had to cancel both classes. I became so dehydrated that I began hallucinating. My husband had been on the phone with my doctors throughout the week, but they couldn't determine how bad I was until the day I started talking earnestly about how mirrors looked against black velvet curtains. I spent one night in the hospital getting hydration. They monitored my vital signs and gave me an x-ray. It revealed that I had an ileus. (This is when the intestine stops working due to non-mechanical causes. I think of it as the stage before an intestinal blockage, but that might not be technically accurate.) The following day, I was able to go to the bathroom again, so I was released from the hospital on a liquid diet. After that week was over, I was ten pounds lighter. From then on, I took high-powered, anti-nausea pills with the Doxil®. The three pills had a co-pay of about one-hundred dollars. They were worth every penny. I didn't throw up from Doxil® again.

Dr. Sure also recommended that I get hydration at the Mansion two or three times a week to prevent a complete blockage. He thought that the vomiting was a result of a problem with my intestine that might be helped by additional hydration. We had talked a lot about my intestines during the tell-me-about-your-side-effects portion of our office visits. Sometimes he would say that I had bad intestines, other times that my intestine had been weakened by all my surgeries. Occasionally, he blamed the English doctors. *They* might not have left a big enough opening where they had done the resection. I remembered that during my blockage after the uterine cancer he had said, "The intestine is the dumbest organ. It doesn't wake from anesthesia very well. When it does, it can't always remember what it is supposed to do."

When I consulted my gastro-intestinal doctor about the ileus, he didn't blame my intestine for it. He considered the job of the intestine one of the hardest in the human body. It had to do so much in such a complex order that a lot could go wrong. He said that it was natural for the intestine to shut itself down as a response to the vomiting and dehydration. It was one of the smartest body parts: it had tried to protect me. He thought that the ileus was an effect of the chemotherapy, not a cause of the vomiting. He took a quick look at the side effects listed on the Doxil® web page and pointed out that ileus was on the list. He didn't think that there was anything wrong with my getting extra hydration, but didn't see an urgent need for it.

I got hydration during afternoons when the Mansion was quiet. The nurses were primarily doing paperwork and giving occasional shots. Getting hydration didn't make me sick, groggy, or anxious. I could use the PowerPort® to get hydration, and so I was able to relax. The nurses seemed to like this version of me. We could chat about normal things rather than symptoms, side effects, and cancer. I became more comfortable with them, too. I recognized their competency and compassion, even though they showed it in different ways. I still preferred interacting with the one who always said she was sorry when she gave me a shot to the one who had more of a suck-it-up attitude. But I could see how her matter-of-fact, teasing approach worked with other patients.

Doxil® also made my blood pressure go up again. I was told to see my primary care physician to get it under control. Once again, I reminded them that I had a cardiologist, and he had refused to change my medication. Dr. Young, the cardiologist, admitted that he didn't understand what was going on. He needed a call from one of my oncologists to explain how the drugs I was taking affected my blood pressure. Again, Dr. Kind promised to contact him. Again, he did not. My blood pressure kept going up. At one point it was so high that the nurse commented, "That can't be right." But it was. She said she'd come back and take it again, but she didn't. I had been monitoring my blood pressure at home, wondering how high it needed to be before I should go to the hospital. I had never gotten a clear answer to that question. The nurses would simply tell me what the range for normal blood pressure was. This was not very helpful, given that I was way above that range. The CA125 also continued to go up while I took Doxil®. I seemed to be in agony for nothing.

Dr. Sure decided to add Cytoxan® to the Doxil®. I received my first dose of Cytoxan® on December 5th, 2008. I thought it was making me more susceptible to germs, because I started coughing a lot and feeling weak and tired. The cough never produced any phlegm. Dr. Sure gave me antibiotics, but they didn't help. I kept coughing, and he gave me more antibiotics. Then, on December 23rd, I got more Cytoxan®. The following day, I was even sicker, and my blood pressure was soaring. I asked to speak to a doctor when I went in for my shot. Dr. Sure was in the office. He sent me to the hospital for a chest scan to see if I had a blood clot. If there was a clot, I wasn't going home that day. The attending doctor said that I didn't have a clot, but I did have fluid in my lungs. That might be because I had the flu. So I didn't have to stay in the hospital. I went home and started throwing up. The next day, Christmas Eve, I threw up more. David phoned the doctor on call. It was the same doctor who had read my chest scan. I hadn't thrown up enough for him to send me to the hospital, but I was free to go to the emergency room if I wanted. I stayed home.

In a few days, I still had the cough, so we called the office again to see if we should cancel our plans to fly to Florida for New Year's Eve. The doctor told us to go; he thought it would be therapeutic to be in warm weather with my family. While I was in Florida the cough grew even worse. My feet swelled. I couldn't sleep without three pillows to prop me up. We called the doctor to see if we should fly home or go to a Florida emergency room. He said that if both feet were swollen, it probably wasn't blood clots. Sometimes fluids seep out of cells during chemotherapy and cause swelling. A few days later, we flew back to Pennsylvania. I could barely walk ten feet without gasping for air.

That evening my husband went on the Internet and diagnosed me. According to WebMD®, I had a clear case of

296

congestive heart failure. The next morning David called the doctors and told them he was taking me to the hospital. They called the hospital to help expedite the admission process. Still, it felt like a long and difficult journey from being dropped off at the door to getting in the bed of my cubicle. I gasped for breath, coughed, walked a few steps, sat and rested, and then did it again. When I was in the cubicle they took some blood from my PowerPort®, gave me hydration, and put me on oxygen. They weighed me, and then they gave me an echocardiogram—a test that uses sound waves to provide images of the heart muscle and valves. We waited.

Eventually one of the cardiologists from Dr. Young's practice confirmed that I had congestive heart failure. All of my symptoms were textbook—the swelling, dry cough, feeling like I was drowning when I slept, and difficulty catching my breath. My heart was not strong enough to pump out a sufficient amount of blood, so fluids were backing up into my lungs and ankles. My echocardiogram showed that 20 to 25 percent of the blood was being pushed out of my heart chamber with each beat. In contrast, a normal person's heart would have pushed out 50 percent or more. I also had valve leakages. The doctor instructed the nurse to take me off of the hydration. I should not be receiving fluids because they made the heart work harder. I thought of all the hydration I had been getting at the Mansion for weeks while I coughed. It had probably not been necessary for my intestines, but it had been putting more pressure on my heart, systematically drowning my lungs. The cardiologist's plan was to use drugs to drain me of fluids. He hoped my heart could rebound and my lungs dry out. I would be peeing a lot. He offered to put in a catheter so that I wouldn't have to walk to the bathroom in my room. That struck me as odd. I could still walk. I knew how to pee. I didn't want to risk a urinary tract or bladder infection, which I knew catheters could cause. I declined his offer.

I realized, once I was on the cardiology floor, why the doctors might have been accustomed to giving patients catheters. Almost everyone there was ancient. The televisions were all at top volume so that the elderly patients could hear them. Wheelchairs crowded the hallways. I did not see my first roommate, so I couldn't say how old she was, but she sounded like she had reached the age of dementia. The curtain was drawn between our beds, but I had heard her talking and yelling, often incoherently. Every time I coughed (which was often that first day), she'd yell, "Stop that! Who is that? I don't have a roommate! Why is she doing this to me?" There was almost always a nurse in the room trying to calm her down and patiently answering the same questions over and over again. After a few hours, when I was wheeled back to the floor after a chest scan, they put me in another room.

I was never sorry that I had declined the catheter. I had always enjoyed peeing, especially when I had a full bladder. I could regulate the speed, and I could easily fill up the toilet hat. This was something that I was in control of, something I was good at, and it wasn't something I got to do much of on chemotherapy. The constant diarrhea had cut down on my peeing, and I missed it. My kidneys had survived the peritonitis in 1980, rebounded quickly after all of my surgeries, and now they were supposed to save my heart and my lungs. I had confidence that my kidneys could do this.

In the first few days in the hospital I peed so much that I lost about fifteen pounds. The drugs were working just like they were supposed to. *Good drugs; great kidneys!* I thought. Apparently, unlike the rest of my body, my bladder and kidneys were people-pleasers. For the five days that I was in the hospital, I had three teams of doctors: the three gynecological oncologists from the Mansion (because they were the admitting physicians); four cardiologists (Dr. Young was not among them); and five pulmonary doctors (they came in teams, so I think some of them were still interns). Each team read the other teams' notes, and sometimes the doctors would ask me what one of the other teams had said to me, but they never talked directly to each other. Since they didn't talk to one another, sometimes they gave contradictory information. One team confidently reassured me that I would leave the following day. The team I saw an hour later asserted that it would be many days before I could expect to be discharged. I had come to expect this, and I didn't let it bother me. I'd leave when they brought me the wheelchair.

In spite of the doctors' disorganization, this was my favorite hospital stay. In large part, this was because one of the biggest causes of stress for me was missing—the need for daily blood samples and IVs. I also preferred the cardiology ward to the orthopedic, cancer, and gastrointestinal wards I had been in. There had been a macho, suck-it-up, that-doesn't-hurt approach on the orthopedic ward. It made me feel like my pain was disregarded. On the cancer ward, there was a silent sadness. Nurses didn't get to feel like they cured you because they hadn't. Maybe you'd survive, but it wouldn't be evident during the hospital stay. The gastrointestinal ward was smelly, depressing, and lacked painkillers. This put patients, nurses, and guests in a bad mood. Here on the cardiology ward, the nurses seemed bright and efficient. They also were personable, and seemed to like spending a few minutes checking in on me. The night I had problems breathing, they were able to help me and reassure me, and they did so quickly. Only one nurse irritated me by waking me up at 4:00 a.m. to do a daily routine that all the others did at 7:00 a.m. She said it allowed her to "get it out of the way." Compared to what I was used to enduring in hospitals, this was nothing. Heart problems would be my ailment of choice. They were kind enough to kill quickly, unlike cancer. I left the hospital feeling much better than when I entered.

I might have also valued that hospital stay more because I finally had some success advocating for myself. After the chest x-ray, the pulmonary doctor came in with her silent sidekick. She explained that the scan showed that my lungs had more fluid in them than they had two weeks earlier. Therefore, she wanted to drain some of the fluid and to test it to see if the cancer had spread to my lungs. I said, "No, I don't want you to do that yet." I counted off the reasons. First, we had just started to treat the problem, so we didn't know if the drugs would drain the lungs sufficiently. I wanted to give them a chance to do that. Second, the lungs should have been worse, since I was suffering from heart failure for an additional two weeks after the test she was referring to was run. Third, I was too weak for more chemo, so finding out that the cancer had spread to my lungs wouldn't change my treatment plan. Fourth, I had had a needle in my lung before. I knew how that felt, and I knew the risks of puncturing the lung. I would only go through that again if my life depended on it. If things got worse, I could have the procedure done later on.

When I finished, I felt surprised that she had listened to my long rationale. I was used to getting cut off by doctors when I spoke. Maybe she had listened because I started by refusing the procedure, or maybe because I spoke in declarative statements instead of questions. Maybe she was just a good listener. For whatever reason, she had listened. She told me how low the risks were that they'd puncture my lung. I said, "Thank you for the information, but I'm not going to do it." She said that she'd need to have me sign off, documenting that she had suggested this and I had refused. That was fine with me. The sidekick continued to say nothing, but his eyes were wider than they were when he first came in. He actually looked scared.

Apparently the one thing that doctors could successfully communicate to each other was when a patient was disobedient. For the rest of my stay, every doctor who came into my room started the meeting by saying, "I see that you have refused to have your lungs drained." After they said this, I would give each of them an abbreviated explanation for my refusal. I had grown tired of justifying this decision by the time the associate doctor on the oncology team saw me. He was an old man I had never seen at the Mansion. There was defensiveness in my voice when I rehashed my justification. He shrugged and said,

"Okay, it's your body. You can decide what to do with it." I had never heard a doctor say such a thing, and it caught me off guard. I could not stop myself from exclaiming,

"Ha! That's not what they said in 1980 when my appendix burst!" He agreed.

"Of course, it wasn't your body then! We thought we had all the answers. Things have changed." I felt vindicated. If only I could hear Dr. Evil and his partner admit that they were *wrong*. That it was *my* body and that I *did* have choices. I hadn't been powerless because of who I was, what I did or didn't say, or do. I was powerless because that's how the medical system defined patients.

Had things *really* changed? On one hand, this week in the hospital seemed to indicate that they had. I might still have been powerless over my cancer, but I wasn't powerless when it came to what had happened to me here and now. I had stopped them from draining my lungs. On the other hand, the surprised reaction of the doctors when I refused the lung draining, and the frequency with which they brought up the subject, indicated that my resistance was exceptional. I was also cogent and fairly comfortable during this hospital stay. This allowed me to be more analytic and active about what was happening. I could think about the procedure suggested to me as a *choice*, rather than something that *had to be done* to save me. What if the doctors had pushed harder to get me to agree to the draining? Would I have been able to resist their authority? Would it ever have occurred to me to refuse treatment if I hadn't already been damaged by doctors?

The first time Dr. Sure came to see me, he seemed shaken. He shook his head and said, "This shouldn't have happened. You're too young for heart failure." Looking at the statistics, I was too young for uterine and peritoneal cancer, too. It didn't have to do with my age. I said,

"It was on the list of potential side effects for Doxil®."

"Yes," he admitted, "but it was so low on the list." He seemed incredulous—talking more to himself than to me. *So what if it was low on the list?* I thought. *It was on the list, I had the symptoms, and you ignored them. Believing that this wouldn't happen to me shouldn't have blinded you to the fact that it did. You didn't take my complaints seriously— just like after the hysterectomy. You were sure then that I didn't have an intestinal blockage; you were sure this time that I didn't have heart failure.* Dr. Sure was always sure, but he wasn't always right.

He continued to be sure—and, nevertheless, wrong— when he explained to me why I didn't want to have my lungs drained. "You are afraid that the cancer has spread, and you don't want to know that it has," he proposed. This was the doctor who I thought had understood me four years earlier when he said that he had seen inside of me and knew why I was scared. But now it seemed like he didn't know me at all. I had never been afraid to acknowledge the truth of what was going on with my body. I had Stage III inoperable, platinum-resistant cancer. I accepted that it would kill me. But I had always been fearful of pain, especially when it was imposed on me by medical professionals, and I had not been shy about admitting it. Why would he think that information from a test would deter me, instead of the actual experience of the test, and my distrust toward those who ordered and executed it?

The priority, said Dr. Sure, was to get my heart back in shape; to do that we'd need to stop the chemotherapy. "Forever, or just for now," I asked, without knowing which answer I was rooting for. He said,

"We'll see." Then he asked me if I had anyone else to talk to about this besides him and John. I thought, I *can't talk to you. You don't understand what I say.* How many times did David have to translate my questions to him, so that he would understand what I was asking? And who the hell was John? Dr. Sure continued, "Because even though we can talk, it's not the same as getting an outsider's opinion. I'm your doctor, and John loves you. You need to talk to someone who doesn't have a dog in this race." I realized then that he thought my husband's name was "John," despite having talked to David over a dozen times. My surprise at the expression he'd used eclipsed any annoyance that he didn't know my husband's name. Was the "race" my battle with cancer? Did I *have* a dog in the race or was *I* the dog? If we were all simply spectators in attendance at the race, was this him telling me that the race would be won, or lost, with or without his interference? I tuned back in just in time to hear him offer to write an order for a counselor to come talk with me. I said that would be fine. He looked relieved and left.

A few days later the psychologist came to my room. At least, I *thought* she was the psychologist, since she asked me a lot of questions about my state of mind. Some questions, like the one about whether I had ever been committed, were easy to answer. Others seemed more complex, and I thought that they were meant to draw me out, allowing me to talk about how I felt. This was what counseling was all about, wasn't it? I hoped that a counselor who worked in a hospital would specialize in end-of-life issues, so I was ready to get to it. Let the openness begin!

So when she asked if I ever thought of suicide, I had a lot to say. I told her that when I had a full life, I never would have considered it. Even now, when I had heart failure and terminal cancer that hadn't yet manifested itself in excruciating pain, I wouldn't consider it. My mother and some of her elderly friends were members of the Hemlock Society, and they believed that they had the right to put themselves out of their own misery (their phrase—not mine) if the time came. I didn't know what I would do if and when there was nothing left but pain. Would I wait for my terminal cancer to choose the moment of my death, or would I take it into my own hands? My sense was that I would let it play out the way it was going to, that to do otherwise was somehow cheating. I also thought that there might be some cosmic penalty for suicide under any circumstances, and that this superstition might be enough to stop me from killing myself. Since I hadn't gotten to that brutal place yet, I couldn't say for sure if or how my opinion might change. I finally stopped talking and looked at the counselor. She said, "So, should I put you down as a 'no'?" That was all she had. *How odd*, I thought. Maybe she was saving her diagnosis and advice for later? Or, maybe I hadn't said anything interesting enough for her to comment on yet.

Then she asked me if I was depressed—another hard question. I told her that I was sad that I had terminal cancer and would live a much shorter life than I wanted. There was so much more I wanted to do, and knowing that my health and my limited time wouldn't allow me to do it weighed heavily on me. I was deeply disappointed that the chemotherapy was so hard on me, and it took away the opportunity to live the rest of this short life the way I wanted. I was frustrated with the medical profession and having to relive the same traumas again and again. To feel misunderstood so often by so many people made me sad, too. I considered depression more of a numb feeling than a sad feeling, so I didn't think I should label myself "depressed." But, I didn't want rejecting the terminology to suggest that I was happy. I wasn't happy, I qualified, but I tried not to dwell on the fun things that I couldn't do anymore and instead to enjoy what I could, when I could. I wasn't always successful at doing that, but maybe I was being too hard on myself? After all, how sad was appropriate for someone in my bleak situation? Was being happy in a sad situation denial or transcendence? It seemed like one of those unanswerable questions. Certainly, I didn't know the answer. Did she? She said, "So, should I put you down as 'yes' or 'no' to the question of whether or not you are depressed?"

This didn't seem like counseling—or, at least, not useful counseling. Maybe it was an assessment that came before counseling? Did I have to earn counseling with answers that indicated I was troubled enough? Or, was this all psychologists had to offer to terminally-ill patients? I gave simple answers to the rest of the questions. At the end of the meeting, she asked me if I thought counseling would be helpful to me. I didn't know because I didn't know what counselors had to offer to terminally-ill patients. If there were specialists who dealt with terminal illness, then I thought I would like to talk to one. She said that she knew counselors who dealt with patients in chronic pain.

"That's not the same," I told her. "That's about learning how to survive despite an obstacle. But that's not about suffering and dying. So, I don't know if they would understand."

"You probably think no one understands you, though," she replied. I wondered whether she meant this as an insight or a judgment. The way she said it, disdainfully and abruptly, led me to think it was the latter. *What a bitch*, I thought. I didn't need this.

"I don't think *you* understand," I conceded. "But I hope that a counselor who listened to me closely and had thought about end-of-life issues would be able to understand me. But I don't really know." She said that she hadn't meant to offend me. I was glad to hear that. She left, and I was gladder still.

* * *

My last meeting with a doctor during that hospital stay was with the lung doctor who had wanted to drain my lungs. By then, it was clear that the medication had been sufficient to drain the fluid. I hadn't needed the procedure after all. She had a different sidekick that day. She introduced me to him as the patient that she had told him about. "It was very instructional for Dr. First Sidekick to hear what you had to say last time" she started. *Here we go*, I thought, preparing to defend myself. "He was a bit rattled by your response." *No kidding.* She continued, "I was able to discuss with him the importance of listening to your patient." *This was a novel idea to him? How sad.* I was glad that it had worked out well for all of us. I didn't have a needle shoved into my chest, and they had a teaching moment.

The day that I was released from the hospital, I was given a pamphlet about heart failure. It had a picture of two, smiling seventy-somethings on the front. It advised me to weigh myself daily. If I gained two pounds or more in a day or five-plus pounds in a week, I was to call my doctor because these were signs of heart failure. *Obviously these people have never been on a cruise before*, I thought. The pamphlet also reminded me to minimize my salt intake, and not drink more than six glasses of beverage a day. It recommended exercise like walking to the mailbox or light gardening. I should never exert myself so much that I felt my heart pound or I could not talk comfortably. I had officially entered the geriatric world.

I was given prescriptions for Coreg®, to control my high blood pressure, and Lasix®, a diuretic to minimize the fluid buildup in my body. I was told to take magnesium oxide and potassium, and I was taken off of Lisinopril. The doctors scheduled a blood test for a week later to assess if these drug levels were working, and warned me that I might be lethargic during my adjustment to them. I was already pretty tired since my heart was still weak, and I was still recovering from the Doxil® and Cytoxan®. So it was hard to know how lethargic was too lethargic. I had to start teaching again in a week.

On the first day of class, I had to rest on a bench after walking about fifty feet from my car to the building that I taught in. Then, I had to rest again after climbing one flight of stairs. I taught sitting on a stool. This was just the go-over-the-syllabus week, so I knew I was in for a hard semester even without the chemotherapy. My digestion was also strange. Instead of my usual diarrhea, I was constipated. Yet my bowel movements had the same urgency as before. One day that week, I felt my anus tearing and saw that I had passed a hard, softball-sized stool. Bleeding followed.

The day after my blood test, a nurse at the cardiologist's office called me eight times, leaving increasingly-alarmed and alarming messages that I should stop taking the drugs and call them back. My bad cell phone habits meant that I didn't get these messages until the following day. When I called, they said that my medication needed to be adjusted before I had kidney failure. I should stop taking potassium and take only half of the Lasix®. I needed to get another blood test the following day and again the following week. They said that my blood tests had reported dangerous levels of drugs in my system and that I must have been exhausted. *Welcome to my world*, I thought. Apparently a normal level of chemo exhaustion is an alarming level of exhaustion in the heart community. The drugs were adjusted again the following week.

The following month, when I refilled my prescriptions, I found out why the drugs had been off. For a month I had been taking two, little, round pills (which were in the bottle labeled

"Coreg®") and one little, football-shaped pill (which was in the bottle labeled "Lasix®"). This time the footballs were in the Coreg® bottle and the round pills were in the Lasix® bottle. Before taking any, I told my husband that I thought the prescription had been filled incorrectly. Again, he turned to the Internet and found photographs of the pills. The prescription had been inaccurately filled the first month. For the first ten days after I left the hospital, I had been taking twice as much of the diuretic as the doctor had recommended. That explained the kidney problems and the stool problems. A pharmacist's mistake had risked my health. The mistake had also caused dehydration that had led to the softball stool, the rectal pain, and anal bleeding.

By April 2009, my CA125 was up to 150. By now I knew that when the tumor marker went up, the doctors would suggest more chemotherapy. Since my heart function had rebounded to 45 percent of the blood being pushed out with each beat, they thought I was strong enough for heart-friendly chemotherapy. I had already tried most of what they had to offer, but Dr. Kind thought Abraxane® might work. The trick, he said, was to find a drug that would fool the cancer into allowing the drug to destroy it without the drug being too hard on the rest of me. Although Abraxane® was a drug that my cancer was familiar with (diminishing the likelihood that it would successfully trick the cancer), it was steeped in a lipid solution that my body hadn't seen before. Dr. Kind was hopeful. Abraxane® was heart-friendly drug; but it wasn't hair-friendly. I would be bald again, and no longer incognito.

I asked for an every-three-week schedule, for Abraxane®, rather than the three-weeks-on-and-one-week-off schedule. It meant that I would have worse side effects for a week or ten days, but then have enough time off to do things. I also wanted to avoid being in a medical setting four days out of every week (one blood test, one chemo treatment, and two shots) and the weekly stress of wondering if my platelets would be too low for me to receive treatment. Having a large-dose schedule would give me more control over my schedule during the summer. I wouldn't have been able to do this if I was still teaching, but since it would start during the week of final exams and continue throughout the summer, it was do-able. I started the Abraxane® on April 7th, 2009.

Although Dr. Kind preferred a weekly dose, he accepted my rationale and endorsed my plan. "If it's going to work, it is going to work," he conceded. I couldn't help but feel more in control of my treatment than I had been before. In part, this was because I was dealing primarily with Dr. Kind instead of Dr. Sure. In part, it was because the doctors had lost some power when they had not taken my complaints about the cough, the blood pressure, and the swelling as seriously as they should have. But mostly, it was because David and I had gained power when David, not the doctors, had correctly diagnosed my heart failure. My husband had done with ease what the doctors never quite seemed to achieve— he had saved my life.

With our newly-found authority, David and I insisted that the oncologists and the cardiologists coordinate my care. I wanted each to know what the other was doing, so each could advise me. I didn't want to sacrifice my heart for my cancer treatment, nor did I want my cancer treatment compromised by my heart problems. The cardiologist thought this was a good idea, and told me that he had called Dr. Kind many times without hearing back from him. When we saw Dr. Kind, he said that he was aware of these calls but hadn't gotten a chance to call the cardiologist back. He would try again. I doubt that he tried, but I know that he never succeeded.

When I realized that this seemingly simple request—for two doctors to talk to each other about my case—was not going to happen, I was reminded of how limited a patient's power is. I couldn't get them to do anything they didn't want to do. The best I could hope for was that I could stop them from doing things that would kill me. We tried to protect my heart by copying the cardiologist on all of my chemotherapy lab work. We also asked him how high my blood pressure could go before I should halt the chemotherapy. My husband was shocked that Dr. Kind never called the cardiologist. Dr. Kind was, after all, a kind man. But nothing that doctors did—or didn't do—surprised me much anymore.

Abraxane's® lipid solution might have made it more likely to fool the cancer into letting the poison inside the cell (like a Trojan horse). But it was particularly hard on my digestion. It felt like I was passing battery acid, a sensation I did not remember having with the other chemotherapies. This was accompanied by anal bleeding and burning, headaches and exhaustion, making for a horrendous first week after chemotherapy. The next two weeks were better. I decided that a 2-to-1 ratio of pretty good to very bad was acceptable.

By now, I had been going to the local hospital for blood tests before each chemotherapy session for almost two years. The admission staff recognized me. The nurses who drew my blood from the PowerPort® knew me. They were friendly. They always asked how I was doing and actually listened to my responses. I seemed to have earned a lot of good will from them because I hadn't gotten upset one day when blood had gushed all over my shirt. Equipment failure, human error—I didn't know what the problem was. I didn't really care, since the mistake only hurt my clothes. The nurse seemed to appreciate that I didn't take it out on her. Pretty soon, I was comfortable enough with them to be friendly, too. The familiarity with the process and the people, as well as the minimal discomfort and uncertainty, made these interactions completely different from what I was used to experiencing with healthcare personnel.

I got to know the nurses while they were sticking the needle into my chest, pulling out blood, putting it into small vials, and putting Heparin (an anti-clotting fluid) into my PowerPort®. One nurse had a father who was dying of cancer. She thought he seemed to be enjoying the attention it brought him. She didn't think that all of the CAT scans his doctors were ordering were justified. Another nurse had a retired husband who wanted to travel, but she didn't have enough vacation time to satisfy his wanderlust. She wanted to retire too, but she had to keep working so they could have health insurance. I got to know some of the women who worked in the laboratory and took me (and my blood) to and from Day Surgery, where the nurses were. One of them had a tattoo of a black tear under her eye. It was for her son, who had been incapacitated in a car accident while he was in high school over a decade earlier. He couldn't move or speak, but he could see and make sounds. She was sure that some of those sounds were laughter. She wondered if he might have been better off if he'd died in the accident with his friends. "I know that sounds bad," she said. I told her I didn't think it did. I didn't feel like these women were on the opposite side of a large chasm—a feeling I usually had with healthcare providers. I felt like we had things in common, and we trusted each other.

The Abraxane® was slowly bringing the CA125 down, but it became increasingly difficult to endure. Soon the ratio of pretty good to very bad days was 1-to-1. After my seventh dose of this drug, my predictably awful ten days led to severe abdominal pain. Unfortunately, it was a familiar feeling that I suspected was an intestinal blockage. I called to ask the gastrointestinal doctor to order an x-ray, which he did. It revealed a partial blockage of the small intestine. While I was in the waiting room of the radiology department, the doctor came out to talk to me. He got out his smart phone and asked me what kind of chemotherapy I was on now. The side effect list for Abraxane® included intestinal blockages. He knew I didn't want to have the nose tube or get admitted to the hospital if it could be avoided, so he sent me home with instructions to remain on fluids until my bowels moved. If that didn't happen in the next day, I would be admitted to the hospital. Fortunately, it didn't come to that.

That week I went seventy-two hours without eating solid foods. I wasn't sure what would happen when I ate solids. When I finally did eat, I was conscious of exactly where in my digestive process the food was. I knew when it would hit my troubled small intestines. *Either I will tolerate this, or the pain will start again,* I thought. *It will start with aches, then more extreme spasms, then I'll start burping, then my abdomen will distend, and I will be back in the hospital.* I waited. Thankfully my intestines grumbled and struggled and eventually, digested the food.

I took a two-week break, unable to face more chemotherapy on the day that it was scheduled. That was the first day I was able to stand long enough to toast a bagel, and was confident enough to eat it without fear.

Chapter 13: "He Never Threw Himself a Pity Party": Reflections on the Media's Ideal Cancer Patient

I have watched a lot of television from my sick bed since my diagnosis. I want to be distracted from my discomfort and the boredom of not being able to do things or even think clearly. I avoid dramas, especially hospital dramas with their obsessive attention to the sex lives of doctors. I also don't want to see the parade of sick guest stars and the plethora of mystery illnesses. Yet I still can't seem to avoid television's version of cancer. Whether it's presented as fiction or reality, on serious channels or silly ones, the messages seem the same. They show me what it is like to live with cancer, and it is not how I am living. They show me the ideal cancer patient, and it is not me. I cannot escape from this feeling even when I shut myself away from strangers and friends. It has infiltrated my bedroom. It is coming in through the television, the magazine in my mailbox, and on web pages on my computer.

The media—whether it is centralized, like television shows, or decentralized, like the Internet—portray cancer as a surmountable challenge and chemotherapy as a cakewalk. Much like a montage, treatment is quick, progress inevitable, and life is back-to-normal before you know it. Media lauds patients who accept individual responsibility for their own survival, exalting the battle metaphor for having cancer, rewarding patients who bravely undergo treatment and refuse to give up. Patients who suffer through treatment, and acknowledge the potential succor of death, are vilified or silenced.

The media cites chemotherapy as evidence that we have over our bodies. It's a deafeningly simple message: we control how our bodies look, what they do, and how healthy they are. All we need to do is follow certain guidelines and buy certain products. As a result, if we are unlucky enough (or irresponsible enough with our own health) to be diagnosed with cancer, we are expected to choose chemotherapy and not complain. Alternative approaches to treatment or stopping chemotherapy are equivalent to abdicating control or giving up.

This dreamy-eyed vision of cancer and its corresponding party-line on how to beat cancer hamstrings the media when real cancer patients lose their battles with cancer. Even the media cannot stand over a corpse and pronounce death deserved. When a cancer patient dies, the media scramble to spin the story as a victory, even when the facts belie that characterization. To facilitate this reframing, the media perpetuates the idea that having cancer somehow makes you a better person. Whether you fight and win, or fight and die, as long as you fight, you are exonerated, purified—defined by fire.

Our national consciousness correlates robust health with hard work, good choices, and selflessness—sickness with indolence, poor choices, and selfishness. This kind of thinking, perhaps unintentionally, positions the chronically or terminally ill as complicit in their illnesses; it seems to congratulate the survivors and blame those who aren't surviving.

I am tired of being vilified for having cancer, or rather, for having cancer in the wrong way—the way that makes healthy people uncomfortable. It seems that I am condemned to be perpetually reproached for my slow, painful, and unwarranted death by the likes of Elizabeth Cohen, a CNN health reporter who claims in her article "5 Mistakes Women Make at the Doctor's Office," (Cohen, 2008) that women get inferior care because of the mistakes that they make when talking to doctors. Cohen (2008) says that women don't assert themselves by challenging doctors and asking questions, often failing to trust their own intuitions.

She ignores the fact that media portrayals of cancer patients *discourage* these behaviors by depicting cancer patients as compliant, positive, and grateful to the medical community. Cohen (2008) also notes that women don't recognize gender bias and even when they do, they are more than male patients likely to remain with the same doctor. Isn't this similar to blaming the battered wife for being beaten and letting her abusive husband off the hook? Shouldn't the reporter be complaining that doctors don't listen to women, and that some continue to allow their sexist attitudes about our credibility to interfere with their treatment of us? When doctors conclude that our problems are due to women being stressed out, pre-menstrual, post-menopausal, or just emotional, how is our intuition that they are wrong going to help us?

Cohen seems to think that changing doctors is easy and effective at increasing the quality of care, but she's ignoring the fact that the problems are systemic. It isn't with this doctor or that one. It's the medical profession that trains doctors to order another test and resist any challenges to their authority. It is the media apparatus that confirms this training, socializing us to receive care in a way that is comfortable for everyone except the patient.

I take this report personally. I don't have any emotional distance from it. I feel like CNN is blaming me for every mistake that my doctors have made when they should have been caring for me. If treatment is a test of my convictions, and cancer is a test of my character, then my obituary would report me as spineless and morally bankrupt.

* * *

Television's fictional portrayals of cancer broadcast innumerable unreasonable expectations for the activities, attitudes, and choices of cancer patients. If all you knew about breast cancer and its treatment was what you saw Samantha go through on *Sex and the City*, you'd think that you could drink champagne while getting a chemo infusion, have enough energy to go to lunch in fabulous hats, and then to film premieres in pink wigs. You wouldn't need to miss work or cut back on your social life.

Samantha never looked tired. She only occasionally seemed scared. And my personal pet peeve—she kept her eyebrows. Actually, all of the television cancer patients get to keep their eyebrows and eyelashes. They put a scarf on the actresses and sometimes shave the actors' heads, but they don't touch their eyebrows and eyelashes. Makeup artists can convince us that people are vampires and aliens, but they can't make it look like someone doesn't have eyebrows? That's hard to believe. I guess they just don't want anyone on television to look that bad. Well, we chemotherapy patients *do* look that bad, and television doesn't prepare anyone for that.

In addition to watering down the side effects of chemotherapy, television also overestimates its efficacy—frequently resurrecting characters from the brink of a cruel death by cancer, always just in the nick of time. In the fall of 2009, the season premiere of the hospital drama *Grey's Anatomy* miraculously revived Dr. Izzy, who had flat-lined on the operating table after having a cancerous tumor removed during the season finale. The actress who played the part explained proudly that this was "a hopeful storyline for people who suffer from very serious cancers."[6] Why on earth would she think that an unrealistic fictional storyline would give hope to real people with real cancers that have high mortality rates? Unfounded hope delays important conversations, thoughts, and preparations that there might not be time for in the end. If the fantasy of Dr. Izzy's recovery did provide people with actual hope, it was a false and cruel one.

Television blames cancer patients for losing hope, portraying chemotherapy as a duty that cancer sufferers should bravely and gladly perform on behalf of their family and friends. Mid-January 2010 on season forty-one of the ABC soap opera *All My Children* (Carruthers, 2010) the character of J.R. saw his

---

[6] Editor's Note: I was unable to locate this source. According to Larson's notes, this interview aired on *E! News*. She cites September 24, 2009 as the date she viewed this interview.

leukemia return soon after his first series of chemotherapy ended. He wanted to take his new wife on a honeymoon before resuming treatment. He said that he wanted to "stop talking about cancer for at least a week" and to make memories "in case something happens" (Carruthers, 2010). His doctor agreed that two weeks on a sunny island wouldn't hurt him; the chemotherapy could wait that long.

J.R.'s wife's reaction embodied the cultural expectations for cancer patients, demanding that J.R. fight for his life and his relationships, at any and all costs to himself. Refusing to do as much, and do so immediately, was the same as turning his back on his family. "If you want to take the trip, fine," she challenged, continuing, "But I won't be here when you get back" (Carruthers, 2010). She was unbending: "If you want to be with me, you'll stay and fight for your and our future" (Carruthers, 2010). There is no discussion of J.R.'s desires or what his body requires. Instead, J.R.'s wife delivers an ultimatum that demands he subsume his individual wants and needs to his familial responsibilities. Never mind that no therapist would ever tell a healthy person, much less a chronically- or terminally-ill one, that it would be healthy to subordinate his or her needs to the needs of his or her family. J.R. admits that he is scared and hugs his wife, telling her that she is right.

The narrative is telling us that cancer patients owe everything to their families and nothing to themselves. Delaying or taking a break from chemotherapy is turning our backs on our families and our futures. Healthy people who love cancer sufferers do not need to consider what *we're* going through and the difficulty of *our* choices. By the end of the scene, it is clear that while the ill have a responsibility to their healthy counterparts, their healthy counterparts do not have a responsibility to consider the feelings, needs, or wants of the ill.

In addition to depicting fighting cancer as a responsibility that a cancer sufferer has to his or her family, J.R.'s storyline also portrayed cancer as a test of character. In another scene, J.R.'s stepfather explains to J.R.'s wife that J.R. is afraid to find out "if he has what it takes to win" (Carruthers, 2010). She should make him see that "he doesn't have a choice" (Carruthers, 2010). Technically J.R. *does* have a choice to reject more chemotherapy, so the dialogue must be referring to some sort of a social contract. I think it goes like this: if people care about you, then you don't have the option to die without a long, drawn-out, painful fight that proves that you love them. I think that's an unreasonable expectation. Love doesn't mean that you owe someone your life. There's not a set amount of pain that is reasonable to assume people should go through before they can die, or in this case, take a short break. How reasonable is it for people who are well and have active, full lives to expect their sick relatives to suffer a little longer? I have trouble with the whole storyline, but J.R. was persuaded by it. He professes his love for his family and his desire to get right back to chemotherapy instead of taking a trip. The lesson seems to be that people with strong characters are able to endure treatment and beat cancer. The implication is that there must be something wrong with those of us who don't continue with chemotherapy until we're cured: we *don't* "have what it takes."

The next plot twist showed stopping treatment as an act of cowardice. As the chemotherapy begins hurting J.R. more than it helps him, he is hospitalized and receives a bone-marrow transplant. His body initially rejects the transplant, and J.R. lapses into a coma. This development allowed the show to bring back his dead mother, Dixie. As an angel, this popular character met her son at the doors of heaven and told him that he didn't belong there yet. He longed to stay in this peaceful setting with her, his uncle, and his first wife. But his mother told him that he was trying to "run away from his problems" like he "always did" (Carruthers, 2010). She reminded him of how selfish he had been during his life. She said that death was another escape, like his alcoholism, which he needed to resist. Dixie's lectures confirm that stopping treatment is a failure of fortitude, a lapse in judgment, and ultimately, an indictment of J.R.'s character.

The morals of this story are multifold. Two unsuccessful cycles of chemotherapy and a bone marrow replacement isn't fighting hard enough. It doesn't matter if you do what the doctors ask and suffer through hard therapies; the determination of whether or not you live or die is how strong your will is. Dixie's haranguing snaps J.R. from his coma, cured of cancer, proving that survival is a choice. If you have the determination and strength of character, you will survive. Peacefully accepting death (even when you are in a coma) is selfish and weak. Life-threatening cancer is presented as an opportunity for a flawed man to redeem himself. No wonder I feel like people are judging me when I tell them I have terminal cancer and that chemotherapy cannot save me.

The cancer film *The Bucket List* was frank about the side effects of chemotherapy, but disingenuous about the comfort of prolonged hospital stays. The film admitted that chemotherapy makes you vomit, causes your blood to seep out of your veins, and gives you leg aches. While I certainly never felt like eating a big meal during a chemo cycle like Jack Nicholson's character did, the film accurately showed why it was a bad idea to try. However, it also showed the characters in a medical system that seemed much more humane than any I have encountered. The most jarringly inauthentic thing about the movie was that the hospital room seemed more like a motel room. The door was always shut, there was a wooden bookshelf, and it was quiet. There was no beeping medical equipment, no announcements over an intercom, no staff coming in and out without knocking. Anyone who has ever been in a hospital would note the falseness of the scene in which Jack Nicholson's character's assistant comes in to wake him up by pulling the curtains to reveal a sunny day. No one is allowed to sleep late in a hospital. Mornings, before guests are allowed to visit, are full of action. After they finish taking your blood, feeding you, receiving a visit from the morning-medication nurse and her squeaky cart, being showered or bathed and visited by a doctor, you *might* be able to doze off for a bit. Might.

Although the film exceeded my low expectations for fictional portrayals of cancer patients, the very feasibility of a bucket list eluded me. Many people had asked me what was on my own bucket list, therefore assuming that I *would* be healthy enough to do the things that I wanted to do and that the things I would want to do would be finite. Neither is true. The bucket list concept is for people who don't know about the gradual adjustments sick people have to make. If I can't be away from a bathroom, how can I put a safari on my list? I can't even look forward to a last meal like a death row prisoner might. What I love to eat has already become impossible to digest. Content of the film aside, the very title implies an ease and predictability to having cancer that I have never experienced.

Why do I get so worked up over these little points? I know that no movie or television show is totally realistic. Yet I think these repeated misrepresentations reinforce and introduce misperceptions about being in the hospital that make it harder for the chronically and terminally ill to feel understood. I know a number of people who expected to rest in a hospital. They didn't get to. I know others who think you're guaranteed drugs that will make illnesses pain free and maybe even pleasant. Not so. People think that if you're in the hospital, you'll either die or get well. No, there are lots of options in between. They think that chemotherapy treatments don't have to slow you down. When it confines me to my bed and bathroom, people wonder if I'm really sick or using my illness to avoid things I don't want to do. People expect us to have eyebrows and eyelashes and to have a full head of hair again in a few months. We won't.

Lately, I've been seeing buzz about a new television show called *The Big C*. Laura Linney plays a woman with terminal cancer. I think she's an excellent casting choice—pale and thin enough to maybe pull this off. I wonder if we'll finally get a recurring character with terminal cancer on television to show an authentic version of what being a cancer sufferer is like. Then, I saw that the show was going to be a comedy. Cancer hasn't made me or the people around me laugh much, so I doubt that this show will either. I can't help but wonder if the terminally ill character will be allowed to die or if her survival will be based on ratings, instead of authenticity.

* * *

The most visible chronically- and terminally-ill patients are celebrities. And media coverage of celebrities with cancer implicitly provides a template for how to be an ideal cancer patient. Ideal cancer patients retain normalcy by continuing to work, refusing to complain, softening reality when they describe their treatment, thinking positively, and emerging from the chrysalis (which I would call a "crucible") of cancer as better, happier versions of themselves. Not only does the media (and our culture) try to deny that dying will be the outcome for many cancer patients, but they celebrate celebrity patients who (at least on the surface) seem to validate this denial. The most ostentatious display of this template is from an article written by Rick Reilly, "George vs. the Dragon" (2010), describing the grueling treatment basketball coach George Karl was undergoing for throat and nose cancer.

Reilly didn't shy away from a forthright depiction of the side effects plaguing Karl. However, the praise he lavished upon Karl for his refusal to allow the side effects of chemotherapy and radiation to derail his normalcy undermined any success Reilly may have had in eroding the model of the ideal cancer patient. The article described the radiation that had charred the inside of Karl's mouth so severely that he could barely talk, the tube inserted in his stomach so he could eat, and the cancer drugs that made him nauseous. Only the morphine patch made treatment possible to endure. In spite of the horrors of Karl's treatment, Reilly's editorializing still suggested an unreasonable standard for the behavior of cancer patients. Reilly (2010) reported a nurse informing Karl that treatment would "only [. . .] get harder." She predicted that he wouldn't "feel like working." But Reilly's follow up cavalierly dismissed the nurse's prediction: "Clearly," he quipped, "she's never met George Karl" (2010).

We all know what Reilly's editorial remark is meant to mean: George Karl's strength, determination, and willpower preclude him from leaving work during cancer treatment. But if the time comes when Karl doesn't feel like working, does Reilly's comment hint at some level of personal failure? Would it have been so bad for Reilly to have simply given Karl his blessing to stay home sick—or if not his blessing, at least his confidence that Karl, an adult, would be able to make the best choice for himself when the time came?

Reilly (2010) validated Karl for his ability to conceal the gruesome realities of cancer treatment, writing about Karl's efforts to "cover [his] tube" and his rash while coaching. (It is not enough, apparently, to note that Karl continues to work at all while undergoing treatment for cancer.) Reilly (2010) categorized Karl's efforts to conceal his pain as a "refus[al] to play the victim card," a phrase I find particularly offensive. It indicates that whether a patient allows cancer to impact his or her daily routine is a mere matter of willpower. It trivializes what cancer treatments put people through. It makes statements like, "I'm too sick to do that" sound like cop-outs when they are really just honest statements of fact, which are usually spoken with sadness and regret.

Why would we want to play the victim card when there is such a stigma in America to being a victim? Maybe it's because we've spent so much time building a culture of denial around cancer and illness, and doctors' abilities to mitigate suffering. Maybe cancer sufferers have hidden their pain, their rashes, their vomiting, and their feeding tubes for so long that healthy people cannot imagine how bad treatment really is. Maybe we've heard so many upbeat, bullshit messages: cancer is not that bad; it's a journey, not a curse; treatment has come a long way; and that we are fine and shouldn't let cancer define us—that saying "I can't do that; I'm sick" is no longer credible? Maybe if we could admit that cancer makes you sick, its treatments are grisly, and survival rates for many cancers are abysmal, sick people would have more credibility.

Karl's deification as an ideal cancer patient is complete by the conclusion of Reilly's article, which ends by confirming that having cancer is a cathartic experience. The article closes with Karl noting that he "never used to think about sunshine" (Reilly, 2010). Reilly (2010) observes that Karl "fairly beams saying [this]," and proposes, "Guess there's more than one way to radiate." This conclusion renders Karl's cancer *comfortable* for readers who are otherwise uncomfortable with the notion that George Karl, a good man, has a bad disease. When a good man has a bad disease, there has to be something to render his suppressed suffering worthwhile. For this reason, Reilly depicts Karl as blessed by cancer: it is not all for naught. But all I can think about is Karl's charred mouth.

The embedded lessons from the article about George Karl are simple: cancer patients who comply with our cancer mythology—that it is treatable, endurable, surmountable, and purifying (all of the traits that make cancer and cancer treatment palatable to the healthy)—are worthy of our attention and praise. Celebrity cancer patients who are not compliant with this model are at risk of being shoved aside or, if they lose their cancer battle, having their images burnished after their deaths. When Patrick Swayze was diagnosed with pancreatic cancer, the subsequent media frenzy, as epitomized in his post-diagnosis interview with Barbara Walters entitled "Patrick Swayze: The Truth" (2009), managed to run the gamut of cancer coverage. First, Swayze was implicitly implicated for his own illness. Walters asked him if he thought that smoking caused his disease (thereby implying she suspected that it had) and Swayze gratified her by admitting that he felt that there was a correlation between his smoking and his cancer (Swayze, 2009). This question allowed the public to comfortably distance themselves from Swayze's diagnosis: he smokes and I don't, so I don't have to worry.

The moment that Swayze died, the media launched its attempt to exonerate him—transforming his loss into a win by emphasizing his fighting spirit. I say, "emphasizing," because Swayze's approach to dealing with cancer was more complex than the media coverage of his death allowed. At many moments in his interview with Walters (2009), Swayze subverted the dominant narrative of cancer treatment. Swayze recognized the likelihood that he would die from cancer, but he also felt that acknowledging that likelihood was not incompatible with living while he could. While he characterized cancer as "a long hard battle" that he planned to "fight," he qualified that this "battle" was "one that I'm going to win according to certain rules—the rules that the cancer isn't going away" (Thomson and Wallace 2008). He challenged the never-say-die mentality so inherent in our culture, pledging that, "One of the things I'm not going to do is chase staying alive. You can spend so much time chasing staying alive that you won't live. I want to live" (Thomson and Wallace, 2009). Without some quality of life, he explained, the fight would not be worth waging. To hear any patient reject so gracefully and confidently the culturally-insistent messages was refreshing.

These moments weren't the clips that the media replayed once Swayze was dead. The parts that I saw replayed on commercials and entertainment news shows were the ones that fit the ideal patient model. He talked a lot about working twelve-hour days during which "nobody on the set ever saw me whine or moan like a girly man" (Swayze, 2009). Swayze was replayed saying things like, "I'm not ready to go yet," and "I want to last until they find a cure" (Thomson and Wallace, 2008). These clips received more airtime than the ones in which Swayze spoke bluntly about the realities of the disease and its treatment. During Swayze's interview with Walters, he confided that "There would be many mornings where I'd be curled up on a bathmat, just this side of a scream, so I didn't wake [his wife] Lisa up" (Swayze, 2009). This Swayze vanished in the coverage that followed his death.

In tribute to Swayze after his death, *In Touch* magazine complimented his bravery, work ethic, confidence, unselfishness, and the fact that "he never talked about dying."[7] I don't think that I believe this, but if it were true, why would it be a good thing? The tribute also included this infuriating statement: "Despite all these tragic setbacks, Patrick was never one to have a pity party for himself and always had a positive upbeat attitude—even when chemotherapy put him through hell." I think it is too much to ask that someone be positive when they've exhausted all of the potential remedies to their terminal illness and they are going "through hell." It is reasonable and acceptable for someone who was healthy, happy, rich, famous, and in a wonderful marriage to sometimes feel sorry for themselves when they were incapacitated by a horrible disease that would kill them at the age of fifty-seven. It is preposterous and offensive to imply that sharing your grief about dying with friends and family could be considered a "pity party." What comes to mind when you hear the term "pity party?" For me, it is spoiled adolescents crying about not getting everything they want. There is no way that the phrase is appropriate for someone dying of cancer.

---

[7] Editor's Note: I was unable to locate this source. According to Larson's notes, this interview was printed in *In Touch* Magazine. She cites September 28, 2009 as the date she read this article.

Of all of the cancer narratives churned out by the media machine, the one I felt the most emotionally close to was Farrah Fawcett's. During one of my treatments that coincided with the end of Fawcett's, I became fixated on news about her. It reminded me of how focused my father had become on Donna Reed during his illness. Reed died of pancreatic cancer in 1986, not long before my father died. Perhaps it is natural to feel a kinship and interest in celebrities who are dying of cancer while you are? It probably also depends upon who the celebrity is and whether their work or persona resonates with you. My father loved westerns and other films that aligned good guys against the bad guys in battles that were sure to be won by those with virtue. His favorite movie was *It's a Wonderful Life*, in which Donna Reed played the loving wife of Jimmy Stewart's upright, long-suffering, small-town hero.

Although I couldn't relate to Fawcett during the heyday of her career, I remember being captivated by her image. When I was in high school, she was the "it" girl. Like other awkward female teenagers, I watched her on *Charlie's Angels* with vicarious pleasure. Beauty, power, close girlfriends, and excitement: it was hard to resist the show's appeal. In real life, she was married to handsome Lee Majors, *The Six Million Dollar Man*. Things got messier for her later, but for a time when I was most impressionable about becoming a woman, she seemed to have it all. Now she had a rare and aggressive anal cancer.

Once Fawcett was diagnosed, the minimizing began: one of Fawcett's doctors appeared on *Access Hollywood* to share his opinion that the "hardest thing about chemotherapy is the hair loss."[8] Could he possibly believe this? Clearly he has never taken the drugs that he dispenses, but hasn't he listened to any of his patients? Or do they just tell him what they know he (and everyone else around them) wants to hear? Maybe he, or whoever edited the interview, is just trying to delude the public so they won't be so frightened? Maybe the culture of blame and the ideology of attitudinal cures make it easier for people, including doctors, to deny how devastating chemotherapy is on patients? I don't know.

All I know is that this is a ludicrous statement. Hair loss is a social stigma; you don't look like people expect you to. You don't fit the conventional version of attractive anymore. You make people uncomfortable by reminding them of their own fragility. That can be hard, but it can't kill you. The doctor's statement marginalizes how sick I feel and how vulnerable chemotherapy makes me to life-threatening problems. It also amplifies the idea that the body's primary value is how it looks. After I watched the interview, I expected all of the coverage of Fawcett's illness would follow the same predictable pattern—reducing cancer treatment to the sum of its most apparent side effects.

When I saw that Fawcett had produced a documentary called *Farrah's Story* (2009) about her experience with cancer, I knew I had to watch it. The documentary gave people who had no experience with fighting cancer a brutally-honest view of what it entailed. I watched the nurses try again and again to find veins in

---

[8] Editor's Note: I was unable to locate this source. According to Larson's notes, this interview aired on *Access Hollywood*. She cites May 14, 2009 as the date she viewed this interview.

her damaged arms and hands. I wondered why she didn't have a PowerPort® and thanked God (again) for mine. I watched her get needles inserted into her tumors, and subsequently get sick in the airport bathroom on her way home. I saw her inject herself and take dozens of pills. I saw her sedated in bed, unable to sit up for her son's last visit. I became emotionally exhausted watching all of her suffering. I understood more than many viewers what she was going through. I knew that all of these painful procedures were an investment in a life that she wasn't getting back. I knew what it was like to torture oneself to kill a cancer that just wouldn't die. I knew the heartbreak, the exhaustion, and the misery.

What I couldn't relate to was the language of war and survival that Fawcett used to interpret the experience. She called the cancer a "terrorist" and the battle with it her "own private war" (Fawcett, Gleysteen, and Nevius 2009). She admitted, "I didn't think it would go on for two years. I thought I'd be cured" (Fawcett, Gleysteen, and Nevius 2009). Despite all evidence to the contrary, Fawcett's family and friends repeatedly claimed that she would win her battle. Her father said, "One more treatment, and she'll probably regain her health and be on the good side of life" (Fawcett, Gleysteen, and Nevius 2009). Her son said, "She'll be all right because she looks good" (Fawcett, Gleysteen, and Nevius 2009). She insisted, "I won't surrender," her nurse agreed, and her doctor told her "We'll win. We'll win. We'll win," after a scan revealed that the cancer had spread to her liver and returned to her anus (Fawcett, Gleysteen, and Nevius 2009). Hearing all that denial took my breath away.

Fawcett was hard on herself over the course of the documentary—hard on herself in ways that suggested she was conditioned to judge her own struggle with cancer through the media-perpetuated lens of the ideal cancer patient. In a nod to the expectation that cancer patients are supposed to be brave and suffer in silence, Fawcett said that she didn't want anyone to pity her. I've heard other cancer patients say that, too. I don't quite understand it. The word must connote something different to them than it does to me. I will gladly accept pity; it feels like acknowledgment for the hard things I am going through. It seems like sympathy to me. Why wouldn't Fawcett and I deserve sympathy? How could anyone watch what she was going through and not? Fawcett suggested that she blamed herself for her inability to recover: "I still haven't learned why I can't will my body to heal itself" (Fawcett, Gleysteen, and Nevius 2009). She must have listened to the positive-thinking/mind-over-matter gurus. She felt like she failed. She said, "I will not go gently into that good night" (Fawcett, Gleysteen, and Nevius 2009). But I thought that to go gently sounded wonderful. I pray for as gentle a death as my disease will allow. I root for it to spread to my kidneys instead of my lungs. I think that Fawcett and I have both suffered too much to be denied a gentle journey at the end. She said in her sweet childish voice that she believed that "the devil makes you sick and God makes you well" (Fawcett, Gleysteen, and Nevius 2009). She asked her father when he thought that God would do that for her. I felt my heart ache for her. I don't want her to wonder why God was letting her down.

She experienced something that has a lot in common with what I am going through. The way she talked about it seemed entirely different until she said something that I try not to think about: "Sometimes this disease makes me feel like a stranger to myself . . . inside a body that once was mine . . . intolerable suffering and pain, I have never known. I miss my life" (Fawcett, Gleysteen, and Nevius 2009). When she said this, I felt connected to her. I felt understood. Every now and then the media does that. They allow something true to cut through the crap. They allow a personal sentiment, one at odds with the bright-sided, can-do culture of survival. I find myself looking for those moments.

After Fawcett's death, the media swallowed her story whole. As though she had made a study of the tributes to Swayze, Fawcett's best friend Alana Stewart told Larry King following Fawcett's death that Fawcett had never talked about dying.[9] In fact, one of the last reports the Associated Press issued about Fawcett noted that Ryan O'Neal still planned to marry her (*USA Today*, 2009). Three days after this press release, on June 25th, 2009, Fawcett died; therefore, she couldn't give us this faux-happy ending. No amount of positive thinking, on Fawcett, O'Neal or anyone's part, could save her. Denial seemed to be layered upon denial.

* * *

---

[9] Editor's Note: I was unable to locate this source. According to Larson's notes, this interview aired on *CNN*. She cites March 10, 2010 as the date she viewed this interview.

When the news networks take time to cover a non-celebrity cancer patient, it is usually to critique a narrative that will not bow to the ideal arc: diagnosis; stoic suffering and treatment; and triumphant remission. The news channels in early 2008 gave continuing coverage to a story coming out of Minnesota that allowed us to see what a non-ideal cancer patient looked like. But because he was a teenager (usually described as a child), the coverage was harder on his mother. The first report I saw said that Danny Hauser had Hodgkin's Lymphoma, but was not undergoing chemotherapy because of his mother's religious beliefs. The story was framed as a religious-freedom-versus-child-welfare issue. The media only feature the reporters, doctors, and legal experts who sided against the mother's choice to prevent her son from getting the treatment that they said would save his life. Since the authorities were able to eventually force Danny into treatment, threatening to put him in foster care if he wasn't treated, the theme for the story was that justice was done. A child was saved by the system!

Aside from some brief sound bites, Danny and his mother had almost no voice in their own story. While the media continuously claimed that Danny's mother opposed chemotherapy on religious grounds, some cursory digging on the Internet revealed that Danny had already had some traditional chemotherapy treatments. It seemed to me that this meant there was more to their decision than a religious choice. If they had opposed chemotherapy entirely on religious grounds, he would not have agreed to the first treatments. I eventually learned that Danny had gotten so sick from his first chemotherapy treatments that even though his doctor said that it had reduced the size of his tumor, Danny didn't want to continue receiving them. His mother supported this decision based on her Native American spirituality, her belief in alternative medicine, and because she had seen her sister die while receiving chemotherapy.

While the national news story ended when the treatments recommenced, the local coverage continued until his last treatment when the media was able to pronounce the end of Danny's story "happy." The media reported that Danny and his mother continued to criticize the drugs, and the fact that Danny had been forced to take them. It reported that Danny stayed with his family during chemotherapy and radiation, that he had bad side effects, and that his cancer was receptive to the treatments. Danny had "beaten" the cancer. Of course it's easier to claim that someone beat cancer at the end of treatments, than it is months or years later when cancer may come back. By then, the news cycle for his story will have ended.

What bothered me about the story was how easily Danny's feelings were dismissed. The rhetoric of the coverage painted chemotherapy as something innocuous that would be good for him. Therefore, he should be made to do it. The coverage didn't explain what the treatments would be like and what their risks were. So I assume that people watching the news reports used the image of chemotherapy that they see in the media. If they did, they would naturally think that he and his mother were overreacting because chemotherapy is not a big deal anymore. They would have concluded that his mother needed to stop being a religious nut and start being a mother and that Danny needed to man up.

I read in an article from *ABC News* that during the hearing, Danny said he believed the chemotherapy would kill him and that if he were forced to have it, "I'd fight it. I'd punch them, and I'd kick them" (Cox, 2009). His words made me think about how many times doctors had told me things that were incorrect, and how my body or intuition often knew that. I remember how it felt to have them ignore me. I wondered if Danny had heard another voice, whether it was God's, his body's, or his soul's, which told him this wasn't the best thing for him. Maybe he would have died if he had been allowed to listen to that voice. I don't know. Doctors and the State don't know either, but they acted as though they did.

In my uncertainty, I am troubled by everyone else's surety. I was struck by how invested the State was in telling Danny what he had to do for his own good, yet how little it was willing to do after it told him. The State wasn't going to sit with him while the nurses stuck needles in his hands. The State wasn't going to hold a washcloth to his forehead while he vomited the next day. The government wasn't even going to be paying for his treatments. If the family was bankrupted by his medical care and the family farm lost, would the State have provided his family with an income? If college funds were emptied, would it have sent his siblings to college? I don't think so. That would be his family's responsibility.

I also wondered how it would have forced him to get treatment if the threat of being placed in foster care hadn't worked.

Would it have put him in the back of a police car and taken him to a clinic? When he got to the clinic, would it have held him down, drugged him, or put him in restraints? What if he'd had a fatal reaction to treatment? Whose responsibility would that have been? Would the State have said, "We're sorry, you were right," to his mother? Would the doctor? No.

I don't know if the State did the right thing making Danny receive chemotherapy. I do know that the media coverage of the situation was lacking. It was contemptuous of him and his mother and, by implication, anyone who chooses not to have chemotherapy treatments. The coverage minimized the horrendous nature of chemotherapy. It did not examine alternatives to chemotherapy. Neither did it interview the doctors who administer these alternative treatments. It didn't offer international comparisons, provide any of the important context about American healthcare policy, nor did it offer a description of the Patient's Bill of Rights and what those rights entail. I heard no debate about when a painful medical procedure crosses a line and becomes abuse. The media didn't ask psychologists what consequences there might be to Danny from forcing him to do this. The doctor got his patient. The State got its justice. The media got their happy ending. And Danny—Danny got his remission. But was it really *Danny's* remission? I don't know. I wonder if he does.

* * *

No matter which media outlet I turn to, someone is talking to, about, or around cancer patients. Because I am essentially house-bound, I read their words back on myself. During the election, President Barack Obama went to New Hampshire for a town hall meeting to answer questions from regular citizens. One of the women there introduced herself as a "three-time cancer survivor" (The White House, 2010). The audience applauded and President Obama replied, "We're proud of you" (The White House, 2010). This response was probably not noteworthy to most of the people who heard it. But most of the people aren't dying from cancer like I am. I am not like the woman at the meeting. The opposite of surviving cancer (her) is "not surviving cancer" (me). The opposite of "proud" is "ashamed." I think the president just implied that he's ashamed of me. I cannot imagine that he would ever actually say that he is ashamed of me for not beating cancer. If he did, he'd have to say it to his own mother, who died of ovarian cancer. So, he should have been more careful with his words. He should have said, "We're happy for you," or even, "We congratulate you." He shouldn't have attributed her survival to *her*, because that implies my death will be *my* responsibility.

Because my illness coincides with the healthcare reform debate, I get to watch clips from town hall meetings that I am too sick to attend. The public has been given a lot of airtime, but as prolific as portrayals of cancer patients are in television and film, actual sick people seemed conspicuously absent from the healthcare debate. The few who appeared were outnumbered and out-shouted by the healthy citizens opposed to universal coverage.

At one of the town hall meetings, I saw clips of a crowd booing a woman in a wheelchair who said she would die if national healthcare wasn't passed. People wondered why she didn't have health insurance and couldn't hold onto a job. No one asked if she was too sick to work, or if the loss of her job had led to the loss of her healthcare. I saw a woman (who had lost her job and been diagnosed with cancer) explain that she couldn't afford the surgery her doctor had deemed "urgent." Her congressman told her to find a program to subsidize her surgery, although he couldn't name any besides Medicaid. (She wasn't eligible.) I watched an old lady beg for help from her representative. Her husband was supposed to go from the hospital to the nursing home, but their insurance didn't cover it. Instead, he was sent home to her. She had to care for him because their insurance didn't pay for a home nurse. But she was having trouble feeding him through his tube, and she was too weak to move him. Her congressman told her to ask for help from her neighbors. The crowd applauded. I wondered if any of them got her address, so they could bathe the old man and change his diapers.

Although most of the people on television talking about healthcare reform weren't sick, many of them were angry. A woman was mad that we were "flirting with socialism." She then said that she didn't want anyone to take her Medicare away. She seemed unaware that Medicare was a government program passed in the 1960s, in spite of accusations that it was a socialist program. People talked a lot about how afraid they were that death panels would kill old people. That's what Sarah Palin had told them would happen. They were unaware that old people already have guaranteed healthcare, and none of the bills proposed taking it away from them. They didn't want to lose their freedom and their choices, but they didn't realize that insurance companies determine what medical care is covered, and can arbitrarily change the rules. They don't realize that people with pre-existing conditions have no choices under the current system.

Middle-class people like me, who aren't old enough to be as sick as we are, are in the most jeopardy under the current healthcare system. We don't have Medicare. We don't have Medicaid. Our health insurance comes from our employers. So when we get too sick to work, we have to hope that we can afford to keep our employee health insurance by paying a lot more for it under the Consolidated Omnibus Budget Reconciliation Act (COBRA). COBRA is hard to pay for the first six months after you stop working, because you don't get paid by most employers while you're establishing disability. COBRA only lasts for eighteen months. It takes two years of being on long-term medical disability from work for someone under sixty-five to be eligible for Medicare. What happens during the six months without COBRA and before Medicare? I don't know. We can't get a private plan because pre-existing conditions make us bad investments. Most of us don't have savings that would cover the full bills.

These are the things that I think about when I watch the hyped-up frenzy of the healthcare debate from my sickbed. People, who have no idea what this is like, and seem to be patting themselves on the back because they are healthy enough not to be worried about it, are doing most of the talking. I keep hoping that a cancer patient will capture the media's attention like Joe the Plumber did during the 2008 campaign. Of course, I hope that he or she is more authentic, thoughtful, honest, and articulate than Joe was. I think of what I would say if I could be "Stephanie the Patient" during this healthcare debate. I find myself making speeches in my head to the town hall meeting audiences, Anderson Cooper, and Larry King. I argue with Rush Limbaugh and lecture Barack Obama. I try to finish a sentence when I'm being interviewed by Chris Matthews. Unfortunately, no one hears these speeches but me. I don't need to be persuaded. I get tired of hearing my own arguments. I don't have any power anyway. I am so tired of listening to it that I switch to the *Food Network*.

Unfortunately, like a bad car accident, I can't keep my eyes off the healthcare debate for long. I watch the stonewalling and the waffling and the misrepresentations and the spinelessness of the legislators. This representative body does not seem like it represents me. I try to leave a message on my senator's voicemail, but a recorded voice tells me that it is full. I am alone again with my thoughts and anger. I email CNN and MSNBC, but I get no acknowledgement that the messages were read by anyone.

Then, I hear something frank and blunt that not only seems accurate, but also makes me laugh. It is said by a congressman from the city I grew up in. Orlando's representative, Alan Grayson, mocks opponents of the House bill by saying that their plan is: "Don't get sick. And if you do get sick . . . die quickly" (Montopoli, 2009). I did get sick. I am dying slowly. I am a problem. Maybe I'm just being defensive to think that this national debate blames me (and other ill people) for allowing ourselves to get sick. Maybe they just want to deny that we exist. A culture of lies and fairy tales helps them do that.

Chapter 14: "Maybe He Doesn't Want to Talk to Me": Trying Alternatives

In the fall of 2009, I had a decision to make. Should I continue to take Abraxane®, even though it had led to a partial blockage of my small intestine? Or should I, again, stop treatment before my CA125 was in the normal range? Unlike many of the women treated at the Mansion, I had not gotten a remission that would earn me a rest from chemotherapy. My breaks from chemotherapies occurred when my body was so broken down that it couldn't continue to tolerate treatment. I didn't know if it was even possible for chemotherapy to bring my CA125 number low enough to be in the normal range.

Dr. Kind was reluctant to blame the blockage on the Abraxane®. He recommended that I move to a less-toxic, weekly dose. I suspected that this wouldn't work—and that my body was done with chemotherapy for now (maybe forever) regardless of the dose. But I didn't have any concrete evidence to support this perception. Nevertheless, after a documented ileum, it felt dangerous to take more of the drug that had digestive disorders on its side-effects list.

The day before I was scheduled for the weekly dose, I was still waffling about what to do. I had made an appointment with a nutritionist to talk about what foods might improve my digestion.

In addition to being a nutritionist, she was a holistic healer, so she asked me to talk about my bigger health picture—what my medical history was as well as what was going on with me. Even though I warned her that my picture was huge and hard to summarize quickly, she urged me to tell her. After hearing it, she asked, "How can you continue to hand yourself over to a medical system that you don't believe in and don't trust?" I thought the answer was simple.

"Because it's the only game in town," I recited. But she didn't believe that. She talked a little bit about how the medical establishment was a business that was protecting its profits by portraying treatment alternatives as illegitimate. She could work with me to help me let go of the cancer that I was holding onto. She didn't like to hear me call the cancer "my" cancer. She thought that words, thoughts, and feelings mattered.

She thought that the key to healing was for people to adjust their bad belief systems in order to let go of hurt, anger, disappointment, and guilt. She thought I needed to put aside my anger over the appendix and doctors' mistakes, and overcome my fear of pain. This thinking was what kept people sick. She mentioned, but didn't talk much about, a spiritual component— that the illness may be the result of something that had happened to my soul in a past life. Unresolved emotions and flawed thinking that resulted from a trauma could have caused the illness. She argued that talking to traditional psychotherapists wouldn't get rid of the anger and bad feelings that allowed the problem to keep hurting me. In fact, the illness could have resulted from a flawed belief system that developed before I was at the age of reasoning. Regardless of the origin, the idea was that I needed to recognize the harmful belief or belief system and let it go. If I could leave it behind, she claimed, my body could heal. She suggested I listen when my body talked, and ask it what it wanted more often—not just in times of crisis.

I enjoyed talking to her and hearing her ideas, even though I didn't find them entirely persuasive. Why would her anecdotes be any more applicable to my situation than the doctors'? I didn't like the blame implied in the idea about belief systems and illness. I didn't know if it was possible to overcome my anger and fears, but it sounded like something worth trying to do even if it didn't cure me.

She suggested acupuncture, meditation, visualization, and a sort of chanting (which she didn't call chanting). She also wanted me to change my language toward more positive terms. Positive language had a higher vibration that was healing. To help me resist fear, I was to remind myself, "The opposite of fear is gratitude; they can't coexist at the same moment in your mind. So, when you feel fearful, try to have an attitude of gratitude." Although I tend to be wary of advice that rhymes, I decided to give it a try.

What about tomorrow's chemotherapy? I knew that she was against it, but she advised me to see what my body thought. "Ask your body what you should do before you go to sleep tonight" she advised. "It will give you an answer," she said confidently. Since my mind was so torn, I decided to give it a try. So before I went to bed, I asked aloud,

"Should I have chemo tomorrow? I will accept and heed whatever the answer is."

I dreamt that I was sitting on a deck in an Adirondack chair looking at a bay. It was a beautiful, clear day. I could hear water lapping, and the lines of a sailboat clanging against the mast. I was calm. I was resting. My conscious self said, *I don't understand this message.* Still in the dream, someone else started to walk up a few steps to join me on the deck. I thought it was an old woman because she was wearing a long, full skirt and long sleeves with lace at the wrists. Her hair was grey and pulled back in a bun. The old-fashioned style and her slow gait made me think she was old. I could not see her face clearly, but I knew that she was me. Was this a reassuring message that I would not die in my fifties?

As she got closer, I could see that what I thought were wrinkles marking her face were actually bones. She was a skeleton, but she was smiling. I was not afraid of her. She was coming toward me—joining me. We were going to sit together on the deck and look at the water. What did this mean? That I was going to die soon, but it would be peaceful? My conscious voice said again, *I don't understand what you're saying. I don't know what this means.* Then a clear, loud voice, which I recognized as my own said, "I can't have chemotherapy tomorrow." Suddenly, I woke up. The spoken message had been clear, but I wondered what the imagery meant. Suddenly, I realized that a skeleton was literally my body and that my mind and my body needed to sit and rest together peacefully. No chemo, just calm. I knew this was the right answer. I decided I would not have chemotherapy. Instead, I would call in *well.* The next day I called the doctor's office to cancel my appointment.

I took the week off and did things that made me happy. I wrote about my feelings. I saw friends who needed to talk to me. I gave one person advice that he needed. I gave another forgiveness that she needed. I wasn't worried about the decision being right or wrong. Not only did it feel right to me, it felt wonderful to make a choice, believe in it, and rest. Of course, a Devil's advocate would say that a fallen alcoholic feels the same way about taking a drink. Was I making a sober decision, or was I too drunk on rest and respite to see clearly?

A week later, I didn't get a clear message from my body or in my dreams, so I followed Dr. Kind's advice and tried a weekly dose of Abraxane®. It caused another intestinal blockage that I was cautious enough to manage without being hospitalized. I had only small sips of water for days. My body had made it clear: no more Abraxane®. My CA125 was in the low seventies, and if I was lucky, a few months off wouldn't elevate it a lot.

I didn't want to waste this break from chemo by just enjoying my poison-free time. I wanted to try to heal my body and my spirit. I would look into some of those alternatives that the nutritionist talked about. I had another meeting with her to tell her about my decision and ask what she recommended. She started by saying that I shouldn't use the term, "break," to describe what I was doing. She said it had a "negative vibration," like something was broken. She wanted me to say "rest." That sounded too passive to me. What's a positive word for embracing freedom?

350

"Probation" connotes a parole officer. "Furlough" makes me think of sailors. I decided to call it a "vacation from chemotherapy." Vacations can be fun, relaxing, and fortifying, but they can also be educational and enriching.

I spent time during my chemo vacation listening to my body, managing my fear, releasing anger, and being thankful. I said the nightly chant that the nutritionist recommended. I was more careful to use positive terminology. Instead of wishing to be cancer-free, I'd wish to be well. Whenever I felt fear, I tried to replace it with gratitude. I tried to be more optimistic, reminding myself that a miracle cure was not impossible. I continued to pamper myself—I got massages and took bubble baths. I took my body to beaches in Cozumel, Mexico and in Florida. I took it to the Chesapeake Bay. I kept my eyes and mind open for other ideas. Some people call this being open to the universe. They say that the universe will provide. Others would say that I was looking for God to show me the path that He wanted me to follow. Some people call it listening to your inner voice. I didn't choose between these paradigms. I was not completely sold on any of these ideas, but I thought they couldn't hurt. I'm an empiricist, so I knew that the proof would be in the pudding.

My attitude of gratitude did not heal me, but it did soothe me. I dwelled on the many things and people that I was grateful for—and in some cases, I developed gratitude for the things and people that I hadn't thought to be grateful for. One thing that I had been thankful for ever since my diagnosis was that I did not have children. I had been saved from neglecting them during this long treatment process. My body's reaction to chemotherapy would have made it impossible to take care of children the way I would have wanted to. I could barely take care of myself. I had also been saved from leaving behind anyone who was dependent on me and irreparably damaged by my absence. I wouldn't have to find a way to explain that dying was not the same as abandoning someone. My childlessness had seemed like a loss, but now I saw it as a blessing.

I've also been extremely lucky in the area that is impersonally referred to as a "support system." My husband went from being a happy, hopeful newlywed on an overseas adventure to being a widower-in-waiting who never thought of himself as such. Saying he was my caretaker simplifies his job. He was my nurse, my chef, my medical record keeper, my chauffeur, and my liaison to health insurance companies, pharmacies, and doctor's offices. He was my confidante, my sounding board, my gatekeeper, and my spiritual advisor. He was endlessly patient—supportive of my choices and tolerant of my moods. He adapted to the constantly-evolving routines and schedules, and also to my diminishing capabilities. When I was well enough to go out, he was thrilled to get out of the house. When I could only manage a day on the couch, he was happy to cocoon. Whatever I thought I could eat, he would cook—singing in the kitchen while he did it. When I went through my mashed-potatoes-only phase, he made them full of love . . . and lots of butter, because he wanted to fatten me up. Nothing he ever said or did, no look that ever crossed his face, made me think that because I could no longer be the woman he dated and chose to marry, that I was no longer the woman he loved. He continued to love me and even more miraculously, he continued to love being with me even when all I could do *was* be.

Another thing that I have remained conscious and appreciative of throughout my illness is that I have a job that has made dying of cancer slowly less horrendous. I have no idea how cab drivers, waitresses, factory workers, and salespeople could have kept working with my chemotherapy side effects. I cannot imagine how they cope. I always knew that being a professor was one of those highly-flexible and secure jobs, but those qualities were never as important or evident until I was seriously ill. Most other employment requires more on-site hours and physical capabilities, while offering inadequate pay and minimal health benefits. I received a five-month, paid medical leave, a reduced teaching schedule, and my husband was allowed to fulfill my non-academic responsibilities in England. Now, I had a half-pay, full-year sabbatical to spend writing about my experiences and pursuing alternative medical options.

Friends recommended a local acupuncturist. After a few sessions, I wasn't sure if the acupuncture itself was working, or if her gentle words and peaceful manner alone made me feel better. At each appointment, I told her another piece of my health story. When I finished, the acupuncturist said that there was a gap in my story that she didn't understand. How could such an assertive woman, who knew her body so well, keep getting pushed into things that she believed were unwise for her? Why didn't I advocate for myself? These were difficult questions to answer.

Sometimes I thought that it was simply my fear of pain that made me reluctant to go forward with a recommended medical decision or procedure. I would instruct myself to rise above that fear and endure whatever was being done for my own good. Other times I was overwhelmed by the doctors' justifications for what they needed to do, their quick dismissal of my concerns, and their confidence that they knew what they were doing. I also feared the consequences of challenging them, because I didn't want to make them mad and be punished for doing so. I knew that they could take it out on me by making examinations more uncomfortable or degrading. At other times, I had tried my best to advocate for myself and had utterly failed.

I had figured out how to make my case effectively as a daughter, a student, a scholar, a teacher, a friend, and a mate. I had never figured out how to successfully make my case to a doctor. My father had taught me early on that if I could present a convincing case, I could prevail. I knew that a because-I-want-to argument was a weak one. If I didn't think my case was convincing, then I wouldn't present it. Dad was particularly open to arguments premised upon fairness and equality. If I could show him that a decision or rule was unfair, I had a good chance of being influential. Those weren't the kind of arguments that had a place in a medical setting. My evidence was too intuitive. My questions were too indirect. People in the medical profession weren't good listeners. I didn't speak their language. They didn't negotiate. What I had come to accept was that they were the only authority figures I couldn't please. After listening to all of this, the acupuncturist shook her head. "You need to reverse your thinking. They're not the authority, you are. They need to make their case about what they want to do with, or to your body, to *you*. You're the one with the power to decide." I recalled the Assistant Dean from Dickinson giving me a similar speech many years before. I wondered if it could be that simple. Had I given doctors blank checks and then criticized and resented them for what they chose to do with the money? Could I just cancel the check and pay them on a case-by-case basis?

Her advice made sense when considering whether or not to get more chemo, but I couldn't stop my mind from flipping through other scenarios that had or would strip me of my agency. What about when I couldn't walk because my hip was broken? Where was my authority then? Was it possible to reject the nose tube? Wouldn't they just say: "No tube, no treatment; go die now." As if she could hear what I was thinking, the acupuncturist said, "As a daughter, sister, and niece of doctors, I can tell you that they aren't going to let you die because you refuse a procedure. They'll try to come up with another way to help you survive." I didn't know if I believed this, but I enjoyed considering it.

I also enjoyed that I could *consider*, without feeling charged to *accept*, the acupuncturist's thinking. She never implied that acceptance of her beliefs were a prerequisite for her particular type of healing to work. She spent our appointments describing the underlying philosophies of Chinese medicine. She said that they believed that every person's body was unique and knew how to heal itself. The role of the doctor in Chinese medicine was to help facilitate this self-healing. I liked the way that this Eastern idea shifted the blame from my body, for not behaving as it *should,* to the doctors, for not listening carefully enough or observing closely enough to be helpful. I was tired of my body being indicted. I liked to think that it held answers.

Chinese medicine relates elements in nature to body parts and function and personality types. Certain characteristics of these types would be a person's greatest strength and potentially her greatest weakness. The acupuncturist told me that she thought I was a "wood" person. That initially surprised me because I have such an affinity to water, but she explained that wood needed water to nurture it. One of the characteristics of wood people was that they are rule-based and structured. That rang true. She said that they could also be adaptive and remain strong. "Think about how a tree will grow around an obstacle and then still grow upward. That's a helpful image for a wood person," she said. "When you feel overwhelmed by something and trapped, think of that tree and ask yourself, how else might this be accomplished?"

After I told my husband about this conversation, he would tease me by calling me "Woody" when I tried to tell him that I couldn't, or wasn't supposed to do something. Once he playfully pointed this out, I saw how often I constrained myself. I almost hadn't voted because I had gotten chemotherapy on Election Day. David took me to the municipal building to vote, but after ten minutes, I was too weak to continue standing in the long line. David suggested, "Let's go up front and ask if you can vote right away." I countered,

"We can't. I have to wait in line. It wouldn't be fair to people who got here before me to cut." He said,

"They didn't all have chemo today. If they did, they could ask to vote first, too. Wouldn't you let them?" Of course, I would let them! He was right. They gladly allowed me to vote next. I needed to think about how rules could have exceptions that made things more equitable. Maybe there was wiggle room in medical procedures, too. I kept my eyes open for chemo-free treatments and an alternative was revealed from a surprising source.

* * *

Suzanne Somers kept popping up on my television set. Not finding any better options on my favorite channels, I stopped flipping long enough to hear what she had to say to Larry King. She was promoting her newest book, *Breakthrough*. In the book, she writes about getting sick, and being told that she had cancer and needed chemotherapy. She didn't want the chemotherapy—and ultimately, it turned out she didn't have cancer. Afterward, she interviewed experts on chemotherapy and discovered how bad their track records were for most cancers. Then she interviewed doctors who did not believe in high-dose chemotherapy, and used alternative therapies instead. She was passionate. She was inspired. She wanted people to open their minds. King seemed to enjoy her enthusiasm and the sparkle in her eye. It was hard to tell if he believed a word she said.

I didn't know much about Somers. I knew she fought for more gender equity in pay for television actresses and was vilified for it. I remember watching her on *Three's Company* reruns in the afternoons when I was trying to write my dissertation. One of my strategies for finishing the research was to work at home and not change out of my pajamas until I had written a certain number of pages. If I had written an additional number of pages, I'd allow myself the mindless pleasure of back-to-back episodes of this silly sitcom on weekday afternoons. Watching Somers' dumb-blonde routine and John Ritter's sexist goofing (before I knew to label it as such) would completely push political science from my head for an hour. Then it would be back to work after dinner. This was during my career-building stage when I refused to allow myself to read fiction or magazines. For about eight years, it was only serious academic reading material for me. So, I guess you could say that I was favorably predisposed toward Somers. She'd helped me out before, and she seemed to have done her research on cancer. Many of the things she was saying about the limitations of chemotherapy I had already discovered in my experiences and research.

A few days later I saw her again, this time on *The Rachael Ray Show*. Surprisingly, Rachael Ray was giving Somers a harder time than King did. The woman who usually told everyone how cute they looked and gave them snacks was implying that Somers was encouraging patients to make choices that would kill them. Rachael Ray might have tried to say this politely and by quoting other people, but it was clear that she didn't understand that chemotherapy isn't a miracle drug. I could see how the dismal data wouldn't fit well with Rachael's upbeat you-can-do-it attitude, and why she wouldn't want to believe Somers' research. Rachael Ray pointed out that some of the doctors that Somers interviewed in the book were taken to court. Somers countered out that they were not convicted of any wrongdoing, and had been targeted by drug companies who were heavily invested in the current system. I was curious, so I ordered the book. The comments posted online about the book were polarized and emphatic.

Since the bulk of the book was about avoiding cancer, I decided only to read the chapters that were about treatment. The chapter that seemed the most interesting was an interview with Dr. Black-Sheep, who had been running a clinic in Texas since 1977. He was a scientist, as well as a doctor, and he had purportedly discovered that people without cancer had livers that produced a certain enzyme that people with cancer didn't have. Dr. Black-Sheep synthetically recreated this enzyme in a lab and gave it to cancer patients. He also used gene-replacement therapy to treat cancer. He would try to identify the genes that had shut down, and help them turn on again. He claimed that treatments were non-toxic and had been successful for even the hardiest cancers. One of the patients interviewed in the book had ovarian cancer.

I sent the chapter to my friend who has a Ph.D. in chemistry, and asked her what she thought. She said that she already knew about Dr. Black-Sheep. She called him a genius and a pioneer of the next wave of cancer treatment approaches, and that if she had my cancer, she would trust his approach over chemotherapy. I called the clinic and set up an appointment in December. I paid for my records to be sent and reviewed. David and I flew down and spent the day at the clinic. I got lots of blood tests. We talked to the doctor. David asked what kind of success the doctor he was having with ovarian/peritoneal cancer. Dr. Black-Sheep said that he had about one-hundred patients with this difficult disease. Most of them had already had a lot of chemotherapy, which created cancer cells that morphed and strengthened to resist all these drugs. Fifty patients had responded to his treatment (which could last for up to eighteen months). "What does 'respond' mean?" my husband asked, knowing that the FDA defines "responding" as shrinking the tumor for a short period of time. Dr. Black-Sheep said,

"The tumors shrink. The CA125 is normal, and it stays that way."

"Isn't that a cure?" my husband asked.

"We don't call it a 'cure' because the cancer might still be there. It is just being managed by the body." This sounded more promising than any of the chemotherapy I had been offered. I could easily be in the unlucky fifty percent, but it seemed like I had a chance.

I also got some bad news at the clinic. My CA125 indicated that the progress that was made during the seven hard months of taking Abraxane® had been reversed during the two months since I stopped taking it. My CA125 was 152, higher than it had ever been. While I had been feeling better, I had been getting worse.

My insurance company classified Dr. Black-Sheep's approach as "alternative," and wouldn't cover the treatment. The drugs he used were FDA-approved, but they were not on Pennsylvania's list of drugs approved for ovarian/peritoneal cancer treatment. David and I decided to convert the financial investments (stocks and bonds) that made up my life savings into cash. We thought that it would be enough money to get treatment for the two to three months that it would take to figure out if this approach was working. If it was working, we could sell the property that we had bought to build our dream house on. If we had to, I could also ask my mother for money. We would worry about whether the liquidated funds would be enough if the treatment miraculously worked. For a few more months, I would not feel trapped in a system that I didn't believe in. I believed in Dr. Black-Sheep's approach philosophically, but I didn't know if it would work for me.

A few weeks later, while my husband started his new job, I drove to Texas. By then, I was starting to have pains in my side after I ate, and the bloating and diarrhea had reached chemo-like levels. I assumed these were caused by the cancer, adhesions, or a combination of the two. But snow, traffic, and digestive distress didn't stop me from making the trip. I reserved my eating until an hour before I would stop at a hotel, so that my intestine wouldn't force me off of the road. By then I was weak. But at least I wasn't as bored as I used to be on long drives. After three years of hanging out in waiting rooms, lying in bed trying to fall asleep, sitting on toilets, and lounging in bathtubs, I had gotten used to living in my own head. Those eight-hour driving days didn't seem so long.

The first day at the clinic, they told me that my CA125 had continued to rise and was at 202. The PET scan showed an active

361

cancer node in the center of my abdomen, where the scan from fifteen months earlier had only shown a shadow. Over the next ten days, they gave me pills, advice on how to take them, and instructions for coping with the anticipated side effects. They observed me after I took them. They gave me blood and urine tests, and checked my vitals. Like most medical offices, there was a lot of waiting. Unlike most other offices, the focus seemed to be on patients rather than procedures, office politics, and routines.

There were lots of restaurants in the area. On good days, I sampled them. On bad days, I got carry-out so that I could be close to my big hotel bathroom after I ate. By the end of my time there, I was taking over fifty pills a day distributed over a twelve-hour period. Six pill-taking sessions were with food, so I was eating small, frequent meals. This diminished the pain in my side. The few times I ate entire (small) meals, the pain returned. I tried to think of this as just another adjustment I had to make. I wasn't alone. Models everywhere ate like this. I could do it, too.

I spent a lot of time in the waiting room of the clinic in between seeing nurses, doctors, the pharmacist, and my account manager. I met a lot of the patients; others I started to recognize, but never talked to. Some of the patients had never had chemotherapy; others, like me, had exhausted the various options. Some were told to come here by their doctors. Others had read Suzanne Somers' book. The walls were full of pictures of her, as though she were the patron saint of the clinic. Interspersed with the photographs of Somers were pictures of children who had survived brain cancer (thanks to Dr. Black-Sheep). Pictures showed them when they first came to the clinic. Then they were young and bald. Other pictures showed how healthy and normal they looked ten years later at their graduations or in their prom gowns.

The waiting room was usually full. There was the frightfully-thin woman with pancreatic cancer. She wanted to talk about wigs. There was a woman with breast cancer who brought her daughter along. She told me I should be taking more vitamin D3. One woman was about my age. She had breast cancer that spread to her bones, making it hard for her to walk and sleep. She said, she was a vegetarian and believed in natural approaches, but had let doctors talk her into a mastectomy and chemotherapy. She blamed these procedures for her cancer spreading. She couldn't forgive herself for going along with them. She and her husband had taken out a loan to pay for her treatment here.

There was a woman with brain cancer sitting in a wheelchair. She looked tired, but at peace. Her sister and the two men with her were not. They were furious about the treatment she had gotten in Boston and Oklahoma City. They couldn't get some of her records and were shocked and disgusted by the inefficiency. They had bought into the patient's rights rhetoric, not realizing until now that such talk was exceptionally cheap in the cancer world.

There was a tired, angry man with brain cancer. He said that he had no idea, before he got sick, of how dreadfully patients were treated by doctors and hospitals. "Did you know that if you walk out of a hospital without them discharging you, your insurance won't pay for it?" he asked me. I hadn't known this, but it didn't surprise me. I assumed that he was speaking from experience. He could not believe he had been given so few choices, and so little freedom, and respect. He was glad to have escaped here, where there was hope and they talked *to* you instead of *at* you. I thought he was lucky to have avoided the powerlessness of being a patient until his late sixties, but I never would have said that to him. Much of his anger seemed to be directed at his doctors for having told him that his cancer was highly treatable before his treatment had failed. But in the same breath he noted that he liked how much more optimistic the doctors were here. This contradiction led me to believe that if this treatment didn't work, he'd be angry at Dr. Black-Sheep, too. I didn't want to be around to see that.

There was a hyper, cheerful woman who wanted to know everyone's name. She credited her work with Mary Kay® Cosmetics for helping her understand that "Strangers are just friends you haven't made yet." She told me, "You look so much better than you did last night. Your coloring is back." I didn't know that I had looked so bad. Maybe it was the lighting. Maybe it was the diarrhea. I thought it was a strange thing for her to say to someone she didn't know, but then she probably thought we were already friends.

Another cheerful woman got everyone's attention by announcing that she'd been coming to Dr. Black-Sheep's clinic for six months and it was working well for her. Her breast cancer was in remission. I could feel the excitement and hope this produced among those in the room. Someone asked her about the payment plan. She didn't have insurance, "But I've gotten really good at fundraising," she chirped. I tried to picture myself organizing a Help-Stephanie-Live dinner, walk-a-thon, or silent auction. I couldn't. Amid all of the homework that a sick person gets (eat this, read this, get another opinion, pray, meditate, etc.), this assignment seemed like a major project that was beyond me.

Another woman had ovarian cancer. She said that she wasn't going to let them "cut out more of me and give me chemo again." I assumed that she was stuck in a repeated cycle: operation, chemo, short remission . . . operation, chemo, short remission (which many women at the Mansion were in). But she revealed that after her original diagnosis, a hysterectomy and chemotherapy had been followed by a three-year remission. Then it was back, and she had another operation and chemo. That had been four years ago. Now they wanted to do it again. I would have let them. Six months of hell for three years of health sounded like a great deal to me. But she was tired of it. At least she was able to share her fatigue without being berated for it.

One afternoon, as I waited to see if a new drug would raise my blood pressure, I overheard a woman talking on her cell phone. Either she was clueless as to how loud she was or she wanted everyone to overhear her. I gathered that she was talking to her sister about her father:

I tell you, this is like a used-car lot. They get you in an office and take all of your money. . . .He said he didn't care what I said; he was going to do this. He's worried because he hasn't had treatment in three months. It's only cancer, how fast could it grow .

. . ? He read about this in that stupid bimbo, Suzanne Somers' book. Daddy said he did all the research, but it was just a bunch of spam and mail-order magazines. We've got to see if we can get him on a no-spam list and get him off of the mailing lists . . . . Medicare won't pay for this. He said he can afford it, but he's going to end up in a home. That's what I told him. . . .We can use this. He's obviously here to hurt himself. If they try to hurt themselves or others, you can get them institutionalized.

Good God. If she were my daughter, I'd tell her not to worry about losing her inheritance, because I'd already cut her out of the will for being such a cold-hearted witch.

I was treated at the clinic for ten days. When my treatment concluded, I drove to my mother's condominium on the beach in Indialantic, Florida. It wasn't an easy trip. I had to stop frequently to deal with digestive problems and take pills. But it was good to be near family and water, and in fifty-degree weather, instead of the three feet of snow that Carlisle, Pennsylvania was getting. I quickly established a routine—sleeping, writing, pill-taking, eating small meals, going to the bathroom, television, watching the water, and more writing.

At night David and I would talk on the phone. I suggested to him that maybe the cosmic purpose of the Dr. Black-Sheep adventure was not to cure me, but to make it easier for him to adjust to my dying. He kept busy with his new job while I was out of town, so he wouldn't even realize that he was practicing living without me. He would be spared from watching the daily disintegration of my health. Yet, he could still hear my voice on the phone and know that I was not gone yet. Maybe I was supposed to die here in Florida.

David had a completely different narrative. He said he didn't see my story as being about him. He said, he thought that this was a new beginning for both of us. It was a New Year and a new decade (2010). He had a new job. I had a new treatment. Both could work out and allow us to have a long, happy life together. It was a nice story. I liked it a lot more than the one I had told. But neither story was true. I returned to Pennsylvania for tests, Valentine's Day and my fiftieth birthday. That's when I learned that my CA125 had gone up to 322 after the first month of alternative treatment. The cancer was more active, and the rate of increase from month-to-month was increasing too. The expensive alternative drugs hadn't stopped the cancer. It looked like I was in the unfortunate 50 percent.

The doctor wanted me to have the gene tests done again. She wanted to compare these to the results from January. If they'd changed, that would help them come up with other drugs that might target the cancer better. These were expensive blood tests needed to be analyzed in the Texas lab. Was this the approach that I was paying so much for? It sounded a lot like the approach used by conventional doctors—the let's-throw-this-against-the-wall-and-see-if-anything-sticks method. Since I had decided to give the alternative approach two months and I still had some life savings left, I agreed to get the tests. If they led to other drugs, I'd take those. If they didn't indicate a change in treatment, I wasn't sure what I'd do.

I took the script for the blood tests to the hospital the following day. Something didn't feel quite right about it. I had a rough night—a nagging headache, bad digestion, waking up in a panic every few hours when my first thought was, *Am I still alive?* The rising CA125 was worrying me. What were my other options? I could get more chemotherapy at the Mansion, even though they had nothing new to offer. Some of the old stuff had at least brought down the CA125 while I was taking it. Friends had sent me lots of links to what they considered useful options. Some were for clinical trials that I was not eligible for—I had had too much chemotherapy, the wrong strain of peritoneal cancer, or too weak a heart. David was interested in another doctor that was in Somers' book. That doctor also thought that liver enzymes were the key. His approach included hundreds of supplements, dietary changes, and daily-coffee enemas. It sounded hard on the intestine and rectum—not my strongest body parts.

The next day when I went to the hospital, the admissions worker returned from the lab with the news that they couldn't do the blood test. They couldn't send blood samples to an out-of-state lab. I told her that the local lab didn't do these tests and I understood that I would be charged out-of-pocket. She insisted that they could only draw the blood. I would need to provide the vials for the blood, and I would need to ship them myself. I had read the instructions for shipping listed on the order. They were elaborate—requiring a certain kind of packaging and dry ice. "Do you have vials you could sell me?" I asked. "Could you mail it and I pay you?" She didn't think so. I tried to picture what I would do once I was handed the blood. Could I just go to a post office and say: "I'd like this packaged with dry ice?" Where do you get dry ice? Could I get it from a butcher shop? Could I pilfer it from the biology department at school? Even if I could get dry ice, I wasn't sure how would I do all of this when I only had a two-hour window of opportunity to be away from my bathroom.

I thought that perhaps this was a sign to stop the alternative treatment. Maybe it was time to admit that it hadn't worked, and either go back to horrible (but by comparison, inexpensive) chemotherapy or to start to accept the possibility that there were no good treatment options left. Maybe this was a sign that I was done with all treatment. I didn't know, but I knew I was overwhelmed by the news from the hospital administrator. I was exhausted. I was sad. I was hungry. I started to cry, apologized for crying, and said that I didn't know how to do what she was asking me to do; I didn't know if I should even try, since the drugs weren't working, the cancer was growing, and chemotherapy hadn't worked. She was a nice woman who didn't know what to say and needed to get back to work. She was trying to be helpful ("I'll have someone from the lab call you tomorrow or the next day"); she was sympathetic ("I know this is hard"); and she was encouraging ("You can't quit. You need to keep fighting"). But how much fighting was I really required, or able to do when the cancer was terminal? Hadn't three years and two months of suffering been enough? Did I have to fight until I was knocked out by the medical options? Couldn't I simply forfeit points and walk to my corner with some dignity? She expected me to continue to fight *and* find dry ice? I cried even harder.

She went back to work, and I called David. He said that he would make some calls to see how we could get the blood to Texas. I needed to get some food and take some pills. As I was leaving the hospital waiting room, a young woman came over to me. She said, "Excuse me; I don't want to bother you. But I overheard some of your conversation, and I just wanted you to know that God has not forgotten you. He has a plan for you." My friend Lydia would have had a fit. She had been shocked and angered when a man had come up to us in a restaurant and asked me what my name was so he could pray for me. She found it intrusive and presumptuous. She said it was all about "him wanting to feel good about himself at your expense." All that anger took more energy and certainty than I had. I always thank people when they say they'll pray for me. But to this woman I said,

"I know. I'm not upset and frustrated with God, just with the medical system. God's plan might be that I'm supposed to stop all this and die peacefully now. I don't know. What I'd like to have is some clarity." She agreed, and said that that's what she'd pray that I find. This surprised me. I was used to hearing people say that God would heal me if I believed in him enough, prayed enough, or figured out what I was supposed to do in His name. But she had recently lost her father to cancer, and had supported him when he turned down operations that might have extended his life, but not saved it. I can't usually say this, but I felt better after talking to this stranger.

As I drove away the song with the repetitive and haunting line: "Say what you need to say" played on the radio. It seemed like a message for me (absurdly from John Mayer, of all people). I remembered that when I heard that the CA125 had gone up so much, I had immediately realized, *I need to get this book finished; I don't have much time.* Maybe I didn't know what treatment I should do or how to ship blood on dry ice, but I knew that I had to tell my story even if it wasn't the one that people wanted to hear. It was something I could do. I would say what I needed to say. That was in my control, and the idea made me feel better. Maybe writing was the alternative medicine that would heal me emotionally.

The next morning someone from the hospital called. They had the right vials. They could draw the blood, and they could ship it to Houston on dry ice. But there was one catch. I braced myself. The catch was that I would need to write a check to FedEx for thirty-five dollars. I almost laughed. I was paying 250 dollars per pill for treatments that didn't seem to be working. My insurance wouldn't reimburse me for any of them. I could certainly write a check for thirty-five dollars.

The following Friday at 7:00 p.m. I got a call from Texas. One of the gene markers had changed. It was now registering as high (out of the normal range). *This seems promising . . . maybe they could treat me more effectively,* I hoped. I waited for the miracle solution and it was (drumroll please) . . . Avastin®—a drug I already had during my conventional treatment. It was the one that had increased my blood pressure, but hadn't seemed to have helped fight the cancer. They knew this, but they said that this time it

371

might work better because the gene performance had changed. The Houston doctor said that I needed to get the Avastin® quickly since my CA125 was going up so rapidly. In order to get the Avastin®, I would either need to fly to Texas and pay them thousands of dollars, or call Dr. Kind and allow my insurance to shoulder the bill. The answer I preferred was obvious.

I needed Dr. Kind to give me Avastin® without chemotherapy while I continued to pay for the expensive pills from the alternative treatment. Again, I would be stuck in Pennsylvania during the winter. Again, I would be back at the Mansion. (Assuming that I could effectively get Dr. Kind to do what I wanted.) Soon my life savings would be gone and I would have to get money from my seventy-five-year-old mother. All of this assumed that I would be able to get quick access to Dr. Kind and that I could be persuasive. *What if he feels rejected by my trying the alternative?* I fretted. *What if he insists that I get traditional chemo with the Avastin®? What if he's out-of-town? What if my heart isn't strong enough?* These were the things I thought immediately when the conversation with the Texas doctors ended. But it was Friday night. I couldn't do anything until Monday.

Monday was spent on the phone and waiting for it to ring. The receptionist indicated that the first available appointment was in June. That wouldn't do. David talked to Dr. Kind's assistant to see if I could get the Avastin® earlier. She would talk to him and get back to us. She claimed that they hadn't gotten any of the paperwork on blood tests and scans that I had asked to be sent to them. Yet I had seen them listed on the hospital forms. Even though I didn't believe her, it was easier to request more records be sent than ask her to look for them in my file. She promised to get back to us by the end of the day. She didn't.

The next day, we were told that they could squeeze me in in two weeks. This would be five weeks after the Texas doctor red-flagged my cancer's increased activity. Now what? We left a message for the Texas doctor explaining where things stood and asking her to call Dr. Kind directly and explain to him why I needed the Avastin®. Given how impossible it had been to get him to talk to my cardiologists a year earlier, I wasn't very hopeful that this would solve the problem. The Texas doctor probably wouldn't check her messages until that afternoon. Then she might try to call and he'd be gone. They might play phone tag the next day and then he'd be gone to a conference. I doubted that even that much effort would be put forth.

A few days later, the Texas doctor called to report that she had tried to reach Dr. Kind many times. She never got through, and he never called her back despite his assistant's frequent assurances that he would. "Maybe he doesn't want to talk to me," she suggested. Was it her Polish accent that made her sound like a hurt little girl, or was it the tone in her voice? I told her not to take it personally: Dr. Kind wasn't good about returning phone calls. By then I had an appointment to see him and to get the Avastin® in two weeks. It was not the timing that the Texas doctor and I would have preferred, but it was the one we were stuck with. She reminded me that I could get Avastin® in Texas at any time.

I decided if that week's CA125 result was five-hundred or higher, I would fly to Texas and pay the ten-thousand dollars for Avastin®. My decision was arbitrary. There is no range for CA125 scores that indicates what degree of danger I was in. There doesn't seem to be a consensus among doctors about what to make of CA125 numbers. The number doesn't correspond to the size or spread of the cancer. Some patients have scores in the tens of thousands. Some are in surgery for grapefruit-sized tumors that accompany numbers in the double digits. I remember being told by one doctor that if the number doubles in a few weeks' time then it is likely to be out of control and treatment is no longer an option. Another doctor told me that whenever the number rises, I should have more chemotherapy. But a study I read in a cancer magazine said that patients that got chemotherapy when the number went up did not live any longer than those who waited to get chemotherapy when symptoms of cancer manifested themselves. Dr. Sure had scoffed at me once when I suggested that we wait until my number exceeded one hundred, quipping that this was a fine approach "if you want to die." Yet, Dr. Kind commented that CA125 scores in the two-hundred to six-hundred ranges were nothing to panic about. It all depended upon the direction the numbers were moving in.

Even though I knew I was just rolling the dice, I decided that if the number was less than five-hundred, I would wait for the appointment with Dr. Kind and try to stop worrying about it. I joined David at a hotel in Valley Forge, Pennsylvania. It is near a wonderful mall. I didn't eat that day so that I could leave the bathroom long enough to get a haircut to tame my short curls and buy an overpriced purse. The Texas doctor called to tell me that my CA125 had gone up again. At 440, it was perilously close to my self-imposed panic point.

During the two-week wait, I tried to keep myself distracted. I saw some friends. I wrote. I had a Long Island Ice Tea at a restaurant. The dry cough from the bronchitis had lingered, but it was far less violent. Yet a pain had developed in my chest on the right side. At first, I noticed it only when I coughed, then it seemed to bother me whenever I sat up or tried to turn in bed. The discomfort eased a little when I pressed on it, like I had when my ribs were cracked after the car accident. David thought I had pulled a muscle in my chest. A friend told me that coughing could actually crack your ribs. I wondered if the cancer might have spread to my lung. Maybe that's what I would have to show for trying something new. I tried to put it out of my mind, but it became the elephant in the room.

After the two-week wait, my husband and I had an uneventful meeting with Dr. Kind. He said that he didn't have any idea what the Texas doctors were doing, but he understood my desire to give something else a try. He had no problem giving me the Avastin®. He had already gotten my insurance to authorize it. *So why did I have to wait so long to receive it*, I wondered. *So that we could have this five-minute meeting?* I told him that I would want whatever chemotherapy he recommended if Avastin® alone didn't bring down the CA125. He said that I shouldn't worry about the number, because it was small compared to the levels he'd seen among other women. This was made less reassuring by my memory of him telling me that everyone's levels were different and what was dangerous to one person wasn't to another. I should only compare my own scores to each other. I also remembered how emphatic he was that I keep getting chemotherapy when my numbers had still been in the double digits. These comments didn't add up. Did he think I forgot everything he said to me before and only heard what he said each week? Is that how the other women remained so reassured by him? Or did he simply forget what he said from week-to-week? Did doctors know so little about this cancer and the chemotherapy that all of his statements had the same chance of being correct?

Two weeks after I got the Avastin®, my CA125 was 670. I had completely skipped the five hundreds: the level that I thought would be a deal breaker for the alternate treatment. The Texas doctor called and proposed that it might have been too early to see an effect. They thought I should continue with the pills that they prescribed and get another Avastin® treatment. The CA125 level after that was the crucial one. I couldn't fathom spending another five-thousand dollars for drugs that didn't seem to be working. The two-month trial period I had expected for the alternative approach had gone on for almost three months. Maybe it was time to go back to the traditional chemotherapy to try and get the number down? I was too worried about the CA125 and the money to continue with the alternative treatment. I called Dr. Kind's office and left him a message that I was finished with the other approach and wanted him to think about what other chemotherapy he

wanted to give me with the Avastin® the following week. It was
Thursday, and my appointment was for Tuesday.

On Tuesday, I went to the appointment alone. He had not
considered which chemotherapy to use yet. Dr. Kind said he
needed time to think about which chemotherapy to add to the
Avastin®. This week I would get the Avastin®, the following week
we would have a consultation, and the week after that I'd get a
different chemotherapy. The idea of more waiting frustrated and
worried me, but I didn't think there was anything I could do to
change that. I was at the mercy of his schedule and the standard-
operating procedures of his practice.

The tone of our next meeting was different than usual. I
am not sure how precisely to describe the approach he took toward
me that day. The words—combative, aggressive, patronizing—
probably hyperbolizes the way he spoke to me, but they come close
to characterizing his tone. His problem was with the Texas clinic,
not me. Yet I was the only other person in the examining room
that day, and I was the one who had turned to him for help. So, I
felt like the target of his criticism.

Dr. Kind said that he didn't like how doctors like that
encouraged patients like me into thinking that they had something
to offer when they didn't. He thought that charging patients for
treatments that were not FDA-approved, and therefore would not
be reimbursed by health insurance companies, was unforgivable. I
shared that I understood his concerns, but I believed that a lot of
the approved drugs didn't have a very good record and vested
interests in traditional medicine made it more difficult for

alternative approaches to get accepted into the mainstream. He argued that they took advantage of desperate people. He looked at me quizzically, "Surely you can't believe that this clinic could know something that all the other cancer research doesn't?" I indicated that I thought the alternative approach would be the future in cancer treatment and the fact that it hadn't worked out for me didn't dissuade me from thinking this, even though it did disappoint me.

"The system is stacked against scientists who challenge dominant paradigms," I said. He wasn't pleased:

"It sounds like you think he's Galileo!" By invoking Galileo's name, he was acknowledging that scientific breakthroughs often came from outsiders who were stigmatized by those who believed in and profited from the status quo. But he didn't seem to realize that he had conceded my major point. This wasn't a debate tournament. We weren't in the classroom. I wasn't here to argue with him. I was here to get the Avastin® that the Texas doctors had wanted me to continue, and hoping to get some conventional chemotherapy.

The following week we had a friendlier appointment with David by my side. Dr. Kind suggested that we revisit Cisplatin, a platinum-based chemotherapy that I had been on during the fall of 2007. He thought that since my cancer hadn't seen it in a while, it would be our best bet. The advantage for me was that Cisplatin did not result in hair loss, and it was not as hard on platelets. I would get another CA125 test prior to starting the chemotherapy.

When I arrived the following week, Dr. Kind announced that my CA125 had dropped to 270. He couldn't believe it. He was so surprised at the improvement that he double-checked to make sure it was my laboratory report. He didn't understand what the Texas clinic did, but he advised me to call them and let them know how successful their plan had been.

It was a relief to have the CA125 drop so dramatically. It was a larger percentage decrease from one treatment than I had ever had before, *and* it was from a treatment that hadn't made me sick. I hoped that this result had persuaded Dr. Kind to continue with Avastin® only, but he still thought that adding Cisplatin would be best. It was important to keep the cancer "on the run," he said. Maybe I should have run—back to Texas. But I didn't. I knew that I might be giving up too soon on something that might have just started working. I knew that Cisplatin wouldn't cure me, or work well enough to get me a remission. The weeks of struggling to get back into treatment at the Mansion, the inconvenience of getting treatment from across the country, the months of losing faith in the alternative approach while watching the CA125 climb, and most of all, the prohibitive cost of the treatment kept me at the Mansion. So did inertia. It didn't even feel like I was making a decision. Within minutes of hearing the miraculous news about my CA125, I was in a reclining chair getting pumped full of the drugs that blurred my eyesight, parched my mouth, and muddled my thinking.

Chapter 15: "Did You Get a Double Mastectomy?": Reflections on Strangers and Assumptions about Female Cancer Patients

When I started my chemotherapy adventures, I knew I'd lose my hair, my health, and my time. I hadn't realized that I would forfeit my privacy too. I didn't know that strangers would interpret my baldness as an invitation for conversation. (I guess they assumed that if I didn't want to talk, I'd be wearing a wig.) I didn't think that my blood test results would be announced in front of so many people in a sorority of the sick that would include competition, personality clashes, and so many reminders that I didn't fit in. I hadn't anticipated that strangers on prayer chains would be kept up-to-date on my symptoms. Even though I'm not a particularly private person (as demonstrated by my writing this book), it bothers me that I am not in more control of what people know about me. Chemotherapy has taken self-revelation out of my hands.

When you're a bald, middle-aged woman, you get a lot of stares from people who look away quickly when you catch their eyes. It's as if I am naked in public, making it hard for people to keep their eyes off me, but too embarrassed at my indecency to get caught looking. Children are different. They always stare unashamedly, even when I stare back. While they don't usually talk to me, they do loudly ask their parents, "Why doesn't that lady have any hair?" or say, "Look how funny that lady looks without hair." The parents usually respond by shushing their children. This actually makes me feel worse, because it presumes that I make people uncomfortable and it was rude for the child to point me out. I've never heard a parent explain that when people are sick they sometimes lose their hair. That would be truthful, and it might spare the next bald woman the child encounters. Once when I was on a bus in Rome, a little boy (probably four years old) pointed and burst out laughing. He was howling so long that it was hard not to join him. Then his father yelled, "Basta!" (Enough!) Both responses were honest and understandable; bald women look funny, but don't get carried away with it.

I actually prefer the silent stares and sympathetic half-smiles from the women who wear Think Pink® bracelets to the conversations that some of them initiate. I don't want to answer questions and talk to strangers about my condition; it's hard enough keeping my friends up-to-date. My own story bores and saddens me. I don't know how to tell it in a few sentences. Unwieldy stories like mine, which exceed a few sentences in a public place, typically retain their audience out of obligation. Once I get started, I am sure they don't want to hear my tale. But if they approach me, I usually feel like I have to answer their questions and then politely listen to what they have to say. It baffles me that they *want* to have these conversations instead of deciding against interrupting a sick stranger on a day she feels well enough to be in public. I can only assume that when some people initiate conversations with me, they're more interested in talking about *their* experiences with cancer rather than learning about *mine*.

Their stories seem to be of two varieties. There's the I-know-what-you're-going-through-because-my-relative/close friend/neighbor-is-dying-and-I-feel-terribly-about-her-death commiseration story. There's also the I-know-what-you're-going-through-because-I-had-cancer,-but-look-how-well-I-am-now celebration story. When I am in a charitable mood, I can listen and appreciate that people need someone sympathetic to listen to them, and my hairlessness gives them hope that I'll understand. But I'd rather not hear either of these stories. I'm not a shrink. I'm not objective. I don't have the strength or the time to enjoy our new connection.

While they might see talking to me as a good opportunity for them to be heard, listening to them is not good for me, because in a variety of ways, it makes me feel sad *and* guilty. First, listening to strangers' stories about relatives and friends who have died from cancer reminds me of how powerless I am to protect my own family from grief over my dying. Then, because I have no emotional distance from the concrete and bleak ways in which these unknown people died, I begin to superimpose their deaths upon my own. Late at night, I can conjure a variety of horrifying versions of how the librarian's mother lost her dignity before dying, and I picture myself in her place. I wonder: *Will I be put on a respirator, like the man in the coffee shop's wife was? Will I end up like the waitress's mother and need to have my intestines removed?* Next, I remember how awful I felt when my own father was dying of lymphoma. Yet I have to admit that *having* terminal cancer has been harder on me than *seeing* him have cancer was. This might be a natural feeling, but it makes me suspect that I am a selfish, insensitive daughter.

Finally, my own health story is usually worse than the story that I am being told. The stories' subjects are often much older than me, or people who eventually overcame cancer. So I find myself feeling strangely jealous of these strangers and then feeling badly about this reaction. I don't like causing people to relive the pain that they feel from a loved one's cancer. When strangers talk to me and cry, it makes me want to disappear. In some ways I feel like I already have disappeared, because the tears have almost nothing to do with me.

Certainly some of the strangers are coming to me *not* so that *they* can feel better, but so they can make *me* feel better. They seem to think that their survival story will cheer me up. But I'm not like them. When their chemo worked, it got rid of their cancer. When my chemo works, it gives me a few months without chemo before I am back on it again. I can't feel any better about my situation because someone else in a different situation had a good outcome. If anything, I am jealous of positive outcomes. If these strangers were someone I knew, it would be easier to rejoice in their good fortune. But these people are strangers. I am pleased for them in a general, philosophical way as I suppose they would have been for me if the tables were turned. But I never would have gone up to strangers to tell them that I almost died of appendicitis, and then expected them to be enriched by the fact that I hadn't. Why do they assume that our cancers are the same, or that our bodies react in the same way to treatment? They don't consider that I might actually be dying, not just suffering on the way to recovery, like they did. They are the survivors; I will not be.

The Pink-Ribbon people, especially the most enthusiastic breast cancer survivors, will not want to hear that I'd prefer not to talk to them. After chemotherapy has taken my hair or when it has just begun to grow back, they see me in public and assume that I am in their club. They are sure that they can inspire me. They smile, give me the thumbs-up, and often come over to talk. When they say that cancer is no longer a death sentence, I know it would be rude to say that it is for some of us and will be for me. When they insist that every day is a gift, I am tempted to give them details about my bad days or to joke about whether I can exchange some of my gifts for store credit. There's no honest and acceptable way to tell someone when I will finish chemo. "When I'm dead" is too blunt; "When I can't endure it anymore" will elicit a you-can't-give-up pep talk that I don't want to hear. I never know what to say when someone imparts the wisdom that God never gives us more than we can handle. How do they reconcile this belief with the suicide rate? They see me as their sister until they find out that I'm different. I don't have breast cancer. I am not in remission, and I am not cheerful. They wanted to tell me that I wasn't going to die because they didn't. But then I ruined it.

* * *

I remember a woman once yelled at me across a parking lot, "Hey, do you have breast cancer?" I shook my head and kept walking. It was a week after my gallbladder surgery, and I didn't have the energy to endure another intrusive conversation. But she ran after me. She said, "Well, that's a good thing, isn't it?" She was assuming that the worst cancer I could have was the one that she had. I shook my head again. Then I realized that shaking my head might have mistakenly implied that I thought it would be good to have breast cancer. So I added, still walking,

"Mine is worse." It sounded ridiculous, immature, and competitive, even to me. That's not how I meant it. I just wanted to be left alone. But she continued,

"I asked because I have breast cancer."

I felt stalked. I walked faster keeping my head down. David was uncomfortable. He knew I wanted to get away, but he didn't want to be rude, so while walking with me he turned around and yelled back toward her in his booming voice, "She has ovarian cancer." I felt embarrassed and annoyed. Why did he have to announce this to strangers? Why couldn't she leave me alone? *And, by the way, I don't have ovarian cancer. I have peritoneal cancer.* For some reason this distinction felt particularly meaningful that day. She yelled back,

"You'll be all right!" My agitation increased. *How could she say that?* It would have been kind if she'd said: "I hope you'll be all right." It would have been better if she'd said, "I hope *I'll* be all right," because this exchange was more about her than me. Even if she'd said, "I believe we will be all right," she could have her opinion, and I could disagree with it in my head—away from her, away from this. But instead, she replied to my husband's slight shading of the truth with a complete misrepresentation of reality. She said that I would be all right. No, I wouldn't be. I felt misunderstood (again). I was frustrated with David and angry with her. ("Why did you tell a complete stranger my business? Why did you say I have ovarian?") My husband was annoyed. ("Why couldn't you be friendly to a well-meaning stranger? Why does it matter if I said ovarian?") It was another no-win situation in the cancer world, and just another thing to endure as a cancer sufferer.

The longer I had cancer, the more common these interactions seemed to become. One afternoon on a cruise during a break from chemotherapy, I was lying out in the sun on the "Serenity Deck." No children allowed. No loud announcements. No aggressive peddling of the cocktail-of-the-day. I had a beautiful view from the back of the ship of the vast sky and sea. I was peacefully alone, feeling serene and pain-free. A woman in a pink, breast cancer shirt, a pink, breast cancer cap, and a pink, breast cancer ribbon came up to me, drawn like a moth to my almost-bald head. The light down on my head told her that my hair was growing back. She thought she knew what that meant (remission) and was happy for me. She didn't know that this was the third time my hair had started to grow back: I had gotten too sick to tolerate the chemotherapy. If I could get stronger, I would resume chemotherapy and be bald again in two months. But she thought that chemotherapy was behind me, like it was behind her. She wanted us to be happy about that together. She didn't give me room to disappoint her with my truth, quickly launching into her own success story.

She thought that cancer had been a blessing. She was diagnosed with early breast cancer, had minor surgery, and was back at work within the week. She had a little radiation and had tolerated it well. She didn't need chemotherapy. That was ten years ago, and she had no recurrences. As a breast cancer survivor, she wanted to give back and never forget. She told me that she participates annually in the "Race for the Cure®" and always tries to get the word out. She was proud. Cancer had made her more generous, thankful, and knowledgeable.

I did not consider cancer, this one or the last, a blessing in any way. Like her, I had survived an early cancer, but I had never identified myself as a uterine cancer survivor. I didn't know what the color of our ribbon was, nor if we even had one. It had been eight years since I had the hysterectomy. I felt no need to tell that story to a stranger on a cruise. I was thankful that I didn't need chemotherapy then, and that I hadn't had a recurrence of the last cancer (although I would have preferred it to getting this one). Having a beatable cancer hadn't transformed me. It hadn't redefined me. I just went on with my life.

After she left, I wanted to stop thinking about cancer. I wanted to return to the sun, the breeze, and the moment. I needed painless, perfect moments. I planned to tap into my most blissful memories when I was sick in bed. But the man in the lounge next to me had a different idea. He started telling me about his wife's battle with breast cancer. He was a hero in this story. He drove her to the treatments because she was too weak to go alone. He organized her blood results on a spreadsheet when her platelets were demolished. On her behalf, he talked to the doctors, emphasizing to me, "You have to stay on top of them!" Now, she was fine. I said that I was glad. Yet, the conversation did not seem to be over. It was my turn to share. I replied that I have peritoneal cancer and that I was on a break from chemotherapy to allow my body to get stronger for another try. He was appropriately sympathetic, and wished me well before he got up to go to lunch. I was relieved that the conversation had gone so smoothly. It had been honest, brief, and minimally invasive. Then his wife walked over and looked at me. "That chemotherapy," she paused, "it's worse than the cancer." I was relieved. Here was a person that I could speak to honestly.

"I know what you mean," I exhaled.

"It hurt my heart," she said.

"Me too," I sympathized. "I had congestive heart failure."

"I have a pacemaker where my port used to be."

"I'm sorry to hear that," I said honestly.

"So . . ." she began (a typical lead-in to an invasive question), ". . . did you get a double mastectomy, or a single?"

I couldn't help but look down at my breasts. In a bathing suit, they were too big to be missing . . . too sagging to be fake. I couldn't believe she had asked about them. Her husband said, "She doesn't have breast cancer, honey. It's some other kind of cancer."

"Oh," she said, looking disappointed and a bit troubled, but strangely not embarrassed. Her script had run out. I was just a bald stranger who had nothing in common with her now. Without saying goodbye, she walked away. The Serenity Deck had failed to live up to its name. Sunglasses, a hat, and my nose in a book couldn't protect me from these conversations. Whether it was Think-Pink cheer or thank-God-that's-over relief, whether they wanted to celebrate or commiserate, as a bald, middle-aged woman, I was a target for the breast cancer survivors.

* * *

I *should* be a better audience for breast cancer survivors. I understand much of what they have gone through, at least more than most people do. I know what it feels like to hear a distressing diagnosis, and how hard chemotherapy is. I know the fear. I know the pain. I know the nightmare of a hospital stay, how dehumanizing it can be and how relentless. I even know what it is like to be a cancer survivor. The problem isn't that I don't understand *them*. It is that they don't understand *me*. I know that according to 2007 data an estimated 89 percent of women diagnosed with breast cancer live for five years or more. Do they know that only 45.6 percent of women with ovarian cancer do (NCI, YEAR)? They think of cancer as something triumphantly overcome. I have to live with it until it overcomes me. My story is their worst nightmare.

Primary peritoneal cancer is too rare, too difficult to spell, too impossible to pronounce, and too deadly to have its own ribbon. Instead it shares a teal ribbon with a host of gynecological cancers. Like uterine and ovarian cancers, we don't have any good news to galvanize people to raise money for research. We're an advertising firm's nightmare. Think of all the celebrities who can inspire us with stories of their breast cancer survival. Try to name a celebrity who is an ovarian cancer survivor. You can't. I can think of one celebrity who died of it (Gilda Radner), and two deceased mothers of celebrities (President Obama's and Angelina Jolie's).

The peritoneum, uterus, and ovaries are hidden, but breasts are visible. Most people don't even know they have a peritoneum. A uterus and ovaries are only useful when you're trying to conceive, and most of the time we're trying to avoid that. Besides, most of the women with ovarian cancer are past their child-bearing years. Society is fixated on breasts, so it's easy to get excited about them. Everyone loves breasts! "Save the Ta-Tas" is used to solicit donations as funding for "the Cure." I've seen the slogan on billboards and t-shirts. It always makes me mad. Let's save the women's lives, rather than focus on their body parts, shall we? If the ta-tas have to go for a woman to live, so be it.

There are far fewer cases of primary peritoneal, uterine, and ovarian cancers than breast cancer. The National Cancer Institute (n.d.)[10] estimated that there were 177,162 women alive on January 1, 2007 who had (or once had) ovarian cancer. There were 2,414,693 more women alive (2,591,855 total) who had breast cancer (NCI, n.d.). They estimate that one in seventy-two women born in 2010 will be diagnosed with ovarian cancer in their lifetime (NCI, YEAR). One in eight women will be diagnosed with breast cancer. While more women get breast cancer than get ovarian

---

[10] Editor's Note: Larson's notes do not provide an access date or search terms for these statistics, obtained from the Surveillance, Epidemiology, and End Results Program's "Fast Stats" tool. However, as of February 2014, the interactive tool remains available online and is cited on the References page.

cancer, their chances of surviving five years or more after diagnosis are much better. The Institute estimates that 21,880 women will be diagnosed with ovarian cancer—and 13,850 will die of it—in 2010 (NCI, YEAR). For the same year, almost ten times as many women are expected to be diagnosed with breast cancer (207,090), but only about three times as many (39,840) are expected to die of it (NCI, YEAR).

A vital factor for survival is how advanced cancer is when it is diagnosed. Five-year survival rates for both breast and ovarian cancers drop dramatically when the cancer is discovered after "metastasizing," or spreading out from the region close to the primary cancer site. When the cancer has remained "local," or contained within the primary site, 93.1 percent of ovarian cancer patients and 98.1 percent of breast cancer patients live five years or more. When the cancer is "regional," or confined to the area close to the primary site or the lymph nodes, 69 percent of ovarian cancer patients and 83.1 percent of breast cancer patients survive five years or more. If the cancer is labeled "distant," because it has metastasized outside of this region, only 29.6 percent of ovarian cancer patients and 26 percent of breast cancer patients live for five years or more.

Since fewer women get ovarian cancer than breast cancer, it gets less publicity, and less research money. With a small market, it is not profitable enough for drug companies to invest in studies of ovarian cancer. As a result, we are treated with drugs that were designed to treat breast cancer and colon cancer. Like other hand-me-downs, they don't fit most of us very well. But they cover us up, so it isn't obvious how little can be done to cure us. Should I be thanking the Think Pink® campaign for raising so much money for all that research that is helping so many women? Or should I resent that they consume so much of the enthusiasm and money for fighting women's cancers? Could I feel both? Or does that make me, once again, too complicated, too difficult to relate to, and too unlikable for anyone to listen?

* * *

The breast cancer survivor crowd has a lot more to say about their experiences than the ovarian women. Maybe we're too busy being sick to write about it. Maybe no one wants to hear sad stories when there are so many spunky ones told by the breast cancer survivors. Or maybe ovarian cancer sufferers are just less likely to survive to write books. They see the clock running out, and they don't spend their final seconds crafting memoirs. A quick search of *Amazon*'s holdings on February 20th, 2010 under "breast cancer memoir" revealed one hundred and ten entries. There were only three under "ovarian cancer memoirs." Two of these were written by the dead patients' family members. Only one was a survivor's story, and she was also writing about her breast cancer.

I imagine it must be particularly hard to be one of the women dying of breast cancer. Are they black-balled and ignored, vilified and blamed? Or are they martyred as fallen angels? No matter which, I can't see them as retaining much of their individualities, because their stories have to somehow serve the larger, survivor narrative. Like mine, their experiences also contradict the relentlessly upbeat and feisty, mainstream, breast-cancer rhetoric, which has redefined cancer as a challenge that a determined, modern woman can overcome through pluck, hilarity, and bonding. Surviving breast cancer has become a symbol of female empowerment. The subtext says, "You can do it, girlfriend! It's in your control!" The face of breast cancer wears a smile, lipstick, and it shares a clever wink. You can see it in the titles of the breast cancer memoirs.

Titles such as *Adventures of Cancer Bitch*, *Breastless in the City*, and *Cancer Vixen* make breast cancer sound like a hell of a good time. Clearly, I'm missing out on a lot of fun. Frankly, I don't see an upside to having cancer. I can't think of one good thing about chemotherapy. Unlike the author of *I Wore Lipstick to My Mastectomy*, I wore a nose tube to my intestinal resection. The cover of *I'd Rather Do Chemo Than Clean Out the Garage: Choosing Laughter Over Tears* depicts a woman happily reclining in a chair, wearing a bathrobe and slippers, sharing a laugh with her dog, who sits dutifully (and also smiling) next to her. (For the sake of transparency, this memoir *is* about ovarian, not breast, cancer.) Although the cover of *I'd Rather Do Chemo* . . . suggests that chemo is a rest, I would rather clean one thousand garages than have chemotherapy. I am not in the sisterhood full of hope and healing—I am alone in my bathroom with my rising CA125 marker. I don't get *My One Night Stand with Cancer* (another cancer memoir) or even a year with it, like the author of *Humor After the Tumor: One Woman's Look at Her Year with Breast Cancer*. I will have it for the rest of my short lifetime. I don't find this a hilarious and fulfilling journey. I wish that not being upbeat made me a subversive, a maverick, and an outsider. But these titles just make me look like I am a party pooper.

When people ask, "Do you have breast cancer?" my voice in my head sometimes says, *I wish*. Then I quickly admonish myself. Of course I don't want breast cancer! And I know that I could still get it; it would give me a female cancer trifecta. But I would rather have breast cancer than the cancer I have. Then, I would have a chance. Then, all those mammograms might have paid off. Then, I'd be in the right women's cancer club—the one full of winners. I feel guilty about this admission. It seems disloyal. It seems hypocritical. It is probably asking for trouble.

Even if I did have breast cancer, I know that I wouldn't fit into the Think Pink® club because I can accept that bad things happen to good people. They do all the time. I don't have to reevaluate my worth if something bad happens to me. I don't have to pretend that cancer isn't really that bad or that there's some silver lining to it that will make it worth the suffering. I don't need to have a payoff for tragedy: a special bond with other women with aberrant cells in their bodies; a renewed confidence in my endurance; or a new lease on life. I just need to remember that some awful things happen and they have no payoffs. I can hope for the best, but I can't expect it and I can't blame myself if I don't get it. I have no choice but to play the cards I've been dealt, even when they aren't very good ones.

Chapter 16: Somewhere Along the Way

My CA125 went down once more during eight months of treatment. My only break was to undergo surgery for an anal fissure, followed by a few weeks off to regain my strength. During this time, with depleted fervor, I challenged my insurance company's decision to deny me reimbursement for taking Avastin® without first notifying my doctor's office. At the end of the eighth month, tests showed a "significant advancement of the disease": more and larger tumors spread throughout my abdomen. These prompted consultations with doctors from three major cancer research universities. I tried the Avastin® infusion, coupled with low-dose daily chemotherapy pills that they all recommended to slow the growth. After a month of side effects, including soaring blood pressure and indications of kidney damage, we stopped the treatment. I remained on Femara® (an estrogen-inhibiting pill), but knew from experience that its effectiveness was limited.

I say that "we stopped" because Dr. Kind was on board with the decision. Despite being an oncologist who believed in aggressive treatment, he saw what it was doing to me. He knew what the few chemotherapy drugs that I had not tried were likely to do, or more importantly, not do. "These drugs are intended to extend life, not existence," he clarified. "It's your decision when to stop treatment." It was hard to resist the ideology that viewed "stopping" as "quitting." I did want to postpone death, and I had demonstrated that I could endure a lot of suffering in order to do so. I didn't like to disappoint people—I was a rule-follower. So, when it felt like Dr. Kind gave me permission to stop the drugs, I jumped at the opportunity. He seemed as relieved as I felt. "I think this is a good decision," he said, confiding, "I think you've been ready for this for a while."

I had been. Yet, I still longed to know what to expect. How do people die of this? What sort of timetable was I looking at? What should I do and avoid doing? I had gotten vague answers to these questions before. I wondered if stopping treatment would trigger the release of this information. But when I asked, "What's next?" Dr. Kind interpreted the question by describing *his* role in this final stage:

"I don't see any reason to continue to monitor the cancer's growth with blood tests or scans. We don't need to set up additional appointments; you should just call me when you need me."

This response, our agreement, was an abrupt reversal of the last three years: he had wanted weekly chemotherapy, and I had argued for every three weeks; he resisted breaks, and my body insisted on them; he disparaged Dr. Black-Sheep's treatment, and I defended the drugs that had seemed to temporarily help me. He seemed to have two speeds: full-speed-ahead and stop. It made sense if you used a "fighting" and "giving up" dichotomy for what was happening. But I had never subscribed to this paradigm. I had known since the diagnosis that I was dying: sometimes I was dying more slowly; sometimes with more discomfort; sometimes with one chemotherapy or the other; and sometimes without it. The decision to forgo chemotherapy was not particularly distinctive. I would still be dying. I couldn't help but think: *When he believed he might be able to save me, he was relentless. Now, that he has finally admitted that he can't, he wants me out of his sight.* My face must have revealed some evidence of this uncharitable interpretation, because he said, "I don't take it as a personal failure when my patients don't survive. I like to think that I'm here to help them deal with this disease even if I can't cure them. I don't want you to feel like I'm abandoning you. We can set up an appointment schedule if you'd like. I just can't imagine you'd want to spend much more of the time you have left here." He was right about that.

He continued, "I know that somewhere along the way you've come to believe that doctors do things *to* you, not *for* you. That's not how it is; we're trying to help." If another doctor had said this to me, I probably would have assembled all the evidence I had accumulated to justify the belief that he had succinctly articulated. But this was Dr. Kind. He was sincere. He was caring. And he had just revealed that he knew something about how I felt, though I had never tried to explain to him. It was what I had always wanted: to be seen as I am, not how other patients are, or how the doctor wants me to be or fears that I am. My eyes filled with tears, and I would have sobbed if I had tried to say something, so I just nodded.

When I walked out of the Mansion that day into the crisp autumn air, it was easy to clear my nose of the smell of chemicals. Their heaviness didn't linger like they had when I left with them in my veins. I was officially done with chemotherapy. I stood at the edge of the parking lot for a few minutes taking the time to embrace this thought. I looked around making mental photographs of my "farewell." For the first time, I noticed a beautiful, big tree. Its leaves had all changed to yellow, but were still clinging to the branches. I felt free, even though I knew I was not free of the cancer and the death that it would bring. But that future was not here yet. I didn't know how far away it was. I hoped for months, instead of weeks.

Afterword

Stephanie surprised us all—including herself—by living much longer than she originally anticipated she would when she first learned that she had cancer throughout her abdominal cavity in December 2007. Although she ghoulishly joked that she should call her memoir "Still Dying," in reality she spent those four years after her diagnosis still living. She continued to teach courses at Dickinson College and to work with her colleagues in political science and women's and gender studies. With her husband David, she traveled, visited her family and friends, and spent time by the water—pools and ocean—whenever she could.

Between the time when Stephanie returned from England and March 2011, I spent a few memorable afternoons with her at the Hershey Spa, getting our "treatments" and exchanging gossip. On one particularly unforgettable afternoon, as we lounged by Hershey's exotic outdoor pool, lightning struck; we ran up through the gardens in our spa robes, knocking madly on the locked doors for someone to let us in. Our laughter abated, however, as Stephanie started coughing, and nearly collapsed on the bench inside one of the doors. Everything that happened in those last four years—no matter how good—was always lined with the reality that Stephanie was sick.

Despite feeling horrible most of the time, bothered by both pain and exhaustion, Stephanie continued to work on her memoir. She believed that it would be a powerful indictment of the medical industry—an industry that refuses to acknowledge its own limits and the way that its institutions and practitioners fail to listen to or care for patients. After sharing the first draft with friends and colleagues in 2010, she began the painstaking process of revision.

In October 2010, Stephanie and her doctor agreed that continuing chemotherapy might prolong, but would certainly substantially degrade the quality of, the remainder of Stephanie's life. She stopped treatment but continued to work on her memoir. By March 2011, however, she was too tired to work on it anymore. It was at this point that we all knew she really was dying.

Her husband, David, chronicled Stephanie's final months in email updates to her family and friends. When the first of the updates arrived, we assumed that they were temporary—a courtesy until Stephanie was strong enough to write on her own. But as they kept coming, the content of each email made it increasingly clear that Stephanie was unlikely to speak for herself again.

Looking back, I think these emails may have been a transformative experience for David. As he lovingly narrated Stephanie's death, he seemed to take on the responsibility of delivering her voice to the world.[11]

Email Sent March 15th, 2011:

---

[11] Editor's Note: Amy Farrell, the author of this afterword, thought it was important to include the actual texts of David's emails to Larson's family and friends. She felt that they accurately chronicled Larson's final weeks and provide the appropriate closure to Larson's unfinished memoir. For the reader's clarity, all emails are preceded by the date on which they were sent, and the texts of emails are italicized. Emails are separated by asterisk breaks. Amy's periodic commentary on specific emails follows in unformatted text.

Over the weekend—and actually the past few weeks, Stephanie started having more difficulty eating. She would bloat quickly after eating small amounts of food and would spend hours walking the house in pain due to stomach cramps. We also noticed distension in her stomach above the belly button, a place we hadn't noticed it before. Finally, after eating a small late dinner on Saturday night, Stephanie threw up at 6:30 AM on Sunday morning. It looked as though the food wasn't being digested, so we decided that we'd better call the doctor. We did, and he arranged for a hospital room in Harrisburg, so on Sunday evening we checked Stephanie in.

They gave her an x-ray and found that there was more air in her upper bowel than in her lower bowel, a sign of a partial intestinal blockage. We talked to the doctor yesterday morning, and the strategy is going to be to act slowly. They're giving Stephanie very small amounts of fluid by mouth and no food, hoping that the bowel will calm down and start working right again. If that doesn't help, we'll discuss surgery or other options. She tried some fluids last night and had to have some morphine to dull the pain in her gut. It's very sad.

She's getting good care from the nurses, which is a good thing. She had trouble sleeping Sunday night, but we devised a solution to that (long and boring story—no need to tell it here) and she slept better last night.

Other than the eating complications, Stephanie's doing okay. She's very hungry, which the doctor says is a good sign. She's also very sad and scared, as you can imagine. I bought her a portable DVD player last night, and she's watching Ghost Whisperer and the Big Bang Theory. I spent all day with her yesterday and will spend most of today there as well. I plan on camping there until she's out of the hospital.

There's no need to over-worry at this point. I don't think she's in danger of dying or anything like that. It's just another episode that confirms her belief that this road is going to be exceedingly hard. She has her phone there, so you can call her if you want. She might not answer for a variety of reasons, but I know she'll appreciate your call. I'll keep you updated if anything happens.

* * *

Email Sent March 18th, 2011:

Yesterday was a really hard day for her. She didn't feel too well because of the fluid still accumulating in her abdomen. She vomited for the first time since Sunday morning, probably due to the fact that her stomach is being squeezed by the fluid, and the natural fluids inside of her digestive system had nowhere to go but out.

She had to wait most of the day to have a catheter inserted into her abdominal cavity, and she was finally wheeled down to radiology around 4:00 PM. There were some bumps in the road before the surgery (people laughing and joking around, not enough anesthesia initially), but once the doctor started, the procedure went without incident. They drained almost two liters of fluid, and her distension went down noticeably. Stephanie now has a catheter sticking out of the side of her belly so that fluids can be drained as needed. We hope that the relief in pressure will allow her to eat some solid food, but there's no guarantee. The draining of the fluid has made her more comfortable, however, which is good. I left her around midnight, and she was resting comfortably.

At this point, Stephanie will probably get discharged on Sunday or Monday and will come home to our house in Carlisle. She'll be getting hospice care, and we'll need to modify the furniture arrangement to make it work for the extra equipment that will be around. I'm also going to go down to our apartment in Maryland and bring some stuff back that will make things a bit easier and more enjoyable (if this could ever be enjoyable, right?) for Stephanie. We're thinking that the adjustment and modification phase will take about a week in total.

We'll probably try some solid food today, so keep your fingers crossed and say a prayer or two that Stephanie will be able to pass it through her system without too much pain and effort. I'll update you as we know more.

* * *

Email sent March 20th, 2011:

Today was an annoying day, but not a bad day. The nurses on duty weren't particularly good, and her doctor didn't show up (his partner was on call instead of him, but we had hoped he would stop by), so Stephanie got pretty frustrated. However, she was able to eat part of a chicken dish and keep it down. We think that the draining of the ascites [accumulation of fluid in the abdominal cavity] from her abdomen has taken enough pressure off of her bowels to allow her to eat small amounts of food. The lower pressure gives her more comfort, as does the ability to eat solid food. Things are still dire and can (really the correct word is "will") change at any time, so we're happy for these small positive moments.

* * *

The next day, Stephanie was discharged from the hospital. David was managing the move from the apartment in Maryland (where his job was located), arranging a leave-of-absence from work to become Stephanie's full-time caretaker, and adjusting to the new rhythms of hospice care. It was difficult, and they had to change hospice nurses after the first nurse didn't understand how to communicate with Stephanie.

* * *

Email sent March 31st, 2011:

Since Marcus and Sharon [Stephanie's brother and sister-in-law] left on Sunday lots of things have happened.

We continue to settle in as we merge the apartment with the house. I've got movers bringing the last of our stuff from Maryland tomorrow, so it'll be a cramped and busy weekend. Stephanie has been feeling okay, but she has had some digestive pains in the same area that she's been having trouble with. It could be the amount of food she ate, or just a tight area in her intestines. We don't know. We tried draining again and got very little fluid out, so unless the drain is defective she's not producing a lot of fluid and thus excess fluid is not a cause for this discomfort. Her belly hasn't distended too much, though it seems to be a little more distended than when she got out of the hospital.

We found out that we can do home hospice in Florida. However, we need to investigate levels of service in Florida versus Pennsylvania. We'd also have to find a local physician. Stephanie and I are torn, because we'd be giving up the relative comfort of knowing the hospital and personnel and doctors in Pennsylvania. On the other hand, we'd be gaining the benefits of sun and family in Florida. No decisions yet and not sure when we'll make them. . . .

The new hospice nurse is MUCH better than the first one. She seems to listen to what Stephanie is saying and is very sensitive about causing pain. She's also making the effort to "pull through" services by making phone calls to the doctor and to the hospice service. . . .

* * *

A few weeks later, David and Stephanie realized that the abdominal drain was not helping at all; indeed, it had actually decreased her quality of life even further as she could no longer take baths with ease, one of the last pleasures available to her.

* * *

Email sent April 10th, 2011:

Stephanie continues to hang in there, but things are still up in the air. She's eating, but her pain seems to be getting more intense afterwards. She's taken morphine a couple times this week as it seems to help dull the discomfort. We're not sure whether it's the cancer, the food she's eating, or the amount of food. If it's the amount of food, then her cancer's definitely growing because she's not eating a ton.

Despite that, she's had a couple good days. We had a great meal at a new (for us) sushi restaurant in Harrisburg on Friday. She paid for it by not being able to leave her room yesterday. We went out for lunch at another sushi restaurant on Wednesday.

I'm going to put on a couple waterproof bandages today and take a bath to see if our "system" is waterproof. That will allow Stephanie to take baths or even go in pools if it works. Right now, she can only shower, and losing the option to take a bath has been tough. Baths help to equalize some of the pressure in her gut. And speaking of pressure, we're still not getting a whole lot of fluid out of her abdominal drain. What a waste that's turned out to be, as it's also the primary reason she can't take a bath. . . .

We're still undecided about Florida. I think that Stephanie is struggling with the amount of people reaching out to her. She doesn't feel that great most of the time but doesn't want to disappoint her friends that want to say goodbye. Ahhhh . . . one of my Love's great attributes is also a weakness in that she is finding it difficult to be selfish with the time she has left. We talk about it a lot. Everything is logistically possible, but we haven't "jumped."

* * *

David and Stephanie ultimately decided to stay in Pennsylvania to maximize her chances of being heard by her doctors. It would be too hard to find a doctor in Florida and develop a relationship while Stephanie was in hospice care.

By the middle of April, Stephanie was no longer able to eat. While Stephanie and David worked well with the hospice nurses, they both found the restrictions on morphine irritating. Discouraged by the mounting and un-abating pain, Stephanie withdrew into herself. Her care fell almost entirely onto David.

* * *

Email sent April 18th, 2011:

Stephanie had more and more pain during and after eating less and less food as last week went on. Early Sunday morning around 4:00 AM, she threw up for the first time since the day she went into the hospital. This is significant because it probably signals the end of her eating. We had hopes that perhaps she could at least take a bite of food, so she could experience taste, but today she felt pain after sucking (not chewing at all) on one tiny cinnamon heart candy.

I talked to the hospice nurse, and we're trying to figure out a course of action with pain managing drugs. The doctor didn't want to approve pre-measured doses of morphine in syringes because of liability issues (you know, so I could feed my morphine addiction), so we're going to continue with the liquid morphine administered orally until Stephanie can't tolerate that anymore. At that point, we'll switch over to a morphine pump.

Stephanie's been sleeping almost twenty hours a day over the last four days, which is consistent with what happens as the disease progresses. What little waking time she has is usually spent in bed, watching videos or going through old pictures or writing cards. I'd say that in most cases Stephanie has some sort of pain while she is awake. She's lucid and alert and funny and very sad, but ultimately she's incredibly exhausted. Stephanie has decided that she doesn't want to see anyone before she dies, partly because she doesn't want to be remembered looking and feeling like she does and partly because she simply does not have the energy to engage with anyone, including me, for more than a few minutes at a time. You're welcome to call. Just realize that she may not be able to pick up or even return your call if you don't reach her.

I'm holding up physically and mentally, though I get sadder by the hour. Taking care of Stephanie is really a whole lot of down time with intermittent spurts of activity, so physically it's not hard, though the hours are a bit wild. I'll need help once this is all over, so don't worry about me now. The hospice system has been great, so we have the medical support, and there's a social worker who calls weekly to see if we need anything.

* * *

Email sent April 22nd, 2011:

Stephanie's getting weaker as the days go by, and I'm now helping her get out of bed and chairs. She's sipping small amounts of water and has not thrown up since Sunday. I don't know if she's going to throw up again—it depends on whether the moisture is getting through her intestines. I think she has a chance of throwing up one more time before she goes.

Stephanie is lucid and alert but so very tired and dry. I got her lip balm and a mouth moisturizer yesterday, which seems to help.

The home health aide is coming again today to help clean Stephanie. Stephanie enjoyed that earlier this week.

* * *

While David described her care as "a whole lot of down time with intermittent spurts of activity," she was requiring much more care, both physically and mentally. Since she wasn't eating, the doctor suggested that she only had a few weeks left. But the hospice nurse disagreed, telling David that often it takes much longer with a person as young as Stephanie. David didn't know what to believe or anticipate but his care for Stephanie was unwavering.

* * *

Email sent April 24th, 2011:

Things are progressing as you'd expect. Stephanie slept most of the weekend. She got up to brush her teeth and go to the bathroom, and we talked for maybe three hours total besides that.

She doesn't seem to be experiencing too much pain, but she is disoriented at times and is having trouble talking because of her dry mouth. I noticed today that her ankles are swollen. This could be because she hasn't been moving around or because her circulatory system is starting to weaken.

I "hug and lift" Stephanie to get her out of bed, off the toilet, off seats, etc. She's lost a lot of weight, because it's easier for me to scooch her up the bed by lifting her honeymoon style than it was earlier in the week.

I had a hospital bed, hospital table, and a 3-in-1 commode delivered Saturday night. I put the commode over our existing toilet. Basically it raises up the toilet so it's easier to sit down and get up. Pretty ingenious. Stephanie is still managing on our bed, so I decided to put the hospital bed in her room and sleep on it. This way I can hear her easier if she calls out. I'll put her in the hospital bed when it makes sense (i.e., she can't get in and out of our bed anymore).

Last night was sort of fun, like a slumber party. Stephanie woke up about every two hours and wanted to go to the bathroom. So we'd go in and get her situated. I'd give her some privacy and sit outside the door. We'd talk some while she was on the pot, and then again as I was leading her back to bed. I felt like she was "there" for the most part last night. The "spirits" that she thought were trying to get her into the bathroom to torment her the night before didn't make an appearance, presumably because Big David was in the house.

It's been eight days since Stephanie has eaten anything solid. The doctor originally said that it would probably take one to two weeks for her to fade away. The hospice nurse said that she's seen people around Stephanie's age last as long as four weeks with no food and just fluid. We'll see. I think we're probably looking at one to two weeks, but I admit that every time I go in the bedroom I look for the movements in her chest as she breathes.

My time is now being taken up more by tending to Stephanie because of the aid I'm giving her to keep her mobile. I'm getting out of the house when people come over, which is fine. The nurse is here once or twice per week and will probably be here more if we need her, and the health aide will be coming in twice or three times per week to help with Stephanie's cleaning.

* * *

At the end of April, David wrote to update Stephanie's friend Lydia, who had been traveling out of the country. He filled her in on everything she had missed and added, "I don't know how much longer she'll last. She doesn't show any signs of 'imminent' death (as described in the uplifting literature that was left for us by the hospice people), but her condition is very fluid and changes occur rapidly. She's actually declined visibly since three am this morning. This death process is quite bizarre to me at times."

A few days later, David wrote an email to all her friends and family. As he so aptly put it in his message to Lydia, the death process was bizarre . . . and difficult for everyone. The clichés that "no one needs to die in pain" or that "hospice will take care of everything" were simply not true. The dying process was confounding—was it the Ativan or her body poisoning itself that was causing her confusion? Or, did she actually see things that the fully living could not see? The hospice nurses could not do everything, especially as Stephanie looked to David as her primary source of comfort. David himself was becoming exhausted.

* * *

Email sent April 30th, 2011:

Since Tuesday a number of things have happened. I'll summarize using bullet points below.

- *Overall, Stephanie's condition has deteriorated, as can be expected. She hasn't eaten in two weeks and hasn't had any fluids outside of sips of water in a week. That said, she's stronger than I would expect (she's still incredibly weak). She's close to dying, I think, but death doesn't seem to be imminent. Of course, that could change quickly, but as of tonight I'll stand by my statement.*

- *We're seeing hospice people or health aids almost every day of the week, and local friends are coming over as needed so that I can slip out to the store or just get an hour off.*

- *Stephanie's lucidity comes and goes, but has gotten a bit better since we eased her off of the Ativan over this week. It turns out that the pharmacy had given us a stronger dosage per pill than what we had before (2mg instead of 1 mg), so we were giving Stephanie twice the amount of medicine unknowingly. This made her groggy and "out of it" quite often.*

- *She forgets things at certain times (she's called me her friend David and has wondered where her husband David was, for instance) and talks about people that pop in to look at her, especially kids. She doesn't seem threatened by the people, and it's tough to figure out whether she's hallucinating or seeing ghosts or both. She has not seen anyone in her family, though she said that Marty [her deceased father] was waiting outside but wasn't ready to come in. The hospice nurse thinks that some of the confusion could be a result of the body beginning to shut down and not process wastes as efficiently. The wastes in her blood could contribute to confusion.*

- *Stephanie is very weak. I lift her out of bed, put her in a mini wheelchair and roll her to the bathroom, where we reverse the process. I have to help her get her legs in and out of the bed, and I physically move her to change where she is in the bed. It's not that big of a deal, except when she wants to get in and out of bed every hour. I've had to put my foot down a couple of times and tell her that she needed to stay in bed. I figure that as long as I use good form, I'm developing my back muscles again. Gosh, Stephanie as a set of weights. . . . One indication of what's happening with Stephanie is that it's gotten a lot easier to move her around as the days have gone by because she's losing weight.*

- *I can put two hands around her thigh and have my fingers meet, and yet she can still stand.*

- *Stephanie's belly is the only thing not shrinking as she's losing weight. The cancer has definitely grown inside of there.*

- *Last night was a nightmare. Stephanie was up literally every hour trying to get out of bed while not being totally coherent. I doubt I got any REM sleep, and it showed today. We were able to take a few naps so that helped.*

- *Today was actually pretty good. Stephanie was "here" for the most part, though we had some pretty bizarre conversations. We worked well together and had a few laughs, which was nice.*

- *Stephanie is now throwing up every day, or at least she has for the past four days. It's basically liquid and full of bile and very smelly—poison in other words. She's most likely partially or totally blocked, and she could have multiple blockages. Up until yesterday she was pooing, but that hasn't happened today. The only solution to this would be a nose tube, and Stephanie reiterated today that she didn't want a nose tube, even if it meant vomiting every day. I'm fine with that—the less intrusion to her body the better.*

- *Lee [Stephanie's nephew] talked to Stephanie last night. It was sad talking to him afterwards, as he was pretty shaken. Stephanie was able to talk, but wasn't always making sense, which could be very unsettling if you're not prepared for it. I'm talking about statements like "Did you kick the aliens out of your house yet?" or "I'm not sure where my husband is but this guy named David is doing a pretty good job." That being said, it was great that he called because Stephanie knew who it was and she definitely wanted to talk to him.*

- *At the moment I'm doing okay, but I'm very tired. If I can get Stephanie to keep her night-time awakenings to three-hour intervals I'll be okay. I can't take too many of those once-every-hour-awakening nights.*

- *Connie sent some wonderful flowers—irises—and they brought a big smile to Stephanie's face.*

- *Thanks again, Connie, and thanks for sending flowers for the past three years. You've been pretty awesome with that.*

* * *

Almost ten days later, Stephanie continued to get sicker, but her body held on. She and David both worked to be able to keep her at home, away from doctors and the hospital. What continued to come across in David's emails to Stephanie's family and friends was that he still saw Stephanie and himself as a team. When he wrote about Stephanie's "vomit sessions," he reassured us that "*we* [emphasis mine] got everything cleaned up with a minimum amount of fuss." We all knew that David had done the cleaning himself. But to David, Stephanie's suffering was his suffering.

* * *

Email sent May 9th, 2011:

This was a really tough weekend for Stephanie. She threw up multiple times and generally felt pretty bad. Bullet points below as details come to mind:

- *Stephanie hadn't thrown up since Thursday, but she was feeling bloated. She finally threw up on Saturday, but there wasn't a whole lot. Yesterday, the dams burst. Two of the three vomit sessions involved large quantities of bile and thick liquid. It smelled like it had been sitting in her intestines for a bit. It was a mess, but we got everything cleaned up with a minimum amount of fuss.*

413

- *The vomiting didn't help her stomach for very long. The bloating and nausea returned quickly, along with some pain. The pain, I presume, was from air and liquids moving along the temporarily cleared portions of bowel.*

- *I worry that Stephanie's got multiple blockages, and that some of the vomit is coming from an area of the intestine that has a partial blockage at the beginning and end of that section. This could account for much of what Stephanie felt and how she vomited.*

- *Stephanie's very weak and thin. I can count every vertebra in her back by touch—go ahead and try it on a friend, you can't count all of the bones when there's even a small amount of fat covering them. I can actually see the separation between her glutes and quads. I have to help her sit up, move her legs up and down, reposition her legs on the bed, and help her sit down on the toilet.*

- *I asked Stephanie Friday, Saturday, and Sunday if she wanted to go to the hospital, and she said no. She also declined considering a nose tube. I'm with her on both counts. I just hope we can keep her out of the hospital. I'm willing to be Vomit Boy and clean up any messes if it means she can stay at home and be in some comfort.*

- *Stephanie is in bed twenty-four hours a day with the exception of brief trips to the bedside commode.*

- *She's sleeping the same, about eighteen to twenty hours.*

- *Last night was tough because Stephanie didn't feel well. She was restless, confused, and tired.*

- *She kept wanting to get up, but we made a deal that I'd call a hospice nurse this morning if she could remain still. I told her that it would help to calm her stomach, which is not a lie.*

* * *

Stephanie's two biggest fears about the dying process were that she would vomit and that she would be in pain. As the days went on, both fears were realized. As her vital signs weakened, David's emails began to reflect the realization that Stephanie would pass soon and so he increased the frequency of his messages to family and friends.

* * *

Email sent May 12th, 2011:

It's getting closer. Stephanie's blood pressure was down to 80/52 this afternoon from 90/62 Tuesday and 100/62 last Thursday. She's weaker, still in pain, and still vomiting. She vomited last night at 1:00 AM and her stomach continues to be off. Her weight loss has accelerated, and she's beginning to show some common signs of dying such as cold limbs and discoloration in her extremities. Stephanie could go in the next few days, and I wouldn't be surprised if it happened this weekend. I'll keep the updates going on a daily basis from here on out.

* * *

Email sent May 14th, 2011:

No major changes to report. Stephanie continues to decline. Her heartbeat has slowed significantly, down to 52 from 68 last week. She actually slept okay last evening, though she's in quite a bit of pain. She threw up at 6:30 AM this morning and that seemed to help. She was able to sleep from

415

then until noon. I woke up later than I have in years—11:30 AM. Guess I
needed the sleep.

* * *

Email sent May 16th, 2011:

Hospice nurse came today. Blood pressure is 80/50, pulse around
50, and heart rate is getting a bit irregular. Stephanie is in and out of lucidity,
though that isn't exactly the right word. She knows who, what, where in
general, but she gets words mixed up and calls things by different names (she
called her sheets her "brown outfit" and [said] she needed to change it). She's in
constant low-grade pain. We're trying to up the amount of the fentanyl patch
she's now wearing. Hopefully that will help. She threw up twice on Saturday
right after ingesting morphine. I don't think the morphine caused the vomiting,
because I think she was getting ready to vomit anyways. That being said, we
stopped the morphine yesterday, and now she's pooing (though it's not any poo
you or I would recognize. I know, I know—too much information).

* * *

The days went on, and Stephanie deteriorated—
excruciatingly slowly because except for the cancer, she was
healthy. The cancer in her abdominal cavity was slowly starving her
strong heart and beaten, but breathing body. As David described
her struggles and the effects of her starvation, the first signs of his
own fatigue crept into his emails. Sometimes he couldn't recall
what he'd told us in the email before, so he told us again.

* * *

Email sent May 18th, 2011:

Hospice nurse came today. Vitals are the same (Blood pressure:
80/50; pulse: 44).

Stephanie threw up four times yesterday—nothing but greenish-yellow, thick, gooey bile. You can hear it coming up from deep inside her. I'm not sure that I've ever heard such deep toned burps. She hasn't thrown up today, but I expect her to tonight.

The last two nights, I thought I'd wake up and Stephanie would be dead. She slept so quietly and didn't move a muscle. I actually woke up at 4:00 AM yesterday and debated with myself about whether to verify if Stephanie were still alive. I was exhausted and wasn't freaked out if there was a body next to me, so I thought that I could probably sleep until 7:00 AM, call Hospice and get the nurse we usually have rather than some generic on-call nurse. Sounds creepy, doesn't it? But I gave in and got up and saw her chest rise and fall slightly but steadily. She was still alive. I don't know what I would have done if she weren't—perhaps cry for a while and enjoy some final alone time with my love. . . .

Stephanie can still be described by the adjectives I've used in past emails—weak, exhausted, frustrated, confused at times, but very lucid at other times. The hospice nurse admitted to me today that she didn't think that Stephanie would be here today. She also admitted that she is totally flummoxed by Stephanie's condition—she's so weak and yet she just keeps going and going. The nurse is also beginning to understand how medical standards don't necessarily apply to individual patients. Perhaps that will help her in the future.

* * *

Email sent May 25th, 2011:

No significant changes have occurred in the past few days.

Stephanie hasn't vomited since Sunday. Instead she is pooing ten to twelve times a day. It's mostly liquid with fibrous things in it. She's been very bloated and nauseous throughout, and unfortunately we don't have any drug that would address those symptoms.

Stephanie could go anytime, or she could last a week at this point. More as things develop. . . .

* * *

Stephanie began to vomit more often as the cancer completely choked her intestines. David monitored her more, making sure she was comfortable and able to throw up. They developed an intimate routine to deal with Stephanie's need for assistance.

* * *

Email sent May 27th, 2011:

There's one noteworthy change that's occurred in the past two days: Stephanie's heart rate has almost doubled into the 80's. It's a sign that the body is now responding to the dehydration and low blood pressure conditions that Stephanie's endured over the past weeks. This is something normally seen as a person progresses towards death. I envision it as Stephanie finally getting off this plateau and continuing the dying process.

After not vomiting for a few days Stephanie's vomited three times today. Each time it's been the Diet Coke she was drinking about a half hour before. The Diet Coke isn't the cause or catalyst. I think she's now blocking higher up in her digestive system, as the volume of vomit has been quite low.

Stephanie's "here" but not really engaged. She knows who I am, where we are, and she understands what the many emails I read her are saying. She doesn't seem able to communicate that clearly, however, often confusing words and describing people and events that aren't happening.

Through it all, we're doing okay, or at least as well as can be expected. We have a bit of a rhythm and routine. When she says she has to vomit I bring her the "vomit pan" and make sure she's sitting up in bed. As she starts to retch I wet a wash cloth and wipe her face. Once there's a lull she grabs the wash cloth, and I empty the pan. After she's done, she takes a sip of water, swishes it around and spits it out. We call it "swish and spit." Then she takes a swig of water and swallows. Then she rinses with Scope and spits it out. And then she usually asks for Diet Coke.

We've got a few routines like that and some fun terms. "Swish and Swallow" refers to swishing water in her mouth when taking a pill before she swallows. "Plop and drop" is wiping your fanny and immediately dropping the toilet paper into the toilet (no peeking LOL). "Flat or bent" asked as a question refers to whether she wants her legs up close to her body or stretched out. In short, we adapt. I wouldn't say we're making the best of it, because it isn't about making it better. It's more about making it easier to cope. . . .

Anyways, that's what I've got. I can't say whether Stephanie will make it through the weekend. I'll keep you in the loop regardless.

* * *

Email sent May 29th, 2011:

Stephanie continues to vomit—three times in the past twenty-four hours with the latest at 5:30 AM this morning. Even though she's still going to the bathroom, it looks as if most of the liquid she's putting into her system is coming back up mixed with bile. I worry that she's getting blocked higher in her digestive system, which would shorten the time in between vomit incidents.

She's sleeping longer and quieter and not moving much, if at all. She bordered on unresponsive yesterday afternoon but started responding later on in the day.

Hospice nurse is coming later today. I don't expect anything new, but if there is, I'll email.

* * *

The last two weeks of Stephanie's life were characterized by a rapid decline in her physical condition. As her body shut down, it became more difficult to keep the small amounts of liquid she was ingesting from coming back up, and communication became sporadic. She was preparing to die and was waiting for her body to signal that it was time.

* * *

Email sent May 31st, 2011:

Stephanie made it through the weekend, and it looks like she'll make it into June. Probably not very far into June, but heck, I thought that about May. She's definitely going at her own pace.

Catch-22 situation: Stephanie has some pain in her gut. If we give her morphine it takes care of the pain but slows her intestine. Instead of pooing, she tends to vomit more. If we don't give her the morphine, she has the pain, poos quite a bit and still vomits some. The poos are great liquid gushes of bile, which has probably been trapped within the intestines for a while until pressure builds and it's able to force its way through the many partial blockages. Right now we're doing the non-morphine route unless the pain gets too bad.

Stephanie's respiration is slowing, and she stops breathing sometimes for fifteen or twenty seconds. It's a natural part of the body shutting down. Her limbs are like ice, because her heart is in emergency mode and directing all of the blood to her core in an effort to survive. She's super thin—bones are sticking out all over the place. . . . I'd be surprised if she weighs much over one hundred pounds. She's still drinking small amounts of fluid. Her current favorite is Diet Coke.

Stephanie is having trouble communicating, both from exhaustion and confusion. I have to do some instant translating at times to figure out what she wants. Luckily, her wants and needs are pretty simple—change her position, water, Diet Coke, bathroom, vomit. One of her friends called the other day and I put her on speaker phone to say hello. Stephanie could only listen for a minute or so and couldn't say much. I could tell she wanted to cry but she doesn't have enough fluids in her body. That's where we're at . . . more info as things happen.

* * *

Email sent June 4th, 2011:

Stephanie's decline is gaining in momentum. Since the last update, she threw up six, seven, and eight times over the next three days, and has thrown up four times before 8:00 AM this morning. The vomit is yellow-orange, thick, disgusting, and foul-smelling. It coats her mouth, and she has to swish and spit three or four times after she's done to get rid of it. She hasn't pooed in a couple days, though she peed about a gallon yesterday morning.

Stephanie's got a few minor bed sores on her back—minor in the sense that they're not open and infected. They're red, and they sit right over where her bones stick out. The home health aides are doing a good job of washing the areas and keeping them coated with ointments.

* * *

Email Sent June 5th, 2011:

Over the last five days, including today, Stephanie has thrown up at least nine times each day and so far today six times. That's thirty-six times in less than five days. Most of it has been small-ish amounts with a couple mega-

vomits. None of the medications she's received for nausea seem to work. I think that the only thing that would work would be the stomach tube with a big old suction pump. We're not going to do that, of course, as that's one of the things that Stephanie specifically mentioned as not wanting, and I won't go against her word. Actually, I totally agree with her after seeing the equipment and seeing her with a nose tube in operations past. I think our hope was that this wouldn't drag on too long so her agony would be minimized.

Sadly it doesn't seem to be the case, although she continues to grind inexorably to the end. Her heartbeat is very elevated today—in the 90's. At some point, the body will give up and the heart rate will start falling as she begins the final dying process.

As always, I'll keep you posted when I can. I think when Stephanie finally does die, I'm going to call Marcus on the Greco side and Mary Cate on the Srokose side and let those two make the phone calls to the rest of the family. I just picked the names out of the air just now, so don't be mad at me if I'm not the one calling you to announce my wonderful Stephanie's death. I'll then ask for you all to spread the word as necessary.

* * *

Email sent June 8th, 2011:

Nothing incredibly new to report.

Stephanie is restless and has somehow found the energy to stay awake for most of the day the past two days, and well into the night. The problem is that she is "so bored" (her words). She's unable to read, and TV is both confusing and boring. Music is unappealing. I tried reading to her but she loses interest and doesn't always understand what's happening. We've found nothing to keep her occupied and interested. She spends a lot of time staring into space. We also have somewhat interesting, definitely bizarre, conversations about all sorts of subjects. Stephanie has either lost the gag reflex or her vomit is sneaking up on her. She's not vomiting as much as she did a couple days ago, but she tends to vomit with little or no warning. I've walked into the room a couple times already to find her shirt wet. I'm doing a lot of laundry. . . .

Her heart rate is beginning to fall and is definitely weaker and more irregular. It was in the 90s

two days ago, in the 80s yesterday, and in the high 70s a couple minutes ago. This tells me that she's moving forward in her journey.

* * *

Email sent June 10th, 2011:

Death is close. Over the past two days it seems that Stephanie's turned another corner that is bringing her closer to dying.

She remained agitated and awake most of Wednesday evening, sleeping a bit before returning to the same state on Thursday. Around noon on Thursday, she started getting a tic on her upper lip, and she started raising her eyebrows up and down repeatedly. I thought it was a joke at first with the eyebrows, but it just continued. The hospice nurse suggested that Stephanie might be having a mini-stroke, as cancer sometimes throws off clots. There didn't seem to be any other effects other than the facial movements.

Stephanie started to become more agitated and restless as the day went on, asking to leave the bed because she had "to get out of here." It became harder for her to talk and communicate as the day went on. Some of this was due to the fact that she didn't want water and some was due to her physical state.

We gave Stephanie 2 mg of Ativan at 2:00 PM, and it completely looped her out—acting weird and saying odd things. She fell asleep and was pretty much out until about 7:00 PM. I gave her a smaller (1 mg) dose at

8:00 PM, and this just put her to sleep. Stephanie slept through the night until about 10:00 AM today. She woke briefly, unable to talk, but was able to communicate that she wanted her legs moved. She's asleep right now after being awake a grand total of fifteen minutes.

I think Stephanie's entering the final stages of her dying process. It could end today or tomorrow or maybe Sunday. This is just me talking of course, and my track record has been pretty sucky when it's come to predictions on Stephanie. I think this is the real deal, though.

A cute story to leave you by: On Thursday, as I was getting ready to run errands while the health aide was here, I leaned over Stephanie and asked her to "give me some sugar," which is our code word for kisses on the lips. We kissed a few times, and I withdrew to leave, and Stephanie said "Give ME some sugar" and smiled. I smiled too and got the joy of three or four more small kisses from my lovely wife.

* * *

On June 11th, 2011, David sent only one line: "Stephanie made it through the night." Stephanie died on Sunday, June 12. David sent an email the following day announcing her passing.

* * *

Email sent June 13th, 2011:

Stephanie passed away yesterday afternoon around 5:45 PM. Her passing was relatively quiet, but uncomfortable. Her body wanted her to throw up right until the end, but she was too weak. That part was sad. It was also expected given Stephanie's unfortunate medical history. There was no amazing moment at the end, just an expression of exhaustion and a recognition that it was over. Stephanie was lucid until about twelve hours before the end, and then she slowly faded away. I had been sitting with her for a couple hours. I got in

our bed, which sat next to the hospital bed Stephanie was in and started
reading. It wasn't five minutes before I realized that the loud breathing she'd
been exhibiting for the past eight hours had stopped. All was quiet and peaceful
and sad.

Stephanie is going to be cremated. I'm planning a memorial service
for Saturday, July 23rd, at Dickinson (I think in the Great Room at Old
West). We've also set up a Stephanie Larson Scholarship fund at Dickinson
and are asking for donations in lieu of flowers if you're so inclined. Further
information is included below.

Please hold off from calling me for a day or two. I've got support when
I need it and will reach out if I need to. I hope to see you on the 23rd.

Best regards,
David Srokose

* * *

At the end of July, we had a ceremony to celebrate
Stephanie's life. Father Ted Pulcini, a religion professor at
Dickinson, as well as an Orthodox priest, led the service. Many of
us spoke—her department chair Harry Pohlman, who recounted
her many accomplishments, her former student Meghan Allen,
who talked about her as a professor and as a mentor, and many
friends and colleagues, including myself.

Just as Stephanie would have wanted, we ate good meals
that day—a wonderful lunch, and a delicious dinner at a nearby
Italian restaurant. We told stories about Stephanie, and we cried.
We also shared parts of her memoir and talked about what shape it
might take. We agreed that Stephanie's story needed to be told; her
gift to us is an honest and unflinching look at the medical

treatment she endured from her young life until her (too early) death at the age of fifty-one. If it feels "relentless," as one colleague described it, it's because it is. Very few of us have the memory or the stamina to recount in detail our illnesses or the medical treatment that we have received. Stephanie's account means that we cannot hide behind statements that doctors are "doing the best they can," or that science has "progressed so much," or that if we think positively, or "think pink," we will overcome all sickness. Stephanie believed that honesty and dignity would help us all more than these false beliefs. This, then, is her gift to all of us.

—Amy Farrell, August 2013

Acknowledgements

Stephanie Larson was one of the most interesting and complex people I've ever met. That may very well be what attracted me to her. Her relationship with the medical community was similarly complex: fascinating and ultimately illuminating as I travelled the last part of her road with her.

I believe, but am not sure, that Stephanie thought about writing an illness memoir before she met me. She certainly had enough material to draw from, even before the diagnosis of peritoneal cancer in December 2006. I think her last illness spurred a sense of urgency in Stephanie to get her voice out to those who don't quite fit within the confines of the American medical system. Her audience would be those patients, as well as the friends and loved ones who took care of them.

As soon as she started writing, she made me promise that I would publish the book. She subsequently spent hours in coffee shops, in bed, on the couch, and at book stores making notes, writing drafts, firing off letters, and organizing her thoughts. I found notes all over the place after she died—on napkins, placemats, in boxes, and doubling as bookmarks. The physical evidence of the effort she devoted to this book made it apparent that she wanted this to be one of her legacies.

From the time I met Stephanie, I was an intimate participant in her dance with doctors: we were a *team*. We planned strategies, did research, and tag-teamed doctors or nurses when we had to. Because I was so "in" the story, I purposely stayed out of Stephanie's way as she wrote. I didn't read any chapters until the first rough draft was completed in October 2010. When I read the rough draft, I felt like I was being battered with a sledge hammer. It was written engagingly and flowed well, but there was no relief, no break in the narrative for the reader to recover from the horror and the relentlessness of Stephanie's medical traumas. I liked it, and I told Stephanie that. It would need work, which she already knew. What first draft of anything doesn't need work? Stephanie gave the manuscript to a colleague at Dickinson College, who suggested that she reorganize the book anecdotally into a memoir, instead of a chronological narrative. Stephanie worked on a revision right up until March 2011 but never finished the final chapter she'd planned to write. I remember her looking at me early in that month, saying that she wasn't sure she liked how it was turning out. Later that same month, Stephanie entered hospice.

After Stephanie died, Amy Farrell, another friend and colleague from Dickinson, submitted the manuscript to an editing consultant for evaluation, who assessed that the draft was not publishable as written. It was not a feel-good story, and its potential market (people who are sick, people who are close to someone sick) didn't want sad stories. The book would also need to be completely re-worked into a memoir, and the consultant didn't think it would be possible to retain Stephanie's voice and vision if that were done. That stymied me, causing me—and friends who were helping me—to pause. The last thing I wanted to do was lose Stephanie's voice.

I spent some time paralyzed by the possibility that altering the manuscript for publication would mean diluting Stephanie's essence. Then one day—I don't remember the circumstances or where I was—I started to think more like my wife. Stephanie was never one to submit to dominant ideologies: personal, political, or medical. She identified and called out these ideologies where they intersected and reified one another. She would have recognized the gatekeeper mentality of the publishing world, and it wouldn't have stopped her from saying what she wanted to say, however she wanted to say it.

Stephanie had run out of time to supply all the precise words, but the important thing, I realized, was to publish her voice and her story. If a publisher *were* interested in Stephanie's manuscript, it would have to be edited, and there was no guarantee that her voice would be preserved. I started to look outside of the publishing industry—preferably for someone who had been close to Stephanie—to be the primary editor and caretaker of the book.

Shortly after, I had lunch with Susan Feldman, one of Stephanie's closest friends. I was talking about hiring an editor, and she suggested Meghan Allen. Meg was a good friend and former student of Stephanie's. She happened to love my wife, and I thought that she would probably be fantastic at protecting Stephanie's voice. I was so, so right.

The book that follows is alive with Stephanie's voice and spirit. The acknowledgements represent only a fraction of the many hearts and minds that have worked tirelessly to deliver Stephanie's story into your hands today.

Here are some specific people who've touched this project along the way:

Cindy Samet and Susan Feldman were great supports while Stephanie was sick. Cindy has had similar struggles with the medical community and offered perspective and comfort. Susan, in addition to the movie dates and coffees with Stephanie, also suggested that I talk to Meg Allen about editing the book.

Vickie Kuhn and Amy Farrell nurtured this project in its early stages. Vickie called or emailed many times just to see how I was doing and generously donated her time attention as a copy editor. Amy's voice can be heard in a section or two of this book.

Bryan Tramont is one of my MVPs. He was one of Stephanie's best friends, and he embraced me with open arms when she introduced me to him. He has been by my side for this whole process, providing support and advice, admitting me into his inner circle of wonderful friends, and has been....*there* for and with me. Thanks dude.

The Greco clan collectively has been wonderful, trusting me with the care of their daughter, sister, niece, and cousin. I'm a lucky guy to have had them with me the past seven years.

Meghan Allen and her family adopted me into their family as well. Meg was one of the students who became very close to Stephanie and me while we lived in England, and we met her family during one of their visits. We stayed in touch, and Stephanie and I spent a number of holidays with them. Meg is brilliant, thoughtful, beautiful, and talented, and the perfect choice to edit this book. She did all of the heavy lifting, and this book would not have been published – and I don't think I'm exaggerating here – if it weren't for her efforts.

There were other students-turned-friends that were there for Stephanie and me. Chris Eiswerth, Sisi Dong, Jonathan Roberts, Jillian Boland Roberts and Erica Lally served as copy editors of the final manuscript. Chris stepped up at the end and did the lion's share of the final copy editing process. Sisi also helped in the final editing process, and suggested fun dinners and meetings along the way. Jill developed the website for the book. She and Jon have been fantastic friends even if they do beat me regularly in fantasy football.

And finally, I want to mention three people: Albert Baker, Kevin Romano, and Seth Stein. I met Albert and Seth on Xbox Live® while Stephanie was sick. Albert was the guy I was talking to when Stephanie talks about my gaming in the book. Kevin is my nephew and god son who always looks me up when he is online. And Seth was a young kid I met while playing *Call of Duty*® who would ask the sweetest questions about cancer, death, and love after he learned what I was going through. All three of these people were great supports during Stephanie's illness and after. Oh, and they're all incredible gamers.

There are many other people who have floated in and out of my life the past few years and positively affected *Relentless* in some way, and I'm sure I'm forgetting to mention some of them. I could probably write a book of my own thanking them. I'm sure they'll understand, and I'll buy them a pint of great beer as we reminisce about Stephanie Larson.

—David Srokose

About the Author

Professor Stephanie Greco Larson was a part of the Dickinson Community from 1992-2011, and her impact was seen on many levels. She was a member of the Political Science department, and a contributor to many other programs including American Studies, Film Studies, Gender Studies and the Writing Program. Stephanie was innovative in her methods and challenged her students to become better scholars and writers. As her husband, I noticed that Stephanie approached each class as a new opportunity and challenge, whether she taught that class one time or many times over the years.

Professor Larson was a contributor to Dickinson College in more ways than just academics. She was an accomplished and proficient scholar, with numerous published books and journal articles, primarily in on the topic of media and politics. She led study abroad programs in Australia and England participated in faculty intellectual exchanges in Toulouse and Bologna. Professor Larson's wit, perception and analytical skills enabled her to be a successful leader, friend and colleague

About the Editor

Meg Allen is a 2008 graduate of Dickinson College. She had the privilege of being a student of Professor Stephanie Larson's from Fall 2006 until Spring 2008. She is currently a high school English teacher in Maryland and she wishes that Professor

Larson were still around to help her navigate the challenges of teaching and adult life in general.

References

Associated Press. 2009. "Ryan O'Neal says he plans to marry Farrah Fawcettt. *USA Today*, June 22.

http://usatoday30.usatoday.com/life/people/2009-06-22-oneal-fawcett-marriage-plans_N.htm (Access date unavailable).

Carruthers, Julie Hanan, producer. 2010. *All My Children*, season 41, aired January and February 2010, (New York, NY: American Broadcasting Company Studios), Television.

Cohen, Elizabeth. 2008. "5 Mistakes Women Make at the Doctor's Office." *CNN*, May 15.
http://www.cnn.com/2008/HEALTH/05/14/ep.women.mistakes/index.html?iref=newssearch(Access date unavailable).

Cox, Lauren. 2009. "Doctor of Boy Who Fled Chemo Says Hausers Are 'Good People.'" *ABC News*, May 26.
http://abcnews.go.com/Health/CancerPreventionAndTreatment/story?id=7672932 (Access date unavailable).

Swayze, Patrick. 2009. Interview by Barbara Walters. *Patrick Swayze: The Truth*. American Broadcasting Company, 7 January.

Fawcett, Farrah, Alexandra Gleysteen, and Craig J. Nevius, producers. 2009. *Farrah's Story*, aired May 15, (New York, NY: National Broadcasting Company News), Television.

Hallmark, n.d. "Finish all your medicine and get well soon." Greeting card C-529-6.

Hallmark, n.d. "Four out of five doctors want you to get well immediately." Greeting card ZZF-328-1.

Hallmark, n.d. "Get well soon! Meanwhile enjoy the things you see on medication." Greeting card ZF-290-4.

Hallmark, n.d. "Glad your operation is in the past, but don't be afraid to get well too fast." Greeting card 499-GNG-317-8.

Hallmark, n.d. "It can be hard to cope with an illness like this—no matter how strong your faith." Greeting card TOY 867-4.

Hallmark, n.d. "Just sittin' around waitin' for you to get better." Greeting card C-352-4.

Hallmark, n.d. "People who think laughter is the best medicine apparently never had morphine." Greeting card ZF-290-4. http://www.hallmark.com/products/get-well/greeting-cards/the-best-medicine-1PGC8290_DK/?searchTerm=get+well

Hallmark, n.d. "Thanks to modern medicine, you're getting better." Greeting card C-739-6.

Hallmark, n.d. "There's no speed limit on the road to recovery." Greeting card C-253-0.

Hallmark, n.d. "We're thinking of you. Sometimes it's easier to keep a positive attitude when you know that people card about you." Greeting card TOY 225-7.

Hallmark, n.d. "When life hands you lemons, make lemonade." Greeting card ZF 177-2.

Hallmark, n.d. "Why? Somewhere in your heart, you're probably asking this question." Greeting card ECG 8-4.

Hallmark, n.d. "You better get well." Greeting card ZF-181-14.

Hallmark, n.d. "Your operation check list." Greeting card C-738-9.

Montopoli, Brian. 2009. "Alan Grayson 'Die Quickly' Comment Prompts Uproar." *CBS News*, September 30. http://www.cbsnews.com/news/alan-grayson-die-quickly-comment-prompts-uproar/(Access date unavailable).

National Cancer Institute, n.d. "Fast Stats." *Surveillance, Epidemiology, and End Results Program: Turning Cancer Data into Discovery.* http://seer.cancer.gov/faststats/ (Access date unavailable).

Reilly, Rick. 2010. "George vs. the Dragon." *ESPN*, July 14. http://sports.espn.go.com/espn/news/story?id=4997277 (Access date unavailable).

The White House. 2010. "Remarks by the President in Town Hall Meeting in Nashua, New Hampshire." *Office of the Press Secretary.* February 2. http://www.whitehouse.gov/the-press-office/remarks-president-town-hall-meeting-nashua-new-hampshire (Access date unavailable).

Thomson, Katie N., and Rob Wallace. 2008. "Patrick Swayze on Cancer: 'I Want to Last Until They Find a Cure.'" *ABC News,* January 6. http://abcnews.go.com/Entertainment/patrick-swayze-cancer-find-cure/story?id=6586687 (Access date unavailable).

Thomson, Katie N., and Rob Wallace. 2009. "Patrick Swayze Fights Cancer with Wife's Support." *ABC News.* January 7. http://abcnews.go.com/Entertainment/patrick-swayze-fights-cancer-wifes-support/story?id=6589697 (Access date unavailable).

www.ingramcontent.com/pod-product-compliance
Lightning Source LLC
Chambersburg PA
CBHW072105270326
41931CB00010B/1461